"TRY MY PROGRAM FOR 28 DAYS,
AND YOU'LL FEEL SO SENSATIONAL,
YOU'LL ADOPT IT FOR LIFE.
THAT'S A PROMISE!"

—Nathan Pritikin

COL. JAMES B. IRWIN, former Apollo Astronaut: After two heart attacks and triple bypass surgery, he climbed Pike's Peak. "I am indebted to Nathan Pritikin for giving me a new life."

NATHAN MUCHNICK: After four strokes, too sick for bypass surgery, he now runs ten-mile races.

LOUISE TRAIL: Fifteen months after coronary bypass surgery, the one-time cardiac cripple now walk-jogs up to five miles a day.

IRWIN BAKER: Formerly a victim of deadly arrythmia, he now runs ultra-marathons.

———————————————

These are only a few of the success stories inspired by the work of Nathan Pritikin, Founder-Director of the Longevity Center and Pritikin Research Foundation. Twenty years ago, Nathan Pritikin reversed his own serious heart condition with a diet and exercise regimen that achieved almost miraculous results. In his newest best-seller, *THE PRITIKIN PROMISE,* he explains why you may not be as healthy as you think you are . . . and offers the one essential program to keep you fit and trim for life!

THE PRITIKIN PROMISE:

28 Days to a Longer, Healthier Life

Nathan Pritikin

POCKET BOOKS

New York London Toronto Sydney Tokyo Singapore

Acknowledgments
Illustrations by Robin Harris Brisker
Scientific drawings by Nell C. Taylor

Chapter 24 appeared as a guest editorial in *Preventive Medicine II*, 1982.
Copyright © 1982 by Academic Press, Inc. All rights of reproduction in
any form reserved. Reprinted by permission.

POCKET BOOKS, a division of Simon & Schuster Inc.
1230 Avenue of the Americas, New York, NY 10020

ISBN: 0-671-73267-6

First Pocket Books printing March 1985

15   14   13   12   11   10   9   8   7

Printed in the U.S.A.

An Important Note to Readers

This book is intended for active and athletic people who consider themselves healthy. It describes problems common to most people on a typical American diet, and illnesses they may suffer from, often without realizing it, but it is in no way intended as a substitute for medical counseling. If you are on prescription drugs, do not change or modify your medication unless directed to do so by your physician. Changing dosages or schedules for medication on your own could lead to serious illness and even death

While this book is meant primarily for active and athletic people, it should be noted that the Pritikin program has demonstrated extraordinary results in restoring sick people to health. At the Pritikin in-residence centers, we have achieved the following fully documented successes:

1 Of all patients recommended for coronary bypass surgery from mid-1976 to mid-1977, after 5 years more than 80 percent succeed in forgoing the surgery. Most are off all medication, and more than 60 percent no longer have angina

2. Of adult-onset diabetics on insulin (some for more than 20 years), 75 percent can go off insulin within 4 weeks.

3 Of hypertensives (high blood pressure) on medication (some for as long as 25 years), 85 percent are off medication within 4 weeks and maintain normal blood pressures

These and other studies have been documented in medical journals and are available to your physician upon request. As a public service, we are pleased to provide dietary information and printed diets to health professionals (See pages 497 to 498).

Contents

The Pritikin Promise

This is my promise to you: You can banish fatigue, feel more alive and energetic, normalize your weight without hunger, lower your risk of contracting one of the degenerative diseases that are epidemic in our country, and look terrific as well. I know you can do all these things, just as many have.

While excess weight was never a problem for me, in 1955, at age 40, I learned I was seriously ill: I had heart disease. Since then almost 30 years have gone by, and you would expect that if I were still alive at all, I would by now be a semi-invalid at least. Not so. I have completely recovered —without surgery, hospitalization, or medication. I did it with a carefully researched program of diet and exercise. I have never felt better, and medical evidence supports my amazing rehabilitation: my blood pressure, stress tests, cholesterol level, and other tests are well within the normal range for a man half my age, and I have felt *no* symptoms for nearly 30 years.

My lifelong study of nutrition and its effects on the body was put to the test when I learned of my own heart problem. I explored the research into other cultures, and discovered that many primitive peoples, such as the Tarahumara Indians in northern Mexico, have virtually no incidence of heart disease, diabetes, high blood pressure, or cancer. The Tarahumaras have incredible endurance. They can: run 500 miles in 5 days. Play 150–200-*mile* kickball games. Carry 80 percent of their own weight a distance of 110 miles in 70 hours. Their diet, rich in grains, vegetables, and fruits, is as close as science has come to optimal nutritional balance for human beings.

I began to imitate their dietary and exercise habits, and my recovery was under way.

Since 1966 I have written and lectured widely about my program for improving health and vitality and increasing longevity.

The Pritikin Program has now been studied extensively, and the evidence of its effectiveness has been published in medical journals around the world. Since 1970, the program has been widely publicized in newspaper articles and books and on radio and television, and I have lectured to thousands on how to treat people afflicted with heart disease, high blood pressure, and diabetes and on how proper diet greatly reduces the risk of breast and colon cancer.

Now I'm addressing the people of this country who still feel healthy. Most Americans do develop heart disease, and most think they feel healthy until the onset of severe symptoms or sudden heart attack or stroke. I promise to teach you not only how to keep from getting sick, but how to be healthier than you've ever been and to feel happier and more energetic.

This book offers a diet and exercise program for all of you —people of all ages and abilities: walkers, runners, world-class athletes; and especially those of you who have not exercised since you last hopped off the school bus. The same program works for everyone: children, parents, grandparents, and great-great-grandparents.

The how-to-do-it 28-day food plan is more than good-tasting, and is designed for gourmet cooks and for busy people who have very little time for food preparation. In addition, you'll be able to afford a vacation with what you save on your food bill.

You can adapt the exercise part of the program to suit your present level of fitness, then work gradually toward a more invigorating program; but you need *never* work yourself to exhaustion to be fit.

Try my program for 28 days, and you'll feel so sensational, you'll adopt it for life. That's a promise.

NATHAN PRITIKIN

PART ONE

NUTRITION
AND
YOUR
HEALTH

1

CHAPTER

Why a Healthy Person
Should Follow
the Pritikin Program

This book is for healthy people, even those who exercise every day.

But why should YOU, a "healthy" person, bother to change the way you eat? And if you're not already doing so, begin to exercise regularly?

The sad news is, in all likelihood, that you're not as healthy as you may think. If you are over 20 years old, and have been on an American diet all your life, you're undoubtedly not healthy at all; statistically, you are, in fact, well on your way to suffering severe heart disease.

Here are a few basic facts:

The heart is a muscle and requires blood to work. Only three coronary arteries, each no larger than a pencil, supply all the blood to your heart. If these arteries become clogged with cholesterol deposits or "boils" from too much fat and cholesterol in your diet, they will narrow or close so that not enough blood is supplied to the heart. So even though your heart muscle is fine, *you probably have heart disease*.

Are you male and 20? The odds are that all three of your coronary arteries average 20-percent closure. You are in the early stages of heart disease. But you feel fine. For now.

3

Are you female and 30? The odds are that you're as sick as a 20-year-old man with all three arteries 20 percent closed. You're lagging 10 years behind men on the road to heart disease, but you'll catch up after menopause.

Are you male and 35? The odds are that all three of your coronary arteries average 50 percent closure, although you still feel well. Even if all three of your coronaries were 65 percent closed, you could pass the most vigorous stress treadmill test and be told that you are very healthy. Until at least one of your coronary arteries is 90–100 percent closed, you have no symptoms. But now you might have some chest pressure upon activity. Now you might have a heart attack. Now you could suddenly die while running.

Arthur Ashe, world-class tennis player, never knew he had heart disease until, when he was 36, one of his coronary arteries closed completely and he began to feel pressure in his chest.

Why wait until you can be diagnosed as having heart disease? By that time your arteries are so narrowed with cholesterol deposits, you could become one of the 350,000 Americans a year to die without warning from heart disease.

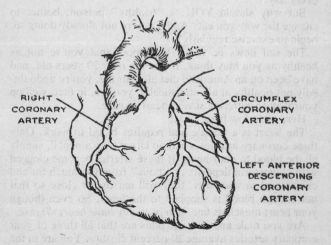

RIGHT CORONARY ARTERY

CIRCUMFLEX CORONARY ARTERY

LEFT ANTERIOR DESCENDING CORONARY ARTERY

THE THREE MAJOR CORONARY ARTERIES

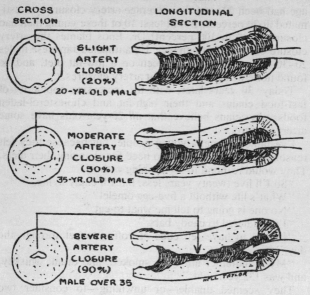

CROSS SECTION • LONGITUDINAL SECTION

SLIGHT ARTERY CLOSURE (20%)
20-YR. OLD MALE

MODERATE ARTERY CLOSURE (50%)
35-YR. OLD MALE

SEVERE ARTERY CLOSURE (90%)
MALE OVER 35

HELL TAYLOR

THREE STAGES OF PROGRESSIVE HEART DISEASE

Most of these people were given clean bills of health at their last physical examinations. Doctors cannot predict whether you will have a heart attack. They can only give you odds based on risk factors, such as cholesterol level, blood pressure, smoking, weight, activity, and heredity. One million Americans, half of all deaths, die from some form of heart disease each year.

It was not until 1953, however, that we learned that for Americans, arteries start closing during our teens.

At that time Dr. William Enos reported on evidence gained from autopsies performed on 300 American soldiers killed in the Korean War. In 77 percent of the men, "gross evidence of coronary disease was demonstrated that varied from minimal eccentric thickening to complete occlusion of one or more of the main coronary branches." Their average

age had been 22, and their average artery closure was estimated at 20 percent. But at least 10 of these young men had closure of 90 to 100 percent! Dr. Enos blames the artery closure on the American diet. He autopsied Japanese males 20–30 years old who had been on a low-fat diet, and he found none with any significant artery closures.

Today, 30 years later, with the increasing popularity of fast-food chains and their high-fat and cholesterol-laden foods, physicians believe that *all* 20-year-olds have some artery closure.

I've talked to many young people, but because they felt reasonably well, most saw no need for changing their diets. They would respond to my probing with:

"So I'll live twenty years less, but I'll enjoy living."

"What's life without a five-egg omelet?"

"No one is going to tell me what to eat."

"I'm addicted to candy bars."

"I have to have ten cups of coffee to get through the day."

"My grandfather ate eggs, smoked, and drank whiskey, and was 132 years old."

They seemed unable—or unwilling—to consider two things:

1) how they would feel in 10 years' time if they continued on their present course, and

2) how much better they could be feeling—and functioning—right now.

In fact, with the Pritikin Program everyone, regardless of age, will notice dramatic changes in a few weeks or less. You will have:

● Less fatigue (especially after lunch!)
● Supercharged energy
● Increased endurance and improved performance in sports
● Much less risk of heart disease, diabetes, and several cancers
● No more constipation
● Better mental acuity
● Virtually no headaches
● Shortened menstrual periods, with less flow, cramps, and premenstrual swelling

- Emotional benefits
- Better sleep habits
- Longer life

In addition, you will look better and younger than ever, and you will save money: the average family of four saves $1,500 per year on groceries with our program.

I hope you will abandon the habits that keep you only half alive and enter the world of vibrant health and well-being. Let's look a little more closely at why you—a "healthy person"—should follow the Pritikin Program.

1. FEEL LESS FATIGUED.

Why are you so exhausted after lunch—on weekends—when you get home from work at night? You will, of course, feel tired if you have not had enough sleep. But fatigue caused by lack of sleep is easily remedied, and it is *not* the most common type. Fatigue is most often caused by an inadequate supply of oxygen to our muscles and brain cells.

If you have a fit of yawning, the deep breathing will increase your oxygen supply slightly for a few seconds. If you want to dramatically increase the oxygen available to your

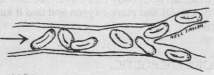

NORMAL RED CELLS EASILY PASS INTO TINY CAPILLARIES

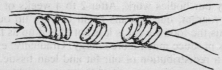

CLUMPED RED CELLS HAVE DIFFICULTY PASSING INTO THE CAPILLARIES

body's cells on a permanent basis, you will have to adhere to a diet low in fat. Tired blood is low-oxygen blood, and low-oxygen blood is too high in fats. Here's what happens.

Blood is a watery substance, called plasma, chock-full of different types of cells, sugar, proteins, amino acids, fats, salts, vitamins, hormones, and many other substances. But the major constituent of blood is red blood cells—5 million per cubic millimeter, an area about half the size of a grain of rice. The red cells are filled with hemoglobin, each molecule of which carries four molecules of oxygen. The red cells look like discs depressed in the middle; they resemble life preservers with a thin membrane stretched across the hole. The arteries carrying the blood become ever smaller as they approach the tissues to be nourished.

The red cells pass, one at a time, by squeezing through the tiniest vessels, called capillaries. The red cells move very close to the cells they nourish, and oxygen diffuses from the red cell to the tissue cell. But after a fatty meal, the blood is greasy for many hours, and as a result the red corpuscles and other blood cells stick together. The more they stick together, the less able they are to pass through the capillaries. Therefore, some tissue is undernourished.

When the brain and the muscles become oxygen-deprived, we feel both physically and mentally tired. A low-fat diet will wake up both body and mind, because the red cells will carry less fat and more oxygen and find it easier to make deliveries.

2. FEEL MORE ENERGETIC.

To be truly healthy, however, we must do more than restrict our fat intake. Exercise is crucial to our well-being and will help us to have more energy by changing our metabolism, or the way our bodies work. After 2 to 4 weeks of a good exercise program, our systems begin to burn up our food faster. Thus the food we eat is less apt to end up as fat, and our bodies produce much more energy. Gradually, exercise promotes a redistribution of our fat and lean tissue. When this happens, even if we remain at the same weight, we'll be thinner, because fat is lighter, bulkier, lumpier, bumpier, and bulgier than muscle. As fat is displaced by increased muscle mass, we become shapelier, smoother, more compact, and therefore slimmer. And because of the increased muscle-to-fat ratio, the food we eat will be burned for energy rather than converted to fat. Muscle cells contain little elongated mitochondria—factories where the workers, or enzymes, interact with the fuel which our bodies metabolize from the food we eat. This interaction produces a chemical form of energy. Exercise causes an increase in the enzymes and enlargement of the muscle cells, so that as our metabolic rate increases, more food is converted faster to energy and less to fat. After we have achieved this exercise-induced increase in lean body tissue, we therefore burn more calories even at rest.

3. IMPROVE ENDURANCE AND PERFORMANCE.

If you are already active in sports, the Pritikin Program will increase your endurance and enhance your performance. Only a regular diet of meals high in complex carbohydrates will provide optimal levels of energy at all times.

Over the years, carefully controlled studies with skiers and with subjects riding stationary bicycles have demonstrated that people on high-carbohydrate diets have more endurance than those on a high-protein diet. These studies show that the benefits of the high-carbohydrate diet include improved work performance and reaction time, increased altitude tolerance, and better control of blood sugar levels.

4. LESS RISK OF DEGENERATIVE DISEASES.

The Pritikin Program can greatly reduce your chances of developing heart disease, diabetes, and several types of cancer, depending on how much at risk you were to begin with. This is determined by evaluation of risk factors. Different diseases are associated with different risk factors, and of course, different diseases have many risk factors in common. Among the risk factors associated with the most prevalent degenerative diseases are high blood pressure, high or low blood sugar, high levels of cholesterol and/or triglycerides in the blood, smoking, excessive alcohol consumption, and overweight. By reducing your risk factors, you will be considerably less likely to develop these diseases.

5. NO MORE CONSTIPATION.

Fiber in our food absorbs several times its weight in water, giving bulk to the intestinal contents and moving waste products through the colon. Because the Pritikin diet contains ample amounts of natural fiber, and because the exercise program speeds up a sluggish metabolism, the program prevents the common problem of "irregularity." Constipated Americans spend millions of dollars each year on laxatives. The expense, discomfort, and disorders that can be caused by constipation, such as hemorrhoids, varicose veins, and diverticular disease, can be prevented by a sensible exercise program and a diet consisting mainly of foods as grown.

6. BETTER MENTAL ACUITY.

In 1977, 31 patients at the Longevity Center in California were tested before starting the Pritikin diet and exercise program and again after 3 weeks to determine the effect of the program on mental acuity and personality. The pilot results indicated improvement in both these areas.

7. FEWER HEADACHES.

A frequent unexpected bonus of going on the program is the relief of headaches. This phenomenon has been reported to us by both participants in our rehabilitation centers and in letters from those who have put themselves on the program. We are not certain of the mechanism by which headaches are alleviated, but suspect that the improved circulation resulting from the low-fat diet and aerobic exercise is probably ınvolved. In addition, exercise. which has been shown to reduce stress, may help prevent tension headaches.

8. EASIER MENSTRUAL PERIODS.

Dietary fats and cholesterol also affect reproductive functions. Girls on a high-fat diet start menstruating at an earlier age, and women reach menopause at a later age. Prostaglandin production, which is affected by dietary fat, increases the amount of flow during menstrual periods, the length of the period, and cramping. Women on the low-fat Pritikin diet have had dramatic results with these problems, and they have also found that regular exercise reduces menstrual cramping and low back pain.

9. FEEL BETTER EMOTIONALLY.

Not least among the benefits to be derived from the high-carbohydrate diet and aerobic exercise program are the emotional gains. You will feel terrific about yourself for having taken charge of your health. You will feel great mentally about how well you feel physically. And you will be delighted with your improved appearance. You'll be thinner and firmer, stronger and more alert; have a bounce to your step, roses in your cheeks, and a twinkle in your eye. Watch out!

Although emotional benefits are subjective in nature and difficult to evaluate quantitatively, there is no doubt that you will notice real improvement in how you feel about your life. Easier to demonstrate and measure are some of the mood changes associated with chemical changes in the body. A diet low in fat and sugar and high in unrefined starchy foods effects the maintenance of normal carbohydrate metabolism and prevents the lethargy, depression, and anxiety associated with low blood sugar.

Recently, substances more exotic than sugar which also relate to mood, such as beta-endorphins, have been measured in the blood, and their quantities have been found to change upon exercise. Exercise stimulates the brain's production of these opiatelike substances—one of the reasons for the mood-altering effect of exercise. Some psychologists are finding exercise significantly more beneficial to their patients with moderate depression than the traditional talk therapy, and infinitely preferable to the use of mood-altering drugs. But people who are not depressed also experience an elevation in mood. Immediately after aerobic exercise, many people experience varying degrees of short-term euphoria—and perhaps more important, an improvement in mood that persists.

10. BETTER SLEEP HABITS.

Most people on the Pritikin Program find they need quite a bit less sleep but still have a lot more energy. The exercise and improved metabolism enable you to sleep more soundly. A caution, however. Exercising too strenuously close to bedtime may prevent some people from falling asleep immediately. So it's best to exercise at least 2 hours before bedtime. Also, if you're exercising more strenuously than usual, you may need a little more sleep temporarily until your body adapts itself to your new level of exertion.

11. LONGER LIFE.

Researchers have been demonstrating for more than 50 years that restricting the food intake of animals ranging from one-celled creatures to humans results in a lengthened life-span. Unrestricted feeding, on the other hand, promotes increased rate of growth, a greater amount of body fat, earlier onset of degenerative diseases, and premature death.

More recent studies have shown that it is not only the quantity of food but its composition that affects the aging process. For instance, if a diet is high in protein, it has to be hypocaloric (or low-calorie) to effect increased longevity, but if it is high in carbohydrate, the caloric content is of no consequence. A diet low in protein (8 percent) and high in carbohydrate (83 percent) when fed to rats in unrestricted amounts was as effective as when higher-protein diets were fed to them on a restricted basis. The more protein and fat in the diet, the shorter the life-span. More carbohydrate increased the life-span, sometimes almost doubling it even if calories were not restricted.

We have no reason to believe that the composition of the diet will not have the same type of effect on humans. If it does, then eating a high-carbohydrate diet will enable us to live not only healthier, but longer lives.

Many diet-book authors are rapidly working in the direction of the Pritikin dietary guidelines, and most new cookbooks today sport low-fat, low-cholesterol, low-sodium, sugarless, or vegetarian recipes. They're recommending more use of complex-carbohydrate foods, such as beans, grains and grain products, and vegetables. They're going with the tide, and they are not the only ones. Government agencies are moving in the same direction.

In 1976 and 1977, Senator George McGovern presided over the Select Committee on Nutrition and Human Needs. Typical of the testimony before the Committee was that of Harvard School of Public Health Professor Mark Hegsted. He stated that the increased amount of fatty, cholesterol-rich, and refined foods in the diet was responsible for the high rates of heart disease, hypertension, certain forms of cancer, and obesity. He said, "We cannot afford to temporize. We have an obligation to inform the public of the current state of knowledge and to assist the public in making the correct food choices. To do less is to avoid our responsibility."

The Committee subsequently published its "Dietary Goals." The recommendations approached those of the Pritikin Research Foundation: they urged Americans to increase significantly our intake of carbohydrates; decrease the sugar in our diet; eat less meat, butter, and eggs; and in general decrease dietary fat (both saturated and unsaturated), cholesterol, and salt.

In his 1979 report to the American people, the Surgeon General admonished us, "You, the individual, can do more for your own health and well-being than any doctor, any hospital, any drug, any exotic medical advice." This report also approaches the Pritikin dietary guidelines in its recommendations to eat more complex carbohydrates and less fat, cholesterol, salt, and sugar. The American Diabetes Association, in its earlier years, used to recommend that 30 percent of the calories in the diet of diabetics come from carbohydrates, but recently the complex-carbohydrate allotment was increased to 60 percent. The latest, safest, most efficient way to normalize carbohydrate metabolism in both diabetics and nondiabetics is with the high-carbohydrate, high-natural-fiber diet.

Some organizations are still sitting on the fence. The U.S. Department of Agriculture, for instance, is quite unspecific in its 1981 publication on diet, saying, "Avoid too much fat, cholesterol, sugar and sodium." Of course, too much is too much, but the publication doesn't tell us how much that is. It doesn't tell us whether we should eat less than we eat now or whether "too much" means even more than the quantities of those substances the average American already consumes.

Even though the bread of this department is, in a manner of speaking, buttered by the dairy and beef industries, there is now so much scientific evidence demonstrating the great risks we incur by eating animal products that the Department does at least mention that "too much" fat and cholesterol can be harmful. I believe that as the current of nutritional enlightenment becomes stronger and stronger, even the U.S. Department of Agriculture will dedicate itself to the task of improving the supply of safe, nutritious food for all Americans.

There is a great deal more I could say about the benefits you will derive from the Pritikin Program; but I think you might be interested in hearing from people just like you who have started the program—and who never intend to finish!

2

We Thought We Were Healthy!
(Until We Went
on Your Diet)

Thousands of people write to tell me about the wonderful improvements in their health on my program. The youngest was 10; the oldest, so far, 91! But most were from 20 to 60 years old.

A common thread runs through almost all their letters. Before they started my program, they thought that the way they felt was about normal for their age. After they began their new diet and exercise routine, they were delighted to lose their chronic fatigue, their constipation, headaches, excess weight, and to gain feelings of vitality, increased endurance, clearer thinking, better memory, and a new joy in living. Some of their thoughts:

"I thought I felt well, but now I know what feeling well really is like."

"Until now, I always assumed that it was normal to be half asleep after 2 P.M."

"Rather than walk a block, I'd drive my car. Now, I look for opportunities to walk a mile or two. It makes me feel so alive."

Many had gone on popular weight-loss diets, and had gained back the weight. They felt depressed and frustrated.

15

Several were involved in exercise programs and thought they were doing fine.

Just a few weeks after they adopted my diet, however, all of them were pleasantly surprised at all the good things that were happening.

Here are some of their letters.

● THOMAS CHRISTOPHER, caterer—Studio City, California, age 23

"I have been on the diet for over 2 years now, and, although I am considered quite young to be on any kind of a health program, I have accrued the same startling benefits from your diet as other Pritikin dieters; that is, increased vitality and health. As far as running goes, I find that the high-carbohydrate Pritikin diet is a perfect runners' diet. It changed my endurance so I was turning in the best times ever on the mile run. Although I had never competed on any level before, I was training to enter world-class competition. The problems I had with severe depression are gone. In fact, I sleep less than required before. The Pritikin diet gets high marks from me."

● SETH D. MADELL, medical student—West Orange, New Jersey, age 26

	Before starting the diet	After starting the diet
Weight	196 lb	170 lb
Exercise	None	Walks, racquetball

"As a former fatty, I am well acquainted with the myriad of fad diets to which the American public are perennially subjected (since, of course, in my quest for a miracle cure I have been on many of them). As a senior medical student, about to begin a career in treating that American public, I am dismally aware of how little the average American medical school teaches about nutritional guides for therapy. I am 26 years old and 5′ 10″, and I tipped the scale at 196 pounds before I started the diet. Fellow students suggested

I use an experimental drug to lose weight so I wouldn't have to diet; however, when the drug created serious problems for me I stopped it.

"In desperation I went to the medical school library and looked up 'weight loss.' What I found in the stacks surprised me. It was your book—*The Pritikin Program for Diet & Exercise*. I read it and was quite impressed, not only because its mainstays were actually some of my favorite foods, but because it was the first popular diet book I know of to back its claims with scientific research published in journals which I knew from my schooling to be reputable.

"I immediately started the diet. In 4 months I lost 26 pounds, from 196 to 170, just 5 pounds from my ideal body weight. My waist reduced 4". I am wearing clothes now I haven't fit into for years and I feel terrific. I am full of energy, more alive and never hungry. I now take regular 30–40-minute walks, interspersed with frequent games of racquetball which is new for me.

"When I became a Pritikin dieter, it was not meant as a lifetime change. It was merely a quick and healthy way to get back in shape. However, I have been so pleased with the results that confront me on the scale and the tape measure (not to mention the countless compliments from many of my peers) that I am resolved to try to make permanent changes in my lifetime dietary regimen so as to conform more closely to the theories espoused in the books. As a former fatty, I have been rewarded for my efforts, and I thank you for giving me the courage to attempt such a radical change in my diet. As a medical student, I thank you for not only instructing me in some of the fact and fallacy of dietary therapy, but also for giving me the basis with which to modify the diets of future overweight patients. More important, however, is that, as a man with a need for self-respect, self-esteem and self-confidence, I am now more able to deal with my own life since a great thorn in my side has been extricated. Thank you, Nathan Pritikin, for your work and your eagerness to spread your gospel to the public. Count me among your converts."

● FRAN HARDY, home economist—Los Angeles, California, age 45

"I am a professor of nutrition, home economist, marriage and family counselor, and a single mother who is working full time (and then some) to support my two daughters and myself. A large portion of my time, by necessity is spent working, running a large household (with boarders) and actively involved with my children aged 11 and 15. I have always appeared to be healthy—sometimes "strapping"—and physically active and strong and sort of appeared to live up to the 'California Woman' image. Until recently I labored to live up to the super woman, super mother, super teacher, super wife, super entertainer image. I was also super harried and a super martyr a portion of the time.

"When I started the Pritikin program I weighed 160 lbs., and now I weigh 135 lbs. I had some problems with arthritis and high blood pressure, both of which have now subsided. And I felt depressed. Since beginning the program, I have been more relaxed, healthier, more optimistic, trimmer, had more stamina than at any other period in my life. Interestingly, I have had more reasons to feel bad (job stress, parenting stress, financial stress, etc. etc.) in a cumulative fashion than at any other period. I am, instead, working more, have more energy, have more perseverance and more interest in life than I have ever demonstrated. That is saying a lot.

"Sure I had my share of ups and downs with the program. At first I found it very difficult to incorporate an exercise program into my life what with time demands, work load and our very warm climate. I have slipped off the diet—as an inveterate reader and follower of gourmet cookbooks it took me a while to appreciate dishes that weren't loaded with butter, cream, cheese, whatever. Sometimes I felt inadequate and discouraged when I compared myself to other Pritikin program followers—people who had REAL health problems and who were *so* good and quick about making the necessary changes in their life styles.

"But now, almost without noticing, I find the program has become intrinsic to me. The concepts of proper nutrition and exercise are simply a way of life that I enjoy, something I just do with pleasure and without having to think about it much anymore.

"I surely have improved my life, and my outlook on life.

I think that the psychological benefits I have experienced are as vital as the physiological improvements."

● RIDGE LAMAR, co-owner and president of oil-exploration company—Douglas, Wyoming, age 34

	Before starting the diet	After starting the diet
½ marathon	Exhausted	PR—quick recovery
Marathon	None	3:30
Palpitations	Bad	Gone

"I am an alcoholic. I quit drinking 5½ years ago. Two things in my life have not only saved me from drinking but have added a quality to my life I never thought possible. These two things are running and your diet. For as long as I can remember, I felt an underlying uneasiness or nervousness. I was miserable. Alcohol was the only thing that relieved that tension. After I shook the habit, I began running. The exercise seemed to relieve some of the tension. However, I still had palpitations and a general feeling of fatigue. It wasn't, however, until I combined the exercise with your diet that I felt really well without alcohol. I no longer have heart palpitations, don't feel the need to nap and have a lot more energy. I used to have to get a good night's sleep after a hard run, or I would die the next day. Now, I seem to start recovering even before the night's sleep, and very seldom do I experience a real sense of fatigue. I finally have trained and completed my first marathon. My time was 3:30:27. I am now toying with the idea of competing in a triathlon next year. I would strongly recommend your diet and the treatment process for recovering alcoholics.

"I have given out dozens of your books to friends as gifts. I notice they are now eating chicken instead of steak."

● VIRGINIA S. MORSE—Carmel, California, age 64
"Four and a half years ago, my husband and I stopped off in Arizona. We were looking for a new place to live and had examined France, Florida, and New Mexico. In our wan-

derings, we had not bothered to have an annual check-up, and we decided that it was high time that we did have one.

"We presumed that we both were in our usual excellent state of health. We were overweight, but that was because we had quit smoking several years earlier and had substituted munching for nicotine. In France, I had taken a great fancy to fried steak with butter and wine sauce. I drank 8 or 10 cups of strong French coffee a day. I adored cheese, nuts, olives, and chocolate. Two or three years earlier, my cholesterol had hit 350 but my doctor had told me not to worry about it; he said it was 'high normal' and I should cut out a couple of eggs a week. Because of our peripatetic life, I had given up tennis, my one athletic activity.

"As part of the annual check-up, Jack was given a treadmill test which he flunked terribly. The doctors expected him to have an immediate and massive heart attack. I was less spectacular. I flunked, but with a diagnosis of oxygen insufficiency. The doctors—by now we had several—wanted to do an angiogram on me.

"They explained they had to know where the blockages were and whether by-pass surgery was indicated, but I was not at all enthusiastic about letting anyone, no matter how well trained, insert a wire into my heart. I had read that an angiogram was major surgery and sometimes fatal.

"As a general principle, I was opposed to surgery and was convinced that subsequent generations would look back on our period of history as a curious time when one human being would lie down on a table and let another human being cut on him with a knife.

"Quite by accident, I came across one of the first news stories written about the work of Nathan Pritikin. Armed with a newsclip, I approached the Great Expert who was pressuring me to have an angiogram and asked what could be done by diet and exercise, and what he thought of the Pritikin program.

" 'Nothing you will know about in your lifetime. It would take 50 years to prove or disprove any of this. We would have to see what condition people are in after 50 years of following this kind of program,' he said.

" 'But don't you think something could be done by diet?' I insisted.

" 'Nothing you will ever know about,' the Great Expert told me.

"That was four years ago. In one month on the diet and exercise program, I passed my treadmill test.

"Since then, I have been in magnificent health. I have lost 25 pounds. I walk every morning. At 64, I play a better game of tennis than I did in my fifties. I adhere to the Pritikin diet. I am primarily a vegetarian and I thoroughly enjoy the food we eat.

"I am confident that Jack and I made absolutely the right choice the day we decided to go the Pritikin route rather than the surgical route. When I look at our lives today and our very excellent health, I have a very warm kind feeling for that persistent gentleman Nathan Pritikin who, in a very short time has done what the Great Expert didn't think could be done in 50 years. Jack and I are both very grateful for Nathan Pritikin, and we feel extremely lucky to have learned about Nathan and his work, just when we needed him."

● J.N.—Naples, Florida, age 41

	Before starting the diet	After starting the diet
Exercise	Walk ¼ mile	Walk 12 miles
Weight	220	182
Blood Pressure	Hypertensive	Dropped 25mm to normal

"Thank you for your fabulous diet. It really put me on the path to good health and happiness. I have never felt better. In January 1982, I weighed 220 pounds and could not walk a quarter of a mile without being dead tired. At 40 years old, I was a mess. I also was drinking quite heavily and looked puffy. I picked up a copy of your book by accident and it made a believer out of me.

"I can walk, because I don't like jogging, 12 miles easily, bike ride long distances, and I weigh a very athletic-looking 182, good for my 6'2". I have all but given up eating meat. I also had high blood pressure, and that dropped 25 points. I feel fantastic and abound with energy. People refuse to believe I am 41 years old. Thank you so much for helping me. Keep making people believe. I'll never go back to the old habits again.''

● JOHN BECKER—Milwaukee, Wisconsin, age 42

	Before starting the diet	After starting the diet
Marathon	3:08	2:57
10K	38 minutes	36.25 minutes
Blood Pressure	124/90	100/70

"In September 1979, I changed to your diet. The most important advantages to me are: (1) I can eat as much as I want —5 bowls of cereal a day, 2 desserts for supper, 1½ pounds of vegetables for lunch; (2) it's easy to keep fit and I don't take any supplements; (3) I save $8.00 a week in food; (4) I have a much more stable blood sugar level; and (5) I don't waste time counting calories.

"Also, I think much of running is psychological. I need an incentive to run hard when I'm out; and my incentive is knowing that I will eat as much as I want without worrying about gaining weight.

"My running times have decreased significantly, my weight has stayed within the normal range and my blood pressure has gone from 124/90 to 100/70.

"I run about 50 miles a week and since starting your diet, my times in all races decreased by eighteen seconds per mile to six minutes at distances from 10,000 to 15,000 meters. I'm always happy to bend someone's ear about your diet.''

● EMILY M. HELLER—Livonia, Michigan, age 74
"YOU have made it possible for me to 'live as I wish,' since November 1976 when I first went on your program. I had been feeling pretty well, but a year prior to that date I was hospitalized for shortness of breath which the doctors called 'coronary insufficiency.' My doctor spoke of a bypass op-

eration, but I said 'no thanks!' Fortunately the cardiologist suggested I was past the GOLDEN AGE for that procedure and suggested trying medication only. During the next twelve months I felt disbelief, then finally doubt and despair. I developed allergies to some of the drugs—Isordil, Inderal, Coumadin, Nitros when needed, then substituted by Nitrol. My whole body, inside and outside, tickled and pricked with no relief except when sleeping. I became allergic to almost all medication except Bufferin, which was forbidden because of the Coumadin. I developed two bladder tumors which had to be removed.

"The emotional upheaval during those twelve months was awful, and I just could not believe all this was happening to me. I hated everyone around me, doctors the most. I felt they were all conspiring against me. I had been giving book reviews for the last thirty-five years on almost every worthwhile book on nutrition, starting with Gaylord Hauser, Pretorius, Kordel, many others, right on down to Adelle Davis with all of her 'Let's' books. Why, my husband and I were living most exemplary lives dietwise—so we thought. Then came the awful awakening! Realization that now, after all of that diet knowledge and effort, here I was, short of breath and not able to walk to the corner—and practically overnight! Just barely enough energy left to get onto the family room couch. All of my wonderful former energy was gone. I couldn't believe it!

"I never smoked (was allergic to it), and only had a slight weight problem of an occasional 5 to 10 pounds.

"While at the Center, I gradually stopped all medication. My walking was slowly increased from one block the first day to 5 miles the last week divided into several walks each day.

"Almost immediately all of my former bouncing energy returned, and I felt marvelous again. I loved everyone around me, including the doctors who were inquisitive about the Pritikin Program and who were simply amazed at my wonderful response to it, and to my renewed energy. They are all very familiar with the Pritikin Program as I speak about it all the time and answer their questions, and relate many facts they did not ask about. There is a very definite interest on their part.

"I do not experience depression or tiredness, I am very happy most of the time and I have terrific energy from 7:30 A.M. to 11 P.M. when I call it a day. I walk approximately three miles five days each week, sometimes dividing it into two walks, do all of our housework, cooking, some garden work, shopping, driving every day, work in my husband's dental office as accountant and part-time receptionist, am active in a local P.E.O. Chapter and several small clubs. On September 25th I will reach my 74th birthday, and—I am still involved in two love affairs—one with my husband George of 44 years, and the other one with Life. I am still 'in love with life,' and I know life 'is still in love with me.' "

● N.R.F., audiologist—Williamsburg, Virginia, age 45

	Before starting the diet	After starting the diet
Minutes/Mile	None	7.5
Run	None	25 miles/week
Blood Pressure	160/98	114/74
Cholesterol	200+	127
Heart Rate	70	54

"In the spring of 1979, I went to my doctor's office, and my blood pressure read 160/98. I then decided to go on the Pritikin diet, and in 2 months' time my blood pressure dropped to 120/86.

"Primarily, I eliminated all sugars and oils after starting Pritikin's program. On other diets, my blood pressure did not normalize, even with a consistent running program of 3–4 miles, 3–4 times a week. My blood pressure now runs about 114/74. In fact, my heart rate used to be up around the high 60s and low 70s before I started this program. Now it's about 54/minute. My cholesterol was always up in the 200s, and I am glad to say that since I have been on the Pritikin diet it's about 127.

"Although I'm not highly competitive, I enjoy running 5–10K runs. I run about a 7½-minute mile, and I'm running

5–10 miles, 3–4 times a week. I find it interesting that nothing really was improving until I eliminated all fats, honey, and molasses from my diet.

"My capacity for work is much greater, I have much more energy, and yet I seem to require less sleep. Can't understand it, but I'm happy for it."

● GLORIA G. ADSUAR—Guaynabo, Puerto Rico, age 44
"I like to think that at the time of my heart attack in February of 1977 I decided to travel further to ask your help than anyone before me. I was a rare medical exception: a female of 37 with no heart history who had a myocardial infarction. I was thin, athletic and had a 16-month-old child.

"The doctors paid no attention to my 284 blood cholesterol level and tried to explain away my infarction as an 'accident.' I was sent to Cleveland Hospital where I went through my first stress test. Incredibly I passed with flying colors! Then I had an angiogram which showed severe coronary artery disease in three main vessels. Bypass surgery was immediately recommended.

"But, I couldn't accept the verdict, because my father had died during bypass surgery two years before. It was then that we decided to investigate your work which a relative had heard about in an Army magazine. It was the best decision I ever made!

"My husband, young child and I attended Session 18 in Santa Barbara while our oldest son went to camp nearby. My life changed, I no longer feared I would die at any moment and I felt better than at any moment in my life.

"Two years after attending the Longevity Center, at age 40 I had another child. I followed your strict diet and adhered to a strict walking-jogging routine until the day of birth. I felt superb throughout the pregnancy and it was the easiest and fastest confinement of my three. I have to chase Irene all over the house since she started walking at nine months. She has been in school since she was two and is the teacher's pet. She has a reputation as a math whiz and for her go-go energy. I can truly say that now at 4 years old, she is a real Pritikin-style baby.

"I don't keep track of my cholesterol but keep to a substantially 'Pritikin' diet and jog some 15 miles weekly. At

44 I feel 25, take care of husband, house and three children plus work part-time as an editor. All this is possible because of your work. Your efforts have truly given me LIFE. Thank you for caring."

● IRWIN BERMAN, car buyer—Des Plaines, Illinois, age 54

	Before starting the diet	After starting the diet
Marathon	Never	4:42
10K	Never	49:02
Run	Never	50 miles/week
Weight	215	155

"I have been on your program since January 1, 1980. Before I started, I weighed 215, smoked 2½ packs of cigarettes a day, and couldn't walk a block without getting winded. The last time I had any exercise is when I was 10 years old, 44 years ago. *The Pritikin Program for Diet & Exercise* book changed my eating habits and exercise. Once I started on the program, everything seemed to fall into place little by little.

"The first year on your program, I did some walking. The second year my walking increased to 12–15 miles a week. After walking so fast, my feet left the ground and I became a jogger. From September to the end of December 1981, I jogged 500 miles. In 1982, I covered 2500 running miles.

"When I went in for my last physical, my doctor didn't believe it. This is the first time he has ever seen anyone reverse the aging process. If I had never read your book, this would never have happened. I have now stabilized my weight, blood pressure, and resting pulse. I haven't had red meat in 3 years, and I don't miss it one bit.

"Since reading your book, I have become a 55-year-old athlete with the body of a 25-year-old athlete. I am proof of what the Pritikin diet can do. It has saved my life and I try to recruit anybody that will listen to me."

3

Your
Nutritional Needs

You have by now read several times that the Pritikin diet will virtually eliminate certain foods from your diet—namely, salt, sugar, fats, and most meats. You may be wondering whether this will somehow upset your body's chemical balance and leave you with some sort of deficiency. Of course all of us, active or sedentary, need certain foods, which nutritionists call large nutrients: carbohydrates, proteins, and fats; and small nutrients: vitamins and minerals. Let me explain how the Pritikin diet ensures that you will have adequate—in fact, abundant—supplies of all the nutrients essential for good health.

CARBOHYDRATE

Carbohydrates (starches and sugars) provide the fuel our bodies burn, or oxidize, to produce the energy for muscular work—breathing, talking, and thinking. Energy is even needed for moving nutrients around in the body and maintaining the many subtle chemical systems that run our bodies.

27

The diet should be higher in carbohydrates than in the other large nutrients. In fact, carbohydrates, mainly in the form of starches, should make up approximately 80 percent of the diet. The exact amount depends on your size, the proportion of body fat to lean tissue, your state of physical and emotional health, your age, your sex, your level of activity, and external factors, such as climate. In any case, most of your food should be energy-providing carbohydrates which are found in foods "as grown," or unprocessed, such as fresh fruits and vegetables. Very lightly processed carbohydrates are also acceptable. Light processing includes light cooking, grinding of grains into whole-grain flour, and drying of fruits, vegetables, and legumes.

PROTEIN

If we became completely dehydrated, we would be made mostly of protein. It constitutes the major portion of our muscles, connective tissue, cartilage, bone, skin, hair, nails, mucous secretions, lubricating fluid in joints, cell membranes, enzymes, antibodies, and our genetic material. It also plays a role in many physiological processes. It probably seems as though we must need a lot of protein! However, although there is a large quantity of protein in the body, we need to eat relatively little of it, because it is recycled in the body quite efficiently. The opposite is true of carbohydrates. The body stores very little carbohydrate, so we have to eat more of it frequently to provide us with the energy necessary to keep us alive and functioning well.

With protein, it is a different matter. We should eat only about the amount we need each day. Proteins, or the amino acids of which they are composed, should not be used as an energy source, because their waste products are so toxic. Proteins will be used for energy only when the body is not obtaining sufficient calories from other sources, as in starvation, or dieting below 500 calories a day.

Most Americans eat far too much protein. The recommended dietary allowance (RDA) for protein of 56 g (grams) for men and 44 g for women* is 60 percent more than the average person needs. People getting exactly the RDA will be obtaining much more protein than they need. And yet the average consumption of protein for 35–50-year-old women is 64 g, and for American males in the same age bracket it is 96 g.

FAT

Energy is stored in the body in the form of fat. Although carbohydrates are the most efficient source of fuel, they cannot be stored in large amounts in the body. Fats also serve as important parts of cell membranes, where they help control which substances leave and enter the cells. As with proteins, we need fats in only very small amounts. The fats in our body do not come only from fats in the food we eat; they are also metabolized from carbohydrates and proteins. Excess food of any type is converted to fat. As with protein, if we consume enough unrefined food to provide us with the calories we need, we will also obtain enough fat.

We need small amounts of proteins and fats in the diet, and the quantity we need remains fairly constant. The need for carbohydrates, however, varies with energy expenditure. Eating a diet consisting mainly of whole or lightly processed foods will ensure our obtaining enough, but not too much, of the three large nutrients.

VITAMINS

The small nutrients, especially vitamins, have been a matter of some concern to Americans since the synthesis in 1947 of vitamin A, the first vitamin to be discovered. Vitamins usu-

---

* These are much higher than the World Health Organization's recommendation of 40 g of protein a day for adults.

ally function by attaching to and activating certain enzymes. They are synthesized by plants, as they are needed to carry on the plant's digestive and other physiological processes, but vitamins cannot be synthesized by humans and must be obtained from external sources.

When a varied diet, as recommended in the Pritikin Program, is eaten, you will get all the vitamins your body can use and then some. Many people, however, believe taking extra vitamins, especially B, C, and E, in the form of supplements will provide additional health benefits. This, however, is simply not the case.

Vitamins of the B complex are found in grains from which the bran and germ have not been removed. If most of the cereal products you eat are made from unrefined grains, you will obtain all the B vitamins you need. The amount of B vitamins you need is proportional to the amount of carbohydrate in the diet. When you eat whole grains, which are a source of both nutrients, the more carbohydrate you eat, the more B vitamins you get. Too much of the vitamins of the B-complex group will do more harm than good. For example, excess amounts of thiamin can cause allergiclike reactions, and niacin overdosing can cause flushing, headaches, cramps, and nausea.

Humans do not have the ability to make vitamin C, or ascorbic acid, as most animals do.

Man, like the guinea pig, the Indian fruit bat, and the red-vented bulbul bird, has lost the ability to synthesize vitamin C. Therefore, some people believe they need to take large amounts in the form of supplements. However, the RDA recommends that you need only 60 mg of vitamin C daily, which you can derive from eating 2 large tomatoes or 1 large orange, either of which contains 60 mg of vitamin C. On the Pritikin diet, you receive more than 5 times this amount.

A diet that contains a wide variety of unprocessed foods —foods as grown—is high in vitamins. Supplements of water-soluble vitamins provide more than the body can use, and the excess is excreted by the kidneys. That makes for very expensive urine.

Vitamin supplements not only are uncalled for, but are potentially hazardous to your health. In the case of vitamin C, the potential dangers are numerous. Vitamin C facilitates the absorption of iron and calcium, but it inhibits the absorption of vitamin B_{12} and copper. Taking large quantities of supplements can cause serious vitamin and mineral imbalances. On our diet you'll have 300 mg/day—5 times the RDA, but not enough to be toxic. Some advocate 10,000 mg/day, which could have dire consequences.

Some people believe vitamin C is good for heart-disease patients, but because it increases the tendency of the blood to clot, it increases the risk of having a heart attack. It has been claimed that in large amounts vitamin C protects against heart disease by lowering a person's cholesterol and/or triglycerides. This claim has been disproved by a study conducted at Stanford University. Nine people with high cholesterol levels were given 4 g a day of vitamin C for 2 months—about 65 times the recommended dietary allowance. At the end of the study, there was no change in cholesterol or triglyceride levels, but the HDL (high-density cholesterol) protective to your heart dropped by more than 20 percent. A study by the U.S. Department of Agriculture found that vitamin C supplementation, by affecting the zinc-to-copper ratio, actually caused elevated levels of cholesterol in the blood.

One of the most prevalent beliefs about vitamin C is that it can prevent and shorten the duration of the common cold. There is some evidence that a regular modest intake of vitamin C (100–200 mg/day), as contained in the Pritikin diet, will be beneficial as compared with a diet abnormally low in vitamin C. On the other hand, there is no proof that megadosages are in any way desirable. In fact, instead of helping prevent colds, taking large doses for prolonged periods of time has been found to have the opposite effect.

Vitamin C supplementation can interfere with certain diagnostic tests, including those for blood sugar levels and diagnosis of liver disease. It can also cause problems in some people on blood-thinning drugs.

Vitamin C supplementation can cause scurvy. If you take the vitamin over an extended time, your body becomes conditioned to the dosage and dependent on an abnormally high intake. This is similar to drug tolerance. Should the dosage then be reduced to a normal intake, you may experience ascorbic acid deficiency symptoms, or "rebound scurvy," until your body readjusts to its normal state. Many cases of scurvy have been seen in infants on a diet containing 60 mg of vitamin C (approximately twice the RDA of 35 mg for infants). Infantile scurvy can result from a baby's mother's ingestion, while pregnant, of only 400 mg a day. For this reason, vitamin C supplements should not be taken during pregnancy. Some adults who have taken large amounts of vitamin C become permanently dependent on larger amounts. A normal diet is no longer capable of meeting their needs, and without supplements, they develop scurvy.

Vitamin C can induce menstrual bleeding in pregnant women, and it is thought that high intakes may terminate pregnancy. In some women, vitamin C supplementation was thought to be responsible for their inability to conceive.

In sensitive people, large amounts of vitamin C can precipitate attacks of gout; in others, it can cause oxalates to be excreted in the urine, increasing the chances of kidney-stone formation in susceptible people; and in persons with other metabolic abnormalities, vitamin C supplementation causes the red blood cells to break down. In at least one such case, the death of a hospitalized patient was due to vitamin C therapy.

Vitamin E is a complex of fat-soluble substances called tocopherols. It is found in almost all foods, but whole grains and leafy greens are especially rich sources. The vitamin combines easily with oxygen, thereby preventing hormones, vitamins, fatty acids, and other substances in the body from being destroyed by becoming oxidized or rancid.

Because of advertising claims, people believe vitamin E supplements will make them sexier, keep them from aging or developing heart disease, and give them more stamina and endurance, although each of these claims has been scientifically disproved. The truth is, there are very few documented cases of vitamin E deficiency in man because vitamin E is so prevalent in common foods. Vitamin E is stored in tissues throughout the body for long periods of time and is therefore available as needed in the system.

Supplementation with the vitamin is less dangerous than with other fat-soluble vitamins, but weakness and fatigue can result from taking large amounts.

MINERALS

Our food also contains minerals that remain in the body after the food has been metabolized, not unlike the ashes left after wood is burned. Maintaining the proper balance of these minerals in the body is of extreme importance. Minerals help regulate the body's water and acid/base balance; serve as components of hormones, enzymes, vitamins, bones, teeth, hair, nails, and blood and other body fluids and play a role in the function of nerves and muscles. Unprocessed foods are the best source of these minerals. In some segments of our population, however, especially among females, the intake of calcium and iron is marginal. The problem is worsened because the high-fat, high-protein diet eaten by most Americans creates an increased need for these minerals, and also because many people avoid eating leafy green vegetables, which are rich sources of these and other minerals, as well as of carotene (vitamin A) and other vitamins.

If your diet contains a variety of fresh unprocessed foods and modest amounts of leafy green vegetables, you have no need of mineral supplementation. Such supplements could, in fact, prove harmful. If, for instance, your daily requirement for potassium were taken at one time, you could become quite ill. And many cases of iron poisoning are seen each year in young children who ingest an excess of mineral-vitamin supplements. Selenium poisoning may become common in the near future because it has recently become a popular supplement, and only a little more than the required amount can cause severe symptoms of toxicity in man and animals.

With the Pritikin Program, your nutritional needs will be met by a well-balanced diet composed predominantly of whole grains, fruits, and vegetables which contain mainly complex carbohydrates, a modest amount of protein, and a small amount of fat. The diet will also supply optimal amounts of the essential vitamins and minerals. The program promises you a future better than you could have imagined for yourself.

4

Popular Misconceptions About Nutrition

Jaguar flesh is eaten by the Abipone of Paraguay to give them speed. The Miri of Assam eat tigers to make themselves fierce. To make themselves faithful, the Kansas Indians eat dog meat. The African Ashanti eat the hearts of their enemies to give them courage. Other primitive peoples believe that eating human brains gives a man wisdom, and that liver, if eaten raw, gives him courage. Primitives are not the only ones who are subject to dietary superstitions. Americans are gullible too. Weight lifters in our country consume drinks made with protein powder to make them muscular. Runners eat candy bars for quick energy. And some not-so-smart people eat fish for brain power.

Following are the most commonly held misconceptions about nutrition today:

Milk is good for everybody.

Twenty percent of white and 75 percent of black adults have some degree of lactose intolerance. They are deficient in the digestive enzyme lactase needed to digest milk and will have cramps, bloating, diarrhea when they drink milk. Only in the last 5 to 8 thousand years, since dairy animals

34

were domesticated, have humans ever ingested dairy products after they were weaned. Milk is a good source of nutrients, especially calcium, but calcium can also be found in abundance in many other foods, especially leafy green vegetables. Milk is a very poor source of other essential nutrients, among them iron and vitamin C. In addition, overconsumption of dairy products will keep your blood cholesterol deceptively low while still allowing cholesterol to be deposited on artery walls to create blockages.

Raw foods are the most nutritious.

While there is some nutrient loss even with light cooking, if you eat enough unrefined foods to maintain your weight, you'll obtain substantially more of all the nutrients than you need. And cooking can actually increase the amount of nutrients available from food. For instance, you will absorb more provitamin A, as well as other vitamins and minerals, from cooked than from raw carrots. Of course, overcooking and discarding cooking water can result in a drastic loss of vitamins and minerals, and should be avoided.

The more protein in the diet, the more healthful it is.

The body's need for protein has been greatly exaggerated. Excessive protein is not only unnecessary—it can be quite harmful. If the above statement were true, we'd have to ban the use of mother's milk for babies, because cow's milk contains 300–400 percent as much protein as human milk.

It is necessary for vegetarians to combine foods, such as corn and beans, to obtain "complete" proteins.

People who eat no meat but are eating enough plant foods to maintain their optimal weight obtain more than the recommended allowances for protein and all the essential amino acids, regardless of how the foods are mixed or combined.

You should avoid certain food or nutrient combinations, such as acids and starches, protein and starches, or acid fruit with sweet fruits.

If a food eaten by itself is good for you, it's good for you if it's eaten with other healthful foods. Almost all foods contain both protein and carbohydrate—wheat, for example. Citrus fruits contain a lot of both carbohydrates and acids (acetic and ascorbic acids). This doesn't mean that oranges and bread are incompatible any more than bread or an orange is incompatible with itself.

Our soil is so depleted, we need to take supplements to obtain enough nutrients.

If the soil is deficient in the minerals they require, plants won't thrive. With the exception of iodine, selenium, cobalt, and zinc, plants need the same vitamins and minerals we need. If the soil contains low levels of one or more of these 4 minerals, the plants grown in the soil will also contain low levels. However, people living in industrialized societies are served by sophisticated transportation systems and eat foods grown in many areas. Deficiencies caused by poor soil conditions are seen almost exclusively in less-developed societies.

Organic foods are more nutritious than those grown with commercial fertilizers.

Plants can absorb only inorganic chemicals through their root system, so the plant will simply break down organic fertilizers into the same inorganic chemicals that are in commercial fertilizers. Organic foods are, however, more desirable because they are grown without the use of harmful pesticides.

Brown sugar is more healthful than white sugar.

Because brown sugar contains a small amount of molasses and small amounts of iron and other minerals, the calories aren't quite as empty. However, the difference in mineral content is insignificant.

Take cod-liver oil as a lubricant for your joints and cure your arthritis.

Any oil you eat adds to your fat intake and gets digested. It does not go to your joints. This is a 9-year-old child's idea of how joints are lubricated.

PUSF (polyunsaturated fats) will save you from heart disease.

The findings of the 7-year, 12,000-man, $115 million MRFIT (Multiple Risk Factor Intervention Trial) study have been published. The 6,000 men on the AHA (American Heart Association) PUSF diet recorded no differences in heart disease or total deaths from the 6,000 men on the ordinary U.S. diet.

Starches make you fat.

Most of the world is on a diet of more than 70 percent complex carbohydrates; and obesity is rare. These carbohydrates do not include refined or isolated sugar. They come almost entirely from unprocessed, whole plant foods which have more bulk and fewer calories than foods from animal sources. Starchy foods are much less fattening than meat or dairy products.

Fish is a brain food.

The brain can use only glucose as a food. Fish has no glucose.

Sugar (soft drinks, candy) gives you quick energy.

It also gives you a quick letdown. Simple sugars stimulate insulin production, which quickly depletes blood glucose and can create hypoglycemia. What follows is lightheadedness, weakness, loss of concentration, and fatigue.

The U.S. diet is one of the most healthful in the world.

If good health is having heart disease, cancer, diabetes, arthritis, etc., then that statement is correct. Populations around the world whose diets served as a model for the Pritikin diet have essentially none of these diseases.

Spinach makes you strong.

A little spinach is good for you. But that famous nutritionist, "Popeye, the sailor man," did a disservice by popularizing spinach. Spinach is high in oxalate content, and oxalates are implicated in the production of urinary stones. They also prevent the absorption of calcium, and in that way contribute to osteoporosis, or brittle bones, if large amounts are consumed on a regular basis.

A soft diet without roughage is the treatment of choice for colon disorders—hemorrhoids, diverticulosis, colitis, etc.

A soft diet without roughage creates all these problems. These colon problems are virtually nonexistent in populations on high-roughage (fiber) diets.

People with ulcers should drink a lot of milk and cream.

Diets that depend on milk may actually aggravate ulcers, owing to the fact that although milk temporarily neutralizes stomach acid, the protein in milk stimulates more acid production. When dairy products are consumed frequently, they can really aggravate the problem. In addition, the dairy diet for ulcers has been found to greatly increase deaths from heart disease, because of its high fat and cholesterol content.

Taking lecithin will prevent the cholesterol in the food you eat from causing heart disease.

Lecithin is very similar to fat. Because it is both fat- and water-soluble, lecithin functions as an emulsifier, preventing the separation of fats and water in foods and in the body. Because of its emulsifying properties, it is used commercially in such foods as mayonnaise, margarine, ice cream, and bakery products. It also has many uses in industry.

Lecithin can lower the amount of cholesterol in the blood. The mechanism is the same as with polyunsaturated fats. It could cause the cholesterol to be driven into the tissues with which it comes in contact, such as the walls of your arteries. It would be better to leave it in the blood.

Lecithin is produced in the liver. We obtain plenty of lecithin from grains and legumes and all other unrefined foods containing oil and should not take it in its extracted form. When it is broken down, most of the molecule will be used as fat, and excessive amounts will cause the same problems caused by the consumption of too much fat.

Lecithin is sold at "health"-food stores in capsules, granules, and so on. These stores often hand out vitamin-supplement catalogs (thinly disguised as nutritional journals) that feature articles on how lecithin can protect you from heart disease and other ailments. Lecithin promotion is the height of dishonesty and irresponsibility, and misleads victims of heart disease so that many of them delay proper treatment of their disease.

Most of the nutritional misinformation you may have heard will have originated in a variety of popular monthly magazines and books. These include:

1. The health-store variety whose purpose is to sell its products;

2. Newsletters from large food lobbies, as well as small groups and individuals promoting food products;

3. Physical-fitness publications, such as those devoted to body building, running, and general health;

4. Uninformed and poorly researched books on diets for weight loss, athletes, pregnant women, and a host of special conditions—everything from avoiding colon cancer to improving your sex life.

In all of these publications, experts and authorities are featured, and most manage to contradict one another completely. It is little wonder the public is so confused about the basic nutritional concepts that control good health and well-being.

In recent years, self-styled nutritionists have had a tremendous impact on the American public. But their books and health magazines are probably more misleading than all the other advertising claims and health writing in the Western Hemisphere.

The publisher of a popular health magazine was a pioneer in the organic farming movement that called attention to the importance of preserving top soil rich in humus, with its natural abundance of micro- and macro-organisms, and free from poisonous pesticides and herbicides. He also advocated foods that had not had their original vitamins and minerals depleted by refining and processing. But in recommending the addition to the diet of nutrients missing from processed foods, he became the guru of a cult which advocated massive ingestion of food supplements. This potentially harmful advice also diverted attention from the real issue: the need for a diet of natural, unrefined food low in fat and cholesterol to which no supplements need be added.

He became the proponent of such ideas as: (1) people do not get enough electricity, and therefore it is beneficial to subject oneself to shortwave radio waves; (2) to cure an enlarged prostate, a man should eat pumpkin seeds; (3) because of the inferior quality of our present food supply and pollution, it is necessary to take 50–70 food-supplement tablets, capsules, or other preparations a day.

After his death in 1971, his son took over the publication business and now publishes numerous books and magazines. His most widely circulating "health" magazine, reaching millions, serves largely as a vehicle for advertisements for vitamins, minerals, and other supplements. The son writes many articles appearing in the magazine, and tells the public he personally takes bone meal, dolomite, fish-liver oil, yeast, and other supplements every morning. There are many advertisements for these products scattered throughout the magazine. This in itself should be enough to warn the wary.

The son is apparently aware of the recent nutrition research, and warns us against the dangers of including excess sugar, salt, and fats in our diet. However, he doesn't follow this advice. On the contrary, he recommends the use of wheat-germ oil, lecithin, avocadoes, full-fat milk, cheese and other dairy products, nuts and seeds, and many other foods and food supplements that are very high in fat.

In the recipe section of the magazine, one finds recipes such as "Pepper and Cheese Custard," which contains, in addition to other fat- and cholesterol-containing ingredients, 4 cups of cheese and 10 eggs, serving 8 people. It provides each person with 387 mg of cholesterol, almost four times the maximum amount of 100 mg per day that may be safely ingested according to compelling scientific evidence. Sixty-five percent of the calories of this recipe are fat calories. Should you happen to have enemies, give them a copy of this recipe.

The best-known of the authors of inaccurate and unscientifically written nutrition books for the lay public was unusual in that she had a professional background in nutrition, having earned her master's degree in biochemistry from a respected university. But she took things out of context, misquoted people, and wrote of her own experiences as scientific facts. Although she did help popularize the use of whole grains and unprocessed foods, she lauded the qualities of cheeses, eggs, butter, liver, and large supplements of vitamins and minerals. She started her career when the study of nutrition was in its infancy and the first vitamins were just being discovered. A great deal of research has been done since then and many of the old ideas have been proven erroneous. Unfortunately, her obsolete and potentially harmful recommendations are still being promoted in her books, 10 million copies of which had been sold by the time of her death in 1974.

Another author of nutrition books who is still propounding outmoded and fallacious concepts began his nutrition career writing advertising copy for a vitamin company. He then graduated to become a popular educator on a daytime radio program advocating the use of vitamin and mineral supplements in the treatment of acne, asthma, dental cavities, "irregularity," rheumatic fever, multiple sclerosis, sexual problems and gray hair.

Obviously, you should approach with great caution the advice of popular writers who advocate the use of extracts of foods. Excessive amounts of food extracts, whether they be vitamins, minerals, oils, sugars, or anything else, can have serious short- and long-range harmful effects on your health. With the Pritikin 28-day diet, you are never dependent on such extracts, and thus never subject to their dangers. Your 28-day diet is based on natural foods which are whole foods, and which supply ample quantities of all your essential nutrients.

5

CHAPTER

Sick and Tired of
Being Sick and Tired

Sick people are angry—at themselves, at the world, at fate. "Why me?" they ask. "Others seem to eat the same foods, smoke, and drink, and they're fine. Why did I become ill?"

Don't get angry; get even! Healthful nutrition is rarely taught in our country, and you're just a victim, like 200 million others, of the American lifestyle. But you can fight back.

You can have a second chance. Read about these people who seized the opportunity after the age of 50 and now have a whole new feeling about life.

● MINNIA BIENER—Margate, Florida, age 69

IN BED FOR 8 YEARS WITH SEVERE ANGINA
NOW WALKS 2 MILES WITH NO SYMPTOMS

"It's hard for me to believe that I am doing as well as I am. As you remember, I was completely disabled before I came to your clinic. Now I have no problem keeping my weight down, and I am so impressed by your lectures I cannot eat fat, salt or sugar. I walk about 2 miles a day, never looked better or had more energy.

42

"I remember when I came to your Center I arrived in a wheelchair. I was unable to walk. Since 1970 I hadn't done any walking—I had been in bed all that time. The last 5½ months before I came to the Center in 1979, I had a nurse at home because I was confined to bed during that time. I wasn't permitted to use the bathroom. I had been in the hospital prior to that period for a month, one week which I spent in the intensive care unit. The doctor wanted me to have angiograms and possibly surgery. When I refused, he said. 'Make up your mind, then—you're not going to get any better.' Well, I thought if that was my life, it was no life. I came to your Center with high hopes, but little expectations. I was 66 years old, but I felt I had some years left. In the first few days Dr. Pritikin and his staff had me walking all the way down to the end of the dining room, about 70–80 feet. They showed me how bent over I was, and encouraged me to stand and walk tall. Even though it was very painful for me to walk at first, I noticed that when the time went on, gradually the pains decreased. I didn't feel as badly as I did when I started, and I started to feel a little better, and they finally got me 10 minutes of walking. And one day, I went down to the exercise room without my wheelchair. I finally got up to a half-mile a day—two 15-minute walks a day. The doctors also gradually got me off my medication for diabetes and high blood pressure. My blood pressure had started at 200/110—it actually got down to 118/66 without any medication. Now my doctor at home told me that once you start taking medication for blood pressure, it can keep you under control, but you have to take it for the rest of your life. I also had been taking a lot of Demerol at home when the pain was getting excruciating, and I was getting attacks of coronary insufficiency. Now I put away the Demerol, I put away the Donnatol bottle; I put away the Valium bottle. It's been a marvelous experience for me. You have no idea what it means to wake up every morning without pain. I used to wake up every morning with such pain that my husband just couldn't bear to see it. There were times when I was so depressed that I felt I couldn't go on suffering like that.

"I had 8 years lying in bed watching TV, just sort of distracting me from the pain. Well, I won't be in bed anymore. For the first time since 1970, I sit down to the breakfast table with my husband, and I have dinner with him.

"My doctor went into heart failure a couple of times and had to be revived. In fact, he died once, and they revived him. He's working again, but all the doctors keep warning me to go to another doctor, because he isn't going to last much longer; he's a very sick man. I wish he would follow the Pritikin Program."

● NATHAN MUCHNICK—Miami Beach, Florida, age 73

FOUR STROKES, TOO SICK FOR BYPASS SURGERY NOW RUNS 10-MILE RACES

"In the early 1970s, I had a number of severe angina attacks. In December 1975, I had a severe stroke, and lost control of my speech and was disoriented. My speech slowly came back, and the numbness from my head and feet disappeared. While I was in the hospital, I was started on Coumadin, in addition to Inderal and Isordil which I had been taking. In January 1976, I started to get severe chest pains which just completely immobilized me. I couldn't walk or step without shooting pain. At that point I was hospitalized. In April 1976, my doctor suggested I have an angiogram taken.

"The same evening after the angiogram, I had severe head pains, and again, I had a minor stroke. My speech was garbled and I was completely disoriented. My doctor decided I was in no condition to have bypass surgery, and after a while, I was sent home. They told me to take it easy, not to walk, but sit up for half an hour after eating. They also increased all my medication.

"At this point, I thought I had better retire and gave up my business. I left my son in charge and moved to Miami Beach. When I was in Miami, I suffered 2 more strokes. I heard about you and decided to come to your Center in January 1977.

"During my stay at the Center, I was taken off all medication except for the Coumadin. I stayed on it a while longer upon the insistence of my Philadelphia doctor until my toes turned purple. I was taken off Coumadin 3 months after I left the Center. About a year after I left the Center, I decided I would start running, I was feeling so well.

Today I run—6 miles every morning...

...been an inspiration for many people in the area. For my doctors, with whom I some times...tests are no... and in fact I just finished a 10K run in West Chester, Pennsylvania. It was a long course of long hills, no short races, one sharp position. I like to see that I conquer run those hills and survive like a real...You keep up your splendid work, and keep talking about you.

After 4 weeks...and such that he...strong enough to grow...to pass...the tests...of treatment...I know that I like...someone...that this diet program is not one of many systems of life chosen...our program is the best they've seen...ical products...

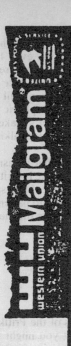

15 ADVISE WITH CONFIDENCE...A...GAMUT CHAPEL...NOW I CAN WORK UP FOR MILE...

My husband and I are showing the volumes at the Pritikin Program. We are very active, and we feel that you might be interested in a letter that I wrote to a physician in Spokane, Washington, when he sent me the documents to review prior to the operation. The letter follows:

January 1979—Dear Doctor: As simply your question...matte has...in our fondest concerns...have been very heartening...our...out of a rut...and...back after 15 months...the technique will...follow it faithfully...the method or power...the lives...have saved my life...

After...hospital I met a Doctor...

...follows the...As time went on...I was...climbing up the...more...and...the short sentences...to the edges...

We began to...in...understanding...needed to...and exercises...and...assumptions...also...needed to take part in the...The program...at the Pritikin Center in Santa Barbara...

My husband went on the program for 27 days...

MAILGRAM

western union

NATMAN MUCMNICK
301 176 ST
MIAMI BEACH FL 33160

4-0253678131 05/11/82 ICS IPMMTZZ CSP LSAB
2155640209 MGM TDMT PHILADELPHIA PA 30 05-11 1250P EST

RECEIVED MAY 12 1982

NATMAN PRITIKIN
1910 OCEANWALK
SANTA MONICA CA 90401

I DID IT I DID IT THANKS TO YOU I COMPLETED TEN MILE MARATHON WITH
DAUGHTER LISA AND SON CHUCK
NATMAN MUCMNICK

12:50 EST

MGMCUMP

'Today, I run 5-6 miles every morning. My running has been an inspiration for many people in this area, even for my doctor and doctors with whom I socialize. My stress tests are normal, and in fact, I just finished a 10K race in West Chester, Pennsylvania. It was a tortuous run, full of long hills, and short dales, but I felt positively euphoric to see that I could run those hills and survive. So let's make a deal. You keep up your splendid work, and I'll keep talking about you.

'After 4 strokes and such bad heart disease that I wasn't strong enough to even receive bypass surgery—the last rites of medicine—I now feel like someone half my age. I feel sad that this diet program is not offered by physicians to patients like myself. Your program is the best-kept secret in the medical profession.''

● LOUISE TRAIL—Moscow, Idaho, age 71

> 15 MONTHS AFTER CORONARY BYPASS SURGERY,
> A CARDIAC CRIPPLE.
> NOW WALK-JOGS UP TO 5 MILES

'My husband and I are enjoying the benefits of the Pritikin Program. We are very active, and I thought you might be interested in a letter that I wrote to my physician in Spokane, Washington, when he sent me a questionnaire to report on my condition. The letter follows:

'' 'January 1979. Dear Doctor: Although your questionnaire has been in my hands for some time, I have been very hesitant to fill it out and return it, because I chose, after 15 months of not feeling well, to follow an alternative method of post-operative living with impressive results.

'' 'After open-heart surgery in December 1976, I faithfully followed Dr. S's instructions when he dismissed me from the hospital. As time went on, I was not feeling better. In spite of following his diet suggestions, I gained weight. The angina pains began again, not often, but severe enough to worry us. It seemed to us that I was heading back to the operating table and wanted to avoid this possibility. So I decided to take part in the 26-day program at the Pritikin Center in Santa Barbara

'' 'My husband went on the program too, as a preventive

46

measure. We entered the program in March 1978, and, by the end of 26 days were already feeling better. After returning home, we continued to follow the diet and exercise rules set up for us there, and we intend to stay on this way of living, as it is not grim or difficult, and the results are very rewarding. Since last March we both lost 38 pounds and never felt better. I walk and jog almost every day 2½–5 miles. Even today, when the temperature was slightly below zero, I walked 1.6 miles. Walking is done on hilly, graveled country roads.

" 'Before I went on the Pritikin Program, I could not even walk up our hills. Now they don't even faze me. In the summer and fall, I swim twice a week, swimming more than a quarter of a mile each time. In July, I went backpacking— a 10-mile trip—carrying my own pack, and keeping up with the young people was no trouble. Sleeping on the ground, hiking back the next day, and I didn't even have as much as a sore muscle.

" 'A year ago, I could not even drive my car. This last October I drove to the Oregon coast and back—about a 1000-mile round trip. I'm now able to do many things that I could not do at all during the first 15 months following my open-heart surgery operation. Some doctors are recommending the Pritikin Program as an alternate to bypass surgery, and for heart surgery patients after they leave the hospital. You can save them a lot of misery and make their lives worth living again. This, I realize, is the testimony of only one person, but there are hundreds of others who have had the same experience. I have a new life, and my husband has a renewed wife.' "

● JESSIE WARRINGTON—Lincolnville, Maine, age 53

   CARDIAC CRIPPLE, 13 HEART PILLS A DAY
   NOW HIKES HILLS, AEROBIC-DANCES AND
   CROSS-COUNTRY-SKIS

"When I was 51, I was in the hospital 2 weeks with a heart condition and I came out an old woman. A few months later, I was still breathless, tired, shuffling around, and taking 13 heart pills a day. The side effects from all that medication were deep depression, crying jags and very short fuses as far as my family was concerned. After much complaining to my doctor, he told me I'd better learn to live with it.

"After hearing this, I literally went to pieces and determined there had to be another way. My daughter-in-law found a doctor who used the Pritikin diet, and I went to him and he literally saved my life. In 2½ months, I lost 29 pounds and could walk 3 miles a day. I could hike the Maine hills again and even took up aerobic dancing and cross-country skiing. I am actually in better health now than I was before I became ill. When something changes one's life as much as your diet has changed mine, you get almost evangelical about it and want everyone to feel as well as you do."

● IRWIN BAKER—Rancho Palos Verdes, California, age 54

DEADLY ARRHYTHMIA
NOW DOES ULTRAMARATHONS

"Before I went on your program, and in fact, for many years before my heart problem intensified, I was a jogger. I would jog approximately ½ mile a day on a fairly regular basis. Occasionally, when I was feeling particularly strong, I would jog as far as one mile without rest. My recollection as to how I felt in those days when I ran that distance was utter exhaustion. In my mind, jogging a mile was a major accomplishment.

"For about 2 years prior to going on your program, I stopped jogging completely on the advice of my cardiologist who recommended that I walk instead, because my heart problem had become much worse. I was experiencing strings of premature ventricular contractions, or PVC's, and I understood that this could be the sign right before sudden death, and of course it worried me. During this period, I was hospitalized twice, and I was put on medications on a regular basis. But the drugs did not eliminate my symptoms. I felt fluttering sensations in my heart several times a day, and needless to say, I became very depressed. I had to give up running. I also had a lot of stomach upsets and acid indigestion due to my drugs, so I consumed many antacid tablets in addition to the medications. I had frequent headaches, severe constipation. In fact, it was so bad I often woke up from the acid indigestion.

"A former patient of your Pritikin Center who is a very close friend suggested your regression diet about January 1977. My cardiologist said, 'No diet can get you off your medication, but since it won't hurt you either, I can't disapprove.'

"Within days my improvement was uncanny. In 6 weeks time, not only had all the symptoms disappeared, but my doctor agreed to let me stop the medication. Now, my heart problems are only a bad memory. The stomach upsets and the acid indigestion that I had, completely disappeared. The constipation and headaches completely disappeared. I haven't taken any medications or antacids ever since.

"For about 5 or 6 months after starting the Pritikin diet and going off the medication, I continued to abstain from running. I was happy to be free of symptoms, but I was fearful that running might bring the symptoms back. However, after about 6 months of symptom-free living, thanks to your diet, I had enough courage to cautiously try running again.

"In the period of the summer of 1977, when I first started running again, to 1980, I have run 12 marathons and two 40-mile ultramarathons. It has now been about 5 years since I started, and today at age 54, I train about 60–70 miles per week. I run one competitive marathon every 2 or 3 months and an ultramarathon (42+ miles) once a year. My first marathon time was 4:09. My current time is around 3:33. The first ultramarathon was 39 miles in January 1979 and it took me 8 hours. This year I ran 42 miles in about the same time.

"I enjoy my new way of life, and in particular, I enjoy eating the Pritikin way. In fact, even if someone could convince me that my diet was bad for my health (an absurd notion) I couldn't go back to my old eating habits anyway. In short, I am hooked, and I love it! I enjoy better all-around health than I did even as a teenager, thanks to the Pritikin diet. It may have saved my life and it certainly improved its quality. I do not take vitamins, aspirins or any other drug or medication.

"I must admit to one problem however. I cannot overcome my tendency to proselytize for Pritikin, much to the consternation of my friends. I take responsibility for a large number of converts over the years, including two of our friends who happen to be physicians.

"I was close to death, but now I'm so alive, my feet don't touch the ground. I'd like to help you convert the world."

PART TWO

SPECIAL ADVICE FOR RUNNERS AND OTHER ATHLETIC PEOPLE

6

Nutritional Needs
of Athletic People

The Pritikin diet is ideal for runners, hikers, bikers, mountain climbers, spelunkers, and other outdoor-sports fans. If you're active in sports, you need the same nutrients as sedentary people. Your body will require some of the vitamins and minerals in slightly larger amounts, but the Pritikin diet would supply them even if you weren't eating more food for the extra calories you need. As far as the large nutrients are concerned, you do need to increase the amount of carbohydrates you eat, but you *don't* need additional fat or protein. Scientific studies have shown that on a diet high in complex carbohydrates, athletes have up to three times the endurance of those on the conventional high-protein, high-fat diets.

PROTEIN

Many athletes and body builders believe they should eat more protein. This is not the case, however, and the following account illustrates the effectiveness of a low-protein, high-carbohydrate diet. The Hawaii "Ironman" Triathlon is a grueling athletic event consisting of a 2.4-mile swim in the open ocean, a 112-mile bicycle course, and a 26.2-mile marathon. In the October 9, 1982 event, there were 850 contestants. First, second, and fourth places were won by men on the Pritikin diet. Dave Scott set a new record by completing the 3 events in 9 hours, 8 minutes. Many people were astonished to learn that on a diet high in starchy foods, the "ironmen" could survive, not to mention breaking world records. Their skepticism was in large part due to the prevalence of myths regarding nutrition and athletic performance—mainly the big protein myth.

Most athletes have always favored high-protein diets. They believed that because muscles are made of protein they should therefore consume plenty of protein. But it is not quite that simple: think of the bull, who grows big and strong eating nothing but grass all day. Unfortunately, the "eat muscle to make muscle" type of reasoning still motivates some weight lifters, who eat diets high in animal foods and take protein-powder supplements to promote muscle development. The problem is, the extra protein goes to fat —not to muscle.

Even on a strict vegetarian diet which includes no eggs or dairy products, if an athlete eats enough food to maintain his weight, there will be more than enough protein for muscle growth and maintenance. Excess protein will go to fat— unless the diet is deficient in carbohydrate, in which case the protein will be inefficiently used as a fuel source to provide energy.

To build muscle, sufficient calories—primarily from carbohydrates—small amounts of protein, and vigorous strenuous activity are needed. You simply cannot substitute protein supplements for proper diet and hard work. In order to enlarge and strengthen muscles, you have to stress them —increase the demand on them to produce energy. Enzymes in the tiny "organs," or mitochondria, of muscle cells provide the energy for physical work, and as the demand on the cells to produce energy increases, your muscles grow by forming more and bigger mitochondria. Prolonged strenuous exercise is the only way to get bigger muscles. Forget about the extra protein and get to work!

Not only does extra protein not make bigger and better

muscles, it can actually be extremely dangerous for athletes. As you will understand by now, we need small amounts of protein and fat for our body tissues, enzymes, and hormones; but the fuel source for our *energy* requirements should be carbohydrate—a clean-burning fuel. When carbohydrate is converted to energy, only carbon dioxide and water remain, and our bodies excrete these chemicals quite easily. Ideally, our entire energy or calorie requirement should come from carbohydrates.

When there is adequate dietary carbohydrate to provide this energy, excess protein, fat, and carbohydrate will be stored as potential energy in the form of fat in the adipose tissues throughout the body. In the absence of sufficient carbohydrate foods, fats and proteins will be converted to the energy needed to keep the body functioning—breathing, digesting, regulating its temperature, and so on.

The problem is that in order for protein to be digested and converted to energy or stored as fat, it has to rid itself of its ammonia molecules, which are left as waste products. Because ammonia is toxic to the cells and difficult to eliminate, we say that protein does not burn clean. As the process continues, two ammonia molecules are joined to form urea. This is less toxic than ammonia, but harmful enough to require large amounts of water to dilute its toxicity so that it can be excreted without damage to the kidneys. High-protein diets are therefore very dehydrating.

Dehydration is of great concern to athletes, who lose enormous quantities of water through perspiration. The body keeps from overheating via perspiration, and evaporation of moisture on the surface of the skin has a cooling effect. Thus the body keeps its internal temperature from increasing too much during strenuous exercise. However, when you are dehydrated, your evaporative cooling mechanism is adversely affected, and you may suffer heatstroke, which can be—and too often is—fatal to athletes exercising strenuously in hot weather.

In addition, too much protein causes minerals, like calcium, to leave the bones in order to neutralize the acids formed in protein metabolism. We believe this to be the principal cause of weak or thin bones (osteoporosis)—epidemic in the United States for those over 50 years old.

And finally, excess protein can have detrimental effects on your performance and endurance. A number of studies have shown that on a mixed diet one has greater endurance than on a high-protein diet; but on a high-carbohydrate diet, athletes have *3 times* the endurance they have on a high-protein diet. "Carbs" are the fuel of winners. So it is not really so surprising that the best-performing athletes in the Hawaii Ironman Triathlon were those on the Pritikin diet.

I believe you will be interested to know that carbohydrates provide greater endurance for other species as well. Carnivorous animals can run with great speed, but their endurance is minimal. Cats, for instance, have the ability to run faster than almost any other animal. The caracal lynx and the cheetah have been clocked up to 65 mph, but only for short distances. You will recall that cats are also renowned for the inordinate amount of time they spend sleeping. However, herbivores, which make up the bulk of the animal kingdom, have far greater endurance. Giraffes and racehorses can not only run 45 mph, but can sustain this speed for long periods of time. The endurance of man and pig, two of the few omnivorous animals, lies midway between that of the meat- and the plant-eaters.

FATS

Fats are a necessary part of our makeup because energy can be stored in a concentrated form in fat cells. During exercise, large amounts of both carbohydrate and fat from the storage depots provide us with energy. Therefore, some athletes believe they need to eat a lot of fat. But a higher proportion of our energy comes from fat when we're at rest than when we're exercising. The idea that athletes need to eat more fat resembles the myth that in order to be brave you have to eat the heart of a lion; or that in order to make muscle you have to eat muscle. In actuality, the "fat" or fatty acids we burn for fuel do not come directly from our food. They are liberated from fats in the adipose (fat) tissue, and the fats in this tissue have come from carbohydrates, proteins, or fats. It is actually preferable when very little of this fat is derived from fatty foods. In fact, we can get most of the fat we need from whole grains—although I must caution you that the essential fatty acids have been removed from refined flour.

Fats are composed of 3 fatty acids attached to a short skeleton, called glycerol; fats are also called triglycerides, which means "3 fatty acids." In order to be stored in the cells of adipose tissue, fatty acids must become part of a triglyceride. Subsequently, the triglycerides in the adipose tissue must be broken down into fatty acids before being released into the blood and transported to the muscle cells to be burned for energy. Adipose tissue is like Grand Central Station. Free fatty acids are constantly breaking away from the triglyceride (fat) molecules in the adipose-tissue station to travel in the bloodstream. Those which are not used for energy return and become part of a triglyceride so they can enter the station again to be stored until needed.

CARBOHYDRATES

The typical American diet doesn't provide enough carbohydrate for athletes in hard training. As you now know, most of the calories of sedentary people should come from carbohydrates, and athletes need an even larger percentage of carbohydrates.

Carbohydrate is the main fuel for endurance, and it can be the limiting factor if your diet is deficient in carbohydrates. Some ardent athletes, especially runners, adhere to a potentially dangerous and misnamed practice called carbohydrate loading. This is their reasoning: because only a small amount of carbohydrate is stored in muscle cells in the form of glycogen, they believe they should increase the amount of this potential energy. Endurance athletes will therefore exercise themselves to exhaustion 7 days prior to a competitive event. For the next 3 days they curtail severely the amount of carbohydrate in their diets by subsisting mainly on high-fat animal products—dairy foods, meat, and eggs. This causes depletion of glycogen in the muscles. During the next 3 days, they eat high-carbohydrate meals in order to load their muscles with glycogen. After the 3-day depletion phase, the muscles overcompensate and take up an abnormally large amount of glycogen.

Here are the dangers in this scheme:

During the depletion phase of carbohydrate loading, the low-carbohydrate diet causes large amounts of fat to circulate in the blood. Should the athlete have heart disease, this could precipitate a heart attack. It can even cause cardiac irregularities in highly trained individuals without preexisting heart problems.

Also, carbohydrate loading causes enormous amounts of glycogen to be stored in all the muscles that have been worked to exhaustion during the depletion phase—not only the leg muscles, but the heart muscles as well. Glycogen is stored with 3 to 4 times its own weight in water. You can well imagine how difficult it will be for a heart so engorged to function properly.

Carbohydrate loading can cause prostatitis, or swelling of the prostate gland, resulting in very painful urination; it can also lead to potassium depletion and a possible heatstroke during the event. Metabolizing fats in the absence of sufficient carbohydrates can also result in the formation of ketones—toxic substances which when excreted can cause dehydration damage to the kidneys. Less dangerous, but certainly worth considering, is the fact that the weight of the glycogen and the water with which it is stored will make the athlete's legs feel heavy. So much glycogen can be taken up that the muscle tissue can rupture, reducing performance.

The best way to improve endurance and performance is to adhere to the Pritikin diet. That way, you are carbohydrate loading—safely—all the time. Your muscles will have an optimal amount of glycogen without the dangerous side effects of depletion/engorging carbohydrate loading.

On the average, carbohydrates make up 50 percent of the calories in the average American diet. Studies by Dr. David Costill, at Ball State University in Indiana, show that on the 50-percent-carbohydrate diet, it takes 3 days after strenuous exercise to restore the proper glycogen levels, but that it takes only 1 day if you're on a 70-percent-carbohydrate diet.

Thus when only half of your calories come from carbohydrates, you can't perform at your best for 3 days following competitive events or heavy training. On the Pritikin diet, however, you're ready to do your best after a single day of rest. After one day on a high-complex-carbohydrate diet, the muscles are fully loaded with glycogen.

VITAMINS

In spite of numerous studies disproving any ergogenic, or work-enhancing, effect of vitamin supplements, some athletes continue to believe in such effects. Dr. D. L. Cooper, a physician at the 1972 Olympics, said. "Vitamins need to be mentioned as another subject of the 'great drug myths.' We must remember that vitamins act primarily as catalytic agents and are not metabolized. If a person eats a balanced diet of fresh, well-prepared food, he is getting all the vitamins his body can use. . . . There are many salesmen in this country and many gullible people who are victimized financially by vitamin 'pushers.' Americans excrete the most expensive urine in the world because it is loaded with so many vitamins!"

Vitamin E is the vitamin most often taken by athletes to improve their performance and increase their endurance. The fact is that large amounts may actually reduce endurance, and in some people cause weakness and fatigue.

In a 50-day double-blind study of ice hockey players in Canada, scientists set out to determine whether vitamin E might give just that little edge of extra endurance the athletes need toward the end of a game. Twenty hockey players were paired off according to what is called oxygen uptake, a measurement of their maximum endurance. One group received 1,200 IU of vitamin E and the other group only a placebo. They were tested on treadmills before and after the 50 days. Those taking the vitamin E increased the maximum amount of oxygen they could consume by 10 percent. Those on the placebo increased the maximum amount of oxygen they could consume by 30 percent. The researcher, Dr. Good, an associate professor in the Department of Physiology, University of Toronto, wrote. "One facetious observation might be that placebo may result in greater improvement than vitamin E."

Vitamin C has also been tested to determine whether

supplementation would have work-enhancing (ergogenic) effects. Two groups of 20 young (average age 24.5) physical-education majors were given treadmill tests before and after a 5-day ingestion of either 2 g of vitamin C or a placebo. The double-blind test showed no significant difference between those who took vitamin C and those on the placebo.

The B vitamins act along with enzymes as coenzymes, or catalysts in the conversion of food, especially carbohydrates, to energy. Therefore, many people reason that if they're tired, B-complex capsules will give them a boost of energy and improve their work performance. However, the amount of B-vitamin catalysts we need is directly related to the amount of carbohydrates burned. The B vitamins are contained in fresh whole-carbohydrate foods in optimal amounts, and taking extra won't provide any additional benefits. Double-blind scientific studies show no difference in work performance between those taking vitamins and those taking placebos. In fact, excessive amounts of nicotinic acid inhibit the ability of the heart muscle to use fatty acids as a fuel source. Supplements of the B complex of vitamins containing nicotinic acid should not be taken before strenuous activity.*

The Pritikin diet contains a wide variety of unprocessed foods as grown and is rich in vitamins. Vitamin supplements not only are uncalled for, but are potentially hazardous to your health.

MINERALS

Recently athletes have become interested in mineral supplements, especially of the trace minerals known as electrolytes. These supplements have become quite popular now, and athletes are paying premium prices for fancy artificially flavored and colored powdered beverage mixes containing sugar, sodium, and potassium. However, only the *fluid* lost in perspiration needs to be replaced, and electrolyte supplements are unnecessary. Even with up to a 4 percent loss of

---

* Counsilman, J. E. *Competitive Swimming Manual for Coaches and Swimmers.* Counsilman Company, 1977, p. 82.

body weight through sweating, mineral loss is small. Compared with other body fluids, sweat is hypotonic, which means the concentration of sodium, potassium, and other electrolytes in perspiration is more dilute than in the body tissues. In fact, it is the most dilute solution produced by the body. There will be some loss of minerals in prolonged sweating, but they are still more highly concentrated in body tissues after dehydration. In addition, during exercise, glycogen in the liver and muscle cells frees up potassium to increase its concentration in the blood. Supplemental electrolytes would result in too high a mineral concentration in the blood—a disastrous imbalance.

Any potassium lost during exercise is easily replaced at the next meal generous in unrefined foods. Lean, well-trained athletes have especially large potassium reserves, because muscle cells contain more potassium than any other tissue. To reiterate: the main loss in sweat is water, and that is what needs to be replaced. If you drink water supplemented with even small amounts of sugar and electrolytes, it will take longer to pass through your stomach and into the tissues, where the fluid is needed. Plain water is the best thing to drink before, during, and after exercise, and it's important to do so on long runs, such as marathons, whether you are thirsty or not to meet your body's fluid needs. And remember that salting your food or taking salt tablets can increase your need for fluids to a point at which the need cannot be met.

It does not matter whether people are sedentary, active, or champion athletes. If they eat a variety of foods, primarily of plant origin, that have not been highly processed, they will not need or benefit from taking vitamin, mineral, or protein supplements or any other magic potion. In the next section, we will take a hard look at more of the myths held by both athletes and nonathletes.

7

Nutritional Advice
for Athletic People

Runners are especially sensitive to any information on methods that can affect their performance. Some of them are always looking for a "magic potion" to give them an extra edge on their competition, and they eagerly scan nutrition publications for the "experts' " advice.

Tom Bassler, M.D., has been featured widely in most running magazines and regularly writes letters to the editors of many medical journals. Bassler's popularity demonstrates the power of self-proclaimed nutritional experts over the reader. His opinions carry great weight because he has run marathons and is active in the AMJA (American Medical Joggers Association), an association of physicians who run. You can judge the wisdom of the following statements he has made.

Statement: "Beer is a good drink for the marathoner. It replaces the potassium you sweat out during a run which helps prevent heart attacks."

Beware! The carbonation and the bitterness of the beer make it taste good when you are hot and thirsty. However.

it will not only make you feel hotter shortly after the first few quaffs, but will greatly increase your chances of sustaining heat injury.

Your body will absorb the alcohol in beer quite rapidly, so that the sedative-hypnotic effects occur quickly. Some beer-drinking runners support their choice for fluid replacement on its potassium content. However, 8 oz of orange juice or a large banana has 8½ times the potassium of 8 oz of beer. You will recall that there is no need to replenish trace minerals during competitive events. In fact, it can be harmful to do so. Vitally important, though, is that water be replaced. For that reason, beer is the last thing an athlete should drink, especially when performing on a hot day. Alcohol acts as a diuretic (stimulating urination) and causes dehydration. Drinking beer could cause death from heatstroke. Drinking 2 or more beers could put you to sleep forever.

Jay Bock, M.D., of the University of Florida did a crossover study with 20 asymptomatic men, 25–65 years old. On one night, half had orange juice; the other half had orange juice with 2 oz of vodka. Continuous monitoring while they were asleep demonstrated that the alcohol drinkers experienced 110 apneic events in which breathing stopped for 10 seconds or more, compared with only 20 events for those on orange juice. Apneic events are often the cause of death because they could initiate ventricular fibrillation, which leads to sudden death, even while you are asleep.

Statement: "Don Jones, who refuses to take his megadoses of vitamin C, tore his achilles."

The U.S. Air Force studied 286 officers (*JAMA*, 1970, *211*: 105) to see if there was a difference in the rate, severity, and duration of athletic injury sustained by those taking 1000 mg of vitamin C a day compared with those taking a placebo. No difference was found.

Statement: "No cases of death due to coronary atherosclerosis have been recorded in marathon finishers."

Years after evidence appeared in medical journals describing marathon runners' deaths from coronary events, Bassler continued to deny the correlation between running and coronary atherosclerosis in some deaths. (See Chapter 25 on runners' deaths.) Since the evidence is now overwhelming that runners die of heart disease, Bassler has evolved a new theory that the runners' deaths are the result of "nutritional arrhythmia," citing nutritional reasons, especially a low-fat (10-percent) diet.

Some examples follow:

Statement: "When I first saw the death certificate of Arne Richards, I knew it was wrong. . . . I knew that was another nutritional arrhythmia . . . [Arne drank a lot of tea.] *Tea has lots of phytates*—blocks absorption of metals [producing mineral deficiency]. Arne just did not have the nutrients he needed to train in the hot Kansas climate."

Tea has *no* phytates.

Statement: "For marathoners, the Pritikin diet or the 'idealized Tarahumara diet' is dangerous because there isn't enough linoleic acid to protect cardiac function. Marathoners burn about 50 Kcal of linoleic acid for each mile beyond the 20 km (12-mile) mark. Any diet with only 10% fat will have only 5% of the calories as linoleic acid . . . and remember that 5% of 2000 Kcal is only 100 Kcal a day. . . . If anyone tried to run marathons regularly on the 80-10-10 Pritikin diet he should be dead or disabled in 18 months."

By this time Bassler had shifted his position and conceded that marathoners do die, suddenly—but from nutritional arrhythmia, because he claims that on a 10-percent-fat diet there will be a deficiency of linoleic acid, an essential fatty acid.

I must take issue with Dr. Bassler's knowledge of nutrition. I can only conclude that Dr. Bassler must have misinterpreted something he read in medical journals about fat requirements of runners. It is well known that runners require about 300 calories of fat each hour from their fat stores for energy. Dr. Bassler perhaps thought that the 300 calories of fat required was linoleic acid, a fat eaten in small quantities but essential, because the body can't make it.

By his reasoning, a runner would have to eat 300 calories of linoleic acid for every hour of running, or risk death. If a marathoner were to drink peanut oil, which Dr. Bassler recommends, he would have to drink 16 ounces or 1½ quarts for a 10-hour triathlon!

The point again is that the energy you derive from fat for running doesn't come from fat that you eat. It comes from your adipose tissue, where fat is stored after being metabolized from all three large nutrients—protein, carbohydrates, and fats.

The body makes all the fat you need from protein, carbohydrates, and fat, as present in ordinary foods, with one exception. Humans cannot make linoleic acid. However, if you eat at least 1 percent of your total calories in linoleic acid, you will meet the body's requirement. Linoleic acid is called an essential fatty acid (EFA) because it *must* come from the diet. It is found primarily in whole grains—oats, whole wheat, brown rice, corn, barley, millet—and in lesser amounts in other plant foods (fruits, vegetables, and legumes).

Energy for muscular work comes primarily from glucose (carbohydrate) and fat. The fat you eat is not directly used for energy after it is digested and absorbed from the small intestine, but goes to the adipose (fat) tissue in the form of triglycerides, which, you will recall, are composed of three fatty acids, referred to as FFA, or free fatty acids, plus glycerol. When the muscles call for fuel, the free fatty acids are released and provide about 50 percent of the calories used. A runner would probably use about 300 calories of FFA per hour.

Bassler's error was in stating that runners use 300 calories of *essential* fatty acids (EFA). In fact, the research to which Bassler referred stated specifically that runners use 300 calories of *free* fatty acids (FFA).

Bassler also stated that "During prolonged running, linoleic acid is specifically utilized as an energy substrate"—in other words, required for fuel, or energy, during running. Once again, we have determined by checking Bassler's sources that he misread the information he used and thus reported it incorrectly. In fact, burning 300 calories of FFA presents no problem. The average athlete has 15 percent body fat—or at 150 pounds, 22 pounds of fat. Each pound can convert to FFA sufficient to run for 11 hours.

Even if it were true that runners need much more linoleic acid, the Pritikin diet would still be the diet of choice, because it provides 3 to 4 times the amount of linoleic acid you need. Medical studies establish that on a 10-percent-fat Pritikin-type diet, the adipose tissue has 60 percent more linoleic acid than on the 42-percent-fat American diet. This higher linoleic, or essential-fatty-acid, reserve gives one greater protection against any possibility of essential-fatty-acid deficiency.

Another Bassler misreading of a medical study was on peanut butter. Bassler advocates peanut oil because it contains 25 percent linoleic acid. In order to get 300 calories of linoleic acid per hour to meet his recommendation for runners, one would have to eat 1200 calories (⅓ lb) of peanut butter for every hour of running.

If one read carefully the medical study he quotes as his peanut butter justification (Smith, *Lancet* 1980, *1*:534), one would learn the following: "Peanut oil contains about 60% oleic acid (18:1) and 25% linoleic acid (18:2) and so theoretically it should be a 'good' oil. . . . Extensive studies have now been reported . . . and in all the trials the most severe atherosclerotic lesions [narrowing or closure of the coronary arteries by cholesterol and fat deposits] in both aorta and coronary arteries were produced by peanut oil. . . . Serum cholesterol levels remained low on peanut oil."

You would be closing your arteries because of his nutritional recommendations.

I have documented at least 50 errors in Bassler's nutritional recommendations and could write a separate book on this subject.

A remark of Bassler's is fitting: "You've got to make your own decision. After all, I might be wrong."

After the publication in running magazines of Bassler's article on nutritional arrhythmia and other irresponsible reports on nutrition, the Community Nutrition Institute warned that "runners and other fitness enthusiasts who rely on the nation's major running magazines for diet advice are more likely to be confused than helped." The editor of *The Community Nutritionist,* Stephen Clapp, says running magazines do not provide sound, consistent advice on nutrition. In his article "Always Say Diet" (*The Community Nutritionist,* Nov.–Dec. 1982), Clapp summarizes the current national dietary recommendations:

1. The National Academy of Sciences reports that the high amount of fat eaten in the American diet is a principal cause of breast, colon, and prostate cancer. Not only does the Academy advise the substantial reduction of all fats, but it cites evidence that polyunsaturated fats, such as are found in corn oil, vegetable margarines, safflower oil, sunflowerseed oil, and the like, increase the incidence of colon cancer more than the same amount of saturated fats, like butter or lard. Fats are out.

2. The American Heart Association has reconfirmed its position favoring a low-fat and low-cholesterol diet because of "a high correlation between the estimated level of fat [and cholesterol] in the diet and the severity of atherosclerosis."

3. The U.S. Dietary Guidelines and the Senate Nutrition Committee's *Dietary Goals* recommend cutting back on all fats, both saturated and polyunsaturated, and cholesterol.

Clapp continues: "There is nutritional expertise available to the editors of running magazines but they choose not to use it. If the running magazines were as irresponsible in medical matters as they are about nutrition, the readers would be offered cures by orgone therapy and phrenology.

"Readers," Clapp says, "*are* eager for sound nutrition information as part of their fitness programs. Reader surveys show that diet advice ranks with training tips among the most popular features. . . . The running magazines," he says, "should catch up with the times." He urges running magazines to hire nutritional editors who "should either be formally trained in nutrition or have the background and the intelligence needed to separate sound advice from quackery."

To which I can but add a fervent Amen!

8

CHAPTER

Joggers and
Athletic Families

I am inundated with letters and stories from athletic people telling of their enthusiasm for the Pritikin diet. I hear from people who run from three times a week for half an hour to those who compete in marathons or triathlons, and I hear from children and from the elderly. I hear from women and from men. I hear from those who were sick when they started running, as well as from those who were healthy.

Perhaps the most vivid testimonial comes from Col. James B. Irwin, a former *Apollo 15* astronaut. We might well ask why an astronaut, who surely has access to the best in medical care, would independently seek out and follow the Pritikin Program. Individuals selected for the space program must undergo the most rigorous screening and training, and we would expect that their good nutrition and exercise habits would continue to serve them later in life. Irwin's remarks as he describes the splashdown of *Apollo 15* and his own health problems attest to the error in that assumption.

● "We splashed down in the Pacific on August 7, 1971. The medical team was on the carrier, all ready for medical tests. The first thing they said to us was, 'You fellas had a heart

68

problem on your flight.' They said it was probably because my electrolytes were low and I'd lost all my potassium, so my wife started feeding me a lot of bananas. I guess that was the very beginning of the Pritikin Program.

"Then one day when I was playing handball in Denver, I felt a crushing pain in my chest. I couldn't breathe, I felt nauseated. An ambulance took me to the hospital, where the doctor had me in intensive care within thirty minutes. He said, 'Irwin, you've had a heart attack.' I said, 'How can that be? I've been an astronaut, I've been to the moon, I can do anything! People who have heart attacks are people who don't exercise, are overweight and smoke. I've always been a great physical specimen. I've been a health nut all my life. It can't happen to me!'

"But it did happen to me, just as it has happened to thousands of other people who also thought of themselves as 'great physical specimens.'

"When I first entered the Naval Academy, I was actually embarrassed by my slight, small frame. However, on the military diet of high-fat and cholesterol-rich dishes, I started putting on weight. Interested in building up my body, I started weightlifting. After graduating from the Naval Academy, I entered the Air Force, where I continued a rigorous program of weightlifting, as well as handball, racquetball and squash. I remember that the things I was the most proud of at that time were my physical strength and my determination.

"I wanted to participate in space, so they sent me down to the School of Aviation Medicine at Brooks Air Force Base in Texas. There I went through a five-day battery of extensive tests, and the only thing they could find wrong with me was a degree of hypertension, which was waived when it gradually came down.

"Finally in 1966, I qualified for the astronaut program and was flown to Houston, where I underwent a few more medical tests and then entered into a new regimen to prepare for the flight to the moon. They allowed us to choose the exercise program we desired. They thought we were mature, intelligent men and could program our own course. So we spent an hour to an hour and a half a day doing very heavy exercise, and when we weren't running or working with weights or playing ball, we were wearing the space suits, which are exercise in themselves. We had special quarters and our own cook. We were served anything we wanted. We had meat twice a day, eggs for breakfast, steak, desserts, pie a la mode.

"The assumption was that we were working so hard that the food would surely be worked off every day. In fact, the morning of the launch, the crew was assembled and fed a huge steak breakfast. They wanted us to be well-nourished for our flight in space.

"During the actual flight, we ate mostly freeze-dried food and an endless supply of Tang to fight dehydration. However, once we got to the moon and began our work outside, we found we didn't have time to take lunch breaks. I had to go without water for eight hours because my water bag wasn't functioning. The only nourishment I had was a gelatin fruit stick to nibble on. The last day there, the surface heat was 180 degrees, and even though we had good insulation, when we got back into the lunar module, pressurized, and took our gloves and boots off, we found that our hands and feet were immersed in sweat.

"We drank a lot of water, decided we had survived, and left the moon. It wasn't long after that we were finally able to relax—and feel fatigue for the first time. Two days later we headed for home and splashdown, and the warning from the doctor on the carrier that they had picked up signs of heart irregularity in me on our flight.

"Then one day, later in 1976, I noticed that I didn't 'feel right' while playing racquetball with my son. I went for a stress test and was told I had a problem. NASA immediately sent me to a cardiologist in Houston who performed a triple bypass from which I made a quick recovery. Too quickly—two months later, I was skiing in Colorado and I had another heart attack riding on a chair lift.

"After more surgery and recuperation, a friend sent me a copy of *Live Longer Now*, which Pritikin co-authored. I read it and it seemed to make sense to me. Then I ran into my friend Charles Stevens, who had had a stroke and had just gotten back from a program at the Pritikin Longevity Center. I didn't recognize him. He had lost a lot of weight, but he had new energy. He told me how remarkable he felt.

'Jim,' he said, 'this is a program you've got to get on.' So that was my New Year's resolution in 1977.

"And since my wife wanted to keep me around a little longer, I received a wealth of support for my new resolve. In April of 1977, I started on a very slow, progressive jogging program. By that summer I was able to climb Pike's Peak—and jog once I got there.

"I had never felt that good before, and my health continues to improve every day. I enjoy life as I never have before. I still go down to Houston; they encourage me to come down for an annual physical. The doctors are amazed at the results. My weight dropped: I'm thirty pounds lighter than when I made the flight to the moon. My blood pressure is lower than it was when I graduated high school. I don't have hypertension any more and my cholesterol is gradually coming down—it was 300 when I had the first heart attack and 320 at the second. When I was down there last January, the doctor said, 'Jim, this program is good for you—it's working. If we didn't have the evidence that you had bypass surgery and two heart attacks, we'd say you are in better condition than any of the astronauts in the program.'

"I am just one witness to the results and the success that can be achieved when people really understand how health works and that they have it within their power to be well. I know I am indebted to Nathan Pritikin for giving me a new life."

The following letter came from a man who gradually worked up from not being able to run one block comfortably to doing good time in 10K races. He says:

● "I began jogging about two years ago when I realized I could not run a block without stepping on my tongue. It was quite a shock for a 52-year-old, 220-lb. jock—because I had been playing racquetball or handball for the last 20 years 2 or 3 times a week. Apparently any fitness and endurance just slipped away over the years.

"I then began jogging in earnest with a goal of running a mile. It took me about 9 months to run a mile in 12 minutes. My next goal was to get the time down to 10 minutes and then try for 2 miles in 20 minutes. That took about another year to accomplish (the jogging gets pretty spotty for about 3–4 months during our lousy midwestern winters).

"We are now up to November 1981 when my wife and I went to the Pritikin Program on Maui. We went because my physical exam during summer of 1981 showed an elevated cholesterol of 300. I did not know what cholesterol was, and the number 300 had no significance to me. But it was the first time in my life that the doctors pointed out to me any signs of something awry. So we went to Maui to find out what this cholesterol stuff is all about. It changed our lives.

"When we checked in at Maui, I was running 2 miles in 20 minutes and I had been stuck at that level for a few months without much prospect of reducing time or increasing mileage. The jogging was keeping me from going over 220 lbs and I was still enjoying my beer.

"As you can see, the Pritikin diet is changing my cholesterol levels (my original reason for going) and my running performance. I am now running six 9-minute miles a day, 5 times a week (over a very severe winter). I am entering my first race next week—a local 10K.

"I feel that the dramatic increase in mileage and modest reduction in time is due to the weight loss on the diet. I am not hauling all that luggage around. I am happy with the diet and the results it is bringing in improved health and lifestyle."

● When contacted in April 1983, Mr. E. said he had done that race in 54 minutes and had recently run a 10K race in 50 minutes. Needless to say, he's still very enthusiastic about the program.

From the time Mr. E. went on the diet until 2 years later, his weight, blood pressure, heart rate, and blood values showed the following changes:

	Before going on the Pritikin diet	After going on the Pritikin diet
Weight	220	172
Heart Rate	57	51
Cholesterol	300	221

Some people enjoy exercise more if they do it with their families. I've selected the following families from the hundreds I've heard from, because each is very special in its own way. Some were sick, others were well; some are young, others are not; but what impresses me is that people of all ages and conditions can have great fun when they share a common interest—in this case, a new healthful lifestyle.

A letter from Hilda Richardson in Hawaii tells of 3 generations of women on the Pritikin diet who run together. Hilda is a 67-year-old grandmother. She runs with her two daughters and their children. She says:

● "I have run 4 marathons, and have been in relays and fun races. Never did I plan to be a runner: my career started in 1976 because of poor health.

"In 1975, the pain in my back was excruciating. X-rays showed spurs, fused vertebrae, degenerated discs, bone destruction and osteoporosis. My circulation was hampered by a clogged aorta. When my doctor told me that my cholesterol level was 395 mg% and triglyceride, 385 mg%, he warned me about an imminent heart attack, and possible breast or colon cancer.

" 'Keep in mind, Mrs. Richardson,' said my doctor, 'your condition has no cure; resign to your fate. What you have is hereditary, degenerative and progressive. Within a year or so you will be confined to a wheelchair.'

"I determined to fight for my health, and after a lot of research decided that nutrition was the key to my problems. On my own, I started avoiding fats and meats, and my health started to improve. In the first part of 1979, I had the good fortune to be listening to the *Merv Griffin Show*, and you were one of his guests. I followed your advice, and I went on your diet.

"By December 1979, I was doing so well that I ran a marathon in 6:10. By this time my cholesterol had dropped from 395 mg% to 223 mg%. My grandson, at 18 years old, was told by a dermatologist that his psoriasis had no cure, but he went on your diet and it is gone. Besides these wonderful recoveries, our family has other benefits: no more constipation, gas pains, stomach acidity, heartburn, sluggishness, or hemorrhoids."

In December 1981, Hilda ran her fourth marathon with a cracked rib and a broken toe. "I had to finish," she said. "I got my two daughters and my grandson to run this race, so I had to finish."

Gina, her daughter, agreed that her mother had shamed her and her son into entering the marathon. "Here was my mother running a marathon at age 66. I didn't think I had an excuse any more." Tony, the 20-year-old grandson, said, "My mom and grandma were making me look bad." He finished in 3:58.

Hilda has her whole family running and eating the Pritikin diet.

The three letters that follow are from young women who enjoy exercising with their husbands.

A 47-year-old woman from Vermont went from an arthritic cripple to a hiker and now takes dancing lessons and leads an active life with her husband.

● "I am writing you to thank you for the incredible change your diet has made in my life. I am a 47-year-old woman who had polio as a small child, which left me with scoliosis [curvature of the spine]. About 20 years ago, I started to develop arthritis in my spine, hip and knee. I have been in all kinds of therapy with extensive drug therapy—all with only temporary results.

"About 4 years ago, I decided to stop taking all drugs, including the vast quantities of aspirin. I tried in vain to live with the constant pain. Each winter in Vermont became more and more difficult. Last winter was the worst ever. I was on the verge of returning to drugs, when I happened to read an article in *House & Garden* about your diet.

"I decided it was worth a try. Only 4 months later, 15 pounds lighter and feeling 20 years younger, I found that all the stiffness in my back and leg had disappeared and about 80% of the pain was also gone. Every day I walk 3 miles to work. As you know, I live in Vermont, near the Green Mountains. On weekends, my husband and I try to take long hikes of possibly 5–7 miles. I am taking a dance class twice a week. All of this from someone whose favorite expression used to be 'my idea of exercise is getting up in the morning'! I can't believe the energy I have, and neither can my husband.

"Another interesting thing happened. My premenstrual symptoms, which were becoming more intense as I approached menopause, have all but disappeared. No more depression, cramping, and headaches. Fantastic! Again, thank you for your diet. Thank you for giving me a new life to live."

● Thirty-nine-year-old Robert Christensen of West Babylon, New York, runs 60 miles a week and now has improved times in all events. His 31-year-old wife tells their story:

"This is the first diet I have ever been on that I could stay on and not have a weak and faint feeling and lose weight so fast. I lost 7 lbs in 3 weeks, and my husband lost approximately 15 lbs in one month. My husband is a runner and runs about 60 miles a week.

"Since he started the diet, he runs much faster and has placed among the top three in his age group in many races. We love the diet and have never felt better. Before reading your book, my husband would consume a pound of butter or margarine in less than a week, with approximately 21 eggs per week, besides drinking alcohol. I can't tell you what a wonderful change your diet has made in our lives. Thank you."

● The Kochers of Gardnerville, Nevada, are husband and wife marathoners. Patricia is 35 years old and runs a 7:50 mile; before starting the diet, a 9:45 mile. She writes:

"My husband and I are both runners, and I have been running almost 5 years. I am 35 years old, and 5 ft tall, so when I weighed 115 lbs, before starting your diet I was trying to lose weight. Once I went on your diet, I had no problem getting the weight off and am at my present weight now of 101 lbs.

"I noticed a big difference in performance after going on your diet. My average running mile used to be 9:45; now at a racing speed, up to half a marathon, I do a 7:50 mile. In winter, we usually do 20–25 miles per week. Ordinarily, in other seasons, we average 33 miles per week, unless we train for a marathon.

"If I go off the diet for more than one meal, I can tell the difference not only in energy but mood changes. In January 1982, we had an underwater weighing test to see our body fat levels. Mine was 22% and my husband's was 11.5%. We repeated that in December 1982, and were amazed to find that even though both of us gained an extra 4 to 5 lbs, we each lost 2% in body fat. During the periods between the underwater weighing (about 10 months) we each had run 2 marathons, a number of half-marathons and shorter races.

"Our eating habits in the past few months have not been as stringent as they have been in the past. We have both been acutely aware that even a moderate change in our habits has affected our daily feeling of well-being as well as performance. The performance change I am aware of, in slacking off the diet, is speed more than endurance. Your letter came at a good time for needed inspiration."

● Brothers Bill and Frank Beddor and Frank's sons, Steve and David, are a family of runners. Bill, age 54, ran his first marathon after his 50th birthday. Eager to test his endurance, he entered the 100-mile Western States Endurance Run in June 1979. This race involves desert, mountains, snow, heat, and pain. After 64 miles, he had to give up, exhausted in mind and body.

In January of 1980, Bill started the Pritikin Program; and with his new energy, he entered the June 1980 Endurance Run. This time he finished the 100 miles in 29 hours.

But 1982 was Bill's banner year:

- June 1982: Western States 100-Mile Race—22:55.
- October 1982: Ironman Triathlon—Third in his age group, 13:48.

Bill's new goals:

- 100-mile run—less than 20 hours.
- Ironman Triathlon—less than 12 hours.
- Diet—100 percent Pritikin for the rest of his life.

Frank, inspired by Bill's new energy, started the Pritikin Program in September 1980 and persuaded his sons, Steve and David, to go on the diet. Although neither father nor sons put enough time into their training, in June 1981, Steve, 20, ran his first marathon with his father and finished.

October 10, 1982, the *Minneapolis Tribune* ran this story: "Beddors win 50-miler. Frank Beddor, Jr., 58, and son David, 20, finished first in the father-son division at last weekend's Michigan 50-Mile Ultramarathon. Frank was the oldest finisher, David the youngest."

9
CHAPTER

Success Stories
from Athletic People

Even world-class endurance athletes thrive on my diet, although that is not to say that this is a guide only for people who wish to set records.

World-class athletes follow the same diet program as active 10-year-olds, 50-year-olds who have just started a walking program, and 90-year-olds who simply want to feel better. Everyone benefits and can function at his or her optimal level physically and mentally on this nutritional program.

Remember, the best-made car in the world will never perform at its maximum on low-quality fuel, and you will never reach your potential on the low-nutrition/high-fat American diet.

TRIATHLON: 2.4-mile ocean swim
112-mile bicycle race
26.2-mile marathon run
October 9, 1982: 850 starting entrants in the Hawaii "Ironman" Triathlon

THE WINNERS:

		AGE:	TIME:
First: Dave Scott		28	9:08:23*
Second: Scott Tinley		25	9:28:28
Third: Jeff Tinley		22	9:36:53
(Scott Tinley's brother)			
Fourth: Scott Molina		22	9:40:23

* Since the Hawaii Triathlon started in 1978, only 3 other athletes have broken the 10-hour total time for the triple event.

THE GREAT SCOTTS

Dave Scott, Scott Tinley, and Scott Molina were all monitored for the 6 weeks before the race as they trained on the Pritikin diet. In Hawaii, a special Pritikin kitchen was set up for their meals.

On the day of the '82 Hawaii Triathlon, the heat was almost unbearable by noon, and the black asphalt road reached temperatures up to 115°F., devastating for some of the athletes.

To Scott Molina, his fourth-place finish was a great victory. In the 1981 contest he had been running in second place when exhaustion and dehydration forced him out less than 10 miles from the finish. This time, he was a strong finisher. Scott Tinley, who won the February 1982 Ironman in 9:19, was only 9 minutes slower in October. He has the second-fastest time in the world, and he is the one Dave Scott will have to watch in the next competition.

Dave Scott had won the 1980 triathlon in 9:24:33, but lost to Scott Tinley in February 1982 by 17 minutes. To regain first place in October 1982 was a great satisfaction, but to set the course record of 9:08:23, 16 minutes faster than his best time, made it even sweeter. He also won each individual event.

Dave has followed his own version of the Pritikin diet for 7 years and prepares his own food. He cooks up 2 lb. of brown rice and leaves it on the stove, and just eats it all through the day, along with yogurt, vegetables, and fruit—up to 20 pieces a day.

This gives him all the calories he needs for those 8-hour training days, and replenishes the glycogen stores in his muscles for the next day. An 80-percent-carbohydrate diet means continuous carbohydrate loading, and no one uses up more glycogen than Dave Scott, the best endurance athlete in the world.

Dave states: "Over the past 7 years I have been following a strict, but enjoyable diet—I do enjoy eating—of approximately 11% (8–14%) of my total calories in fat, 15% (10–20%) in protein, and 74% (70–80%) in complex carbohydrates. This diet has undoubtedly contributed to my athletic performance in triathlons over the last five years. The total reduction of fat and cholesterol, with an increase in muscle and liver glycogen through a higher carbohydrate diet, has enabled me to train for 5–8 hours daily and to compete at a world class level."

Compare Dave with another triathlon entrant, age 22, 6 ft, 151 lb., who finished in 14½ hours. His diet? Red meat, most days; eggs, whole milk, and, as he says, "typical American" (Interview, *Roanoke Times*, Nov. 28, 1982).

TENNIS, ANYONE?

Martina Navratilova, the world's Number 1–seeded tennis player—$1,476,055 in winnings in 1982—has come back to the top in women's tennis after a few years of not playing as well as she wanted to. Now, even Chris Evert Lloyd can barely keep up with her. Miss Navratilova started a new diet last year. "No fats, no oils, no butter, no red meats, no sugar," she explains. "Plenty of vegetables and carbohydrates."

That means, she said, eating a lot of unadorned pasta, potatoes, and bread, which she admitted was not easy for someone who used to like things "swimming in butter."

After several months on the diet, she said, "I feel stronger." And in world-class competition, you need all the strength and endurance you can get.

RUNNERS: WORLD CLASS!

Robert de Castella, marathoner.

In 3 years, Robert has gone from a promising young runner to, as Ron Clarke, a former world-champion runner, described it, the winner of the greatest marathon yet run—the 1982 Commonwealth Games in Brisbane, Australia.

Last year, he won the Japanese Fukuoka out-and-back marathon in 2:08:18, 5 seconds longer than Alberto Salazar's world record for the one-way-course New York marathon. Although the distance is the same, there is a difference in degree of difficulty. The one-way course of 26 miles in the New York marathon was fast because the runners were given a little extra boost from a favorable wind. In an out-and-back course, you run to the 13-mile mark, then turn back to the starting point. In this way, any favoring winds or downhill advantages are averaged.

Robert set a world record for an out-and-back marathon and is setting his sights on U.S. marathons. In 1982, he beat Bill Rodgers and Frank Shorter, among other great runners. On April 9, 1983, Robert raced Alberto Salazar in a world-class marathon in Holland. It was their first race. Robert won first place, and Alberto came in fifth. Alberto said that he had kept up with Robert for the first 22 miles and that Robert had then taken off like a rocket. A convincing demonstration of the high-carbohydrate diet's effect on endurance. Robert's goal is for an Olympic Gold Medal in Los Angeles in 1984. Because marathons are so stressful, Robert has run only 9 since he started, 10 years ago. Unlike many other long-distance runners, he has had an almost injury-free record, and he recovers quickly from minor injuries.

In 1976 Robert's diet changed radically. His father, Rolet, an ex-Army man, had always been very fit and disciplined about his health. He had run for years. Suddenly in 1974, he had a stroke, and 9 months later a heart attack that completely disabled him.

Rolet read an interview with me in *Runner's World* in 1976 describing my success using diet to restore heart-disease victims to normal function. Rolet contacted me, and I sent him the diet program. Robert describes his father's improvement:

"Dad was always very fit and ran a lot, but when he had his heart attack, he could hardly get out of bed to walk upstairs without bad angina for almost a year. Then he put himself on a very stringent nonfat, nonsalt diet with mainly complex carbohydrates, such as potatoes, pumpkins, and other vegetables, cereals and grains. Since then, he's run 16 marathons, the most recent two weeks ago [October 1982] when he ran 3 hours and 12 minutes, a very good run for a man of 58. Now he gets no angina at all."

Robert adopted his father's diet in 1977—nonfat, nonsalt, with no meat, cheese or eggs, and is not concerned about a heart attack, even if he may have a hereditary tendency. "I think my diet and running will protect me from a heart attack," he says.

This father and son have demonstrated quite clearly that the magic for endurance is simply proper nutrition.

As you know, the Pritikin diet was based on the diet of the Tarahumaras in northern Mexico and 25 other native populations where the degenerative diseases (heart disease, cancer, etc.) are unknown. They have thrived on it for 2000 years. It's no experiment.

I can't guarantee that you will attain the endurance of the Tarahumara Indians, because in this entire population running is second nature:

● They can carry 80 percent of their weight 110 miles in 70 hours.

● They can run 500 miles in 5 days to deliver a letter (faster than the postal service).

● Six-year-olds kick a wooden ball the size of an orange 6 miles in 70–80 minutes. Adult men kick the ball 90–180 miles in 24–48 hours.

● A 43-year-old man has kicked the ball 36 miles in 6 hours, with postrace heart rate of 102.

● They hunt deer by running them into exhaustion in 24–48 hours.

● Whole families walk 180 miles to visit friends.

Women also have a kickball game, but because they are busy with food preparation and raising children, they run for *only* 50 miles!

WORLD-RECORD RUNNER (65—69 AGE GROUP)

Jack Stevens, now 66, holds world records for 400, 800, and 1600 meters.

	Age	Meters	Time	Meters	Time
1974	58	800	2:21:3 (record)	1600	5:11
Jan. 1982	65	800	2:24:3 (record)		
April 10, 1982			Started Pritikin diet		
May 1982	65	800	2:22:9 (record)		
Aug. 1982	65	800	2:20:5 (record)		
Nov. 1982	65			1600	4:50:6 (record)

JACK STEVENS AT 65 HAS MADE AN ASTONISHING DISCOVERY
An interview condensed from *Prime Time,* December 1982,
Melbourne, Australia

His physical prowess is improving. He recently ran 800 meters faster than he did 7 years ago, breaking his own world record in the process. Jack's wife is a remarkable athlete as well, and though she started discus and javelin only 5 years ago when she was 60, she is already an American/Australian champion. Diet, they say, is the magic key to their feats. In April 1982, they decided to try the diet devised by U.S. scientist Nathan Pritikin. It is a low-fat, low-cholesterol, high-carbohydrate eating pattern. Pritikin claims that by sticking to his diet people find new energy and health in old age and in fact at any age.

This diet for Jack and Maisie is now a way of life. Jack was a top athlete in the late 1950s, and at 65, although he had slowed a little he still set a new world record for the 800-meter in the 65-69 age group, 2:24.3.

Half a year later, after starting the new diet, he broke his own world record by a stunning 4 seconds, 2:20.5 in the Philadelphia National Masters Sports Festival. His fellow athletes were awestruck. He said the only thing he had done differently was switch to the Pritikin Diet.

Maisie's story is similar. She took up the discus and javelin 5 years ago after being on angina tablets for 10 years, because she was bored just watching her husband compete. Since starting the Pritikin diet, she gradually reduced the number of tablets for her angina, and now she takes none at all. Her arthritis is gone too, and she has also lost 17 pounds. "It's the healthiest I have been in years," she said. "With angina, I couldn't walk up even a slight hill without being totally knocked out by it." This year she is an Australian/American champion in both the discus and the javelin.

Jack writes his own story:

● "For the past 11 years, I have been competing in Veteran (Masters) athletics, running mainly the 400- and 800-meter races. I turned 65 years old on November 23, 1981. The next 12 months changed my life.

"*December 11, 1981*, I had a stress treadmill test, and the heart specialist said that my systolic blood pressure was too high—whether I was on the treadmill or not—and to come back for treatment.

"*January 23, 1982*, I ran the 800 meters in 2:24.5, a new world's record. The old one was 2:25.3, held by Frank Finger, U.S.A. One week later, I ran the 400 meters in 62.17. This bettered slightly the world record also held by Frank Finger, U.S.A. Having retired on my 65th birthday, I decided to change my diet around that time by a large increase in the number of eggs I consumed and also a big intake in cream. But I didn't feel well after that, and I went to my physician again, and he checked me out and found my blood pressure much too high.

"*April 8, 1982*, I decided to go back to the heart specialist. He told me that something must be done with my blood pressure and tried to figure out what drugs I would have to take, and he would try to choose the ones least likely to affect my running.

"*April 10, 1982*, I found your book *The Pritikin Program for Diet & Exercise*. We were almost immediately on your diet.

"*April 29, 1982*, I saw the heart specialist, and that was only two weeks after I started your diet, and he said my blood pressure was much better, and he would postpone ordering the medication. I told him about my diet change, but he was not impressed. He said I should be having a "balanced" diet, including some meat and eggs. I told him that I would go by the way I feel. I was due to race in Fiji in May of 1982, and he made another appointment to see me after Fiji.

"*May 13, 1982*, in Fiji, I ran a good 800-meter race in 2:22.9, which shaved 1.6 seconds off my previous record. And at about that time, I was finding that in my training I was able to do things that I could not manage for several years before that. The only thing different was the diet change.

"*June 3, 1982*, I saw the heart specialist again. He found my blood pressure now normal. But he isn't convinced that it is due to the Pritikin diet, like I am. He says, 'Well, it's just psychological, just due to a diet change.' It's hard to convince the doctors.

"*August 1982*, we traveled to America to compete first in Wichita, Kansas, and a week later in Philadelphia where I broke records again, the fastest times I have been able to achieve in the last 7 years. I feel I owe it to the diet. I no longer 'die' during the second half of the race, and the improvement was quite noticeable even after being on the diet a little more than a month.

"Now regarding my wife, Maisie, who turned 65 in 1982. She has been in the doctor's hands for angina for the last 15 years. She has had to seek treatment earlier this year for what was diagnosed as a hiatus hernia. She has suffered with arthritis in the knee joints for some years, even though she has been competing in discus and javelin for the last 2½ to 3 years. On her change to the Pritikin system, her weight went from 133 down to 112, and her knees are now practically free of any discomfort and she joins me in many running training sessions. Her hiatus hernia is nonexistent and, over a period of almost 6 weeks, she gradually cut down her angina tablets and in a month after that she was without medication of any kind.

"Maisie and I are both feeling the best we have felt in years. And, after 43 years of marriage, we claim to be the happiest couple in the world and we agree that the Pritikin Program has had a lot to do with it."

IT'S NEVER TOO LATE TO START!

● NOEL JOHNSON—Improves with Age

AGE
69 Recommended for nursing home; denied life insurance
70 Drastically changed diet to Pritikin guidelines
71 Ran a 6:27 mile
73 Pikes Peak Marathon
80 New York Marathon
82 New York Marathon
83 New York Marathon

At 70 years old, despite medical advice not to exercise, Noel began his own rehab program of diet and exercise. He changed his diet drastically: no meat, cheese, eggs, butter, margarine, or oils; essentially a plant-food diet with a small amount of animal protein—fish once or twice a week.

Noel wrote me, "I know that your way of life as stated in your book, free from so many damaging oils, has helped me to obtain the physical condition I have at 83."

● EULA WEAVER, almost 91 years old at her last competition. Record holder for 800 meters (85–89 years old) and 1500 meters (85–89 years old and 90–94 years old) at Senior Olympics events, 1974 to 1979.

Five feet 3 inches tall, Eula had weighed 100 pounds for the last 40 years. She developed heart disease with angina at 67, and at 75 years old she was hospitalized with a severe heart attack. At 81 years old, she had congestive heart failure, angina, hypertension, severe arthritis, and claudication (not enough blood flow to the legs). She could walk no more than 100 feet. Circulation to her hands was so bad that she had to wear gloves in the summertime.

She started the Pritikin diet at 81 years old, and in a year was off all medication, had lost her symptoms, and could walk a mile. When she was 85½ years old, she entered the Senior Olympics, ran the 800 and 1500 meters, and won two gold medals. She ran these races for 6 consecutive years and won 12 gold medals.

It's never too late to start.

IN A CLASS BY THEMSELVES

● MONROE ROSENTHAL, M.D.—Marathon 2:45; Ironman Triathlon, 12:08.
● JOHN SCHEFF, M.D.—Marathon 3:00; Ironman Triathlon, 11:36.

Dr. Rosenthal writes:

"As a doctor in Internal Medicine, specializing in diabetes, I was fascinated by your complete reversal of dietary recommendations for diabetics. From the 50 years of low-carbohydrate, high-fat diets, now studies were demonstrating superior results with high-carbohydrate, low-fat diets.

"In late 1979, I read your book *The Pritikin Program for Diet & Exercise*. It made sense to me, especially after I read the chapter for health professionals documenting the scientific rationale for diabetics.

"In February 1980, not only did I start your diet, but set up a metabolic ward in my hospital for my patients. Dramatic results were achieved with diabetes, hypertension, and heart disease.

"My own performance was improving on the diet. The best marathon time before the diet was 2:59, but after 4 months on your diet, I ran a 2:45, my best time ever, and I qualified for the Boston Marathon, which required a 2:50 or faster time.

"After 3 Boston Marathons, I turned to the ultimate contest, the Ironman World Triathlon in Hawaii. In the February 1982 Triathlon, I was pleased with my 12:42, coming in 175th out of 650 entrants. What surprised me in my close association with the other triathletes and especially the top finishers, was that most of them were generally following the guidelines of the Pritikin diet.

"To bring attention that your diet, although originally for sick people, was indeed the best for overall fitness in endurance athletes, I contacted you in February 1982 to do a study on triathletes training on your diet. Some 850 contestants entered the October 1982 race, and the six you sponsored won the 1st, 2nd and 4th places.

"I and another physician, John Scheff, were two of the six you sponsored. My October time was 12:08, 34 minutes faster than February. John had run marathons for a few years and did the February 1982 triathlon in 13:06. He went on your diet 3 or 4 months before the October event, and made a remarkable improvement in his time—from 13:06 to 11:36, 1½ hours less.

"The consensus of the group was that the diet was significant in their improvements in time.

"I continue to use your diet with my patients and am constantly in wonder of such a simple natural approach proving so effective."

● ED WEHAN—age 39. Marathon, 2:37; 50-mile, 5:53; 100-mile Western States, 18:48.

Ed writes:

"During college, I played competitive tennis on a diet of red meat and French fries. My roommate's father gave him a side of beef every semester, which we devoured. I sure wasn't born to a Pritikin diet. Around 1971, in my late twenties, I weighed too much, and started to run to gain conditioning. After a 1½-mile run, I would go home for a couple of Big Macs and fries which made it difficult for me to lose weight.

"After considerable reading, I decided to cut back on simple carbos, fats and oils. Weight started dropping off, and I was feeling better and was able to increase my running distance.

"In 1976, I read your first book, and was surprised that most of my new food habits were your recommendations. I was about two-thirds on your diet and was ready for my first marathon. It was a nervous experience for me, but I finished in 3:30. The next year, I changed my diet in earnest and by 1978 was a strict follower.

"In 1979, I ran the 100-mile Western States and finished 7th with an 18:48, and I now have run this race three times. Over 350 entrants were in the American River 50-miler, and I finished 4th in 5:53.

"As far as marathons, I now run a 2:37, and two marathons were only 2 weeks apart. I seem to have very rapid recovery. Even my 10K is fast, 33:30.

"I attribute my endurance to my diet. I train minimally, compared to most, and still perform well. As we age, I believe our diets can influence performance more than at a younger age. My company does fitness testing, and many of the older runners that I test tend towards your type of diet. Although I'm 39, I look for my fastest times in the next 15 years.''

SUPERMEN—THEIR NEXT EVENT

ultra triathlon,	20-mile swim
48 to 60 hours,	200-mile bicycle race
continuous—nonstop	100-mile run

- ALLAN KOROLOWICZ, age 29
- CRAIG CHAMBERS, age 34

These runners are planning the ultimate triathlon, and if they pull it off, they will have duplicated the 200-mile-run endurance of the Tarahumara.

Allan, who is one of the top ultramarathoners in the world, recently did a 100-mile run across Death Valley, in 115–119°F. air temperatures, with the roads reaching 180–190°F.

Craig was to run 50 miles to pace Allan, but ran 80 miles instead. Craig's development as a superendurance athlete is interesting to follow.

He started running in 1974, eating the typical high-fat American diet. As his distance increased, he started to eat more carbohydrates; then by 1978, he gave up fish, fowl, and meat and became a lacto-ovo-vegetarian. He had information on the Pritikin diet and gradually began shifting away from dairy products.

In April 1978, Craig ran his first marathon. The 26-mile distance inspired him to longer training runs, and by July of 1978, he was running 20 miles most days. A 50-mile race became a reality September 1978, and his best time is 6:07.

The next big challenge was the Western States 100-mile race. It's a wild run through desert, snow, mountains, etc., but he has run it three times, in 1980, 1981, and 1982, with a best time of 21:14.

By 1980, Craig felt stronger without the dairy products, and as his animal protein ate a few eggs each week. His diet now was 10 percent fat and about 75–80 percent carbohydrates, following the Pritikin guidelines.

He felt so strong in 1981 that he raised his training runs to at least 24 miles a day, 7 days a week, and over the past 2 years has run more than 17,000 miles—two-thirds around the world, or 7 coast-to-coast runs. His greatest mileage week totaled 242 miles, or about 35 miles a day.

With this kind of training, he couldn't resist the Ironman Triathlon in 1981, and did it in 12:27. Now, after 30 marathons, with a best time of 2:47, he's aiming for the impossible, the ultratriathlon.

- Marathon a day (7 days a week) for 700+ continuous days
- 1981–82 24+ miles of running daily without missing a day = 17,520 miles
- Marathon, 2:47
- 50-mile, 6:07
- Ironman Triathlon, 12:27
- Western States 100-mile, 21:14

And this is just the beginning for Craig "Superman" Chambers!

People age 20 to 83 years, selected from the case histories, who were or became marathon (or more) runners while following the Pritikin guidelines for at least a year:

Years on Diet	Name	Age	Marathon Time	Other Events
6	Irwin Baker	54	3:33	42-mile, 8:00
4	John Becker	42	2:57	
3	Bill Beddor	54	3:14	100-mile, 22:55; Ironman Triathlon, 13:48
3	David Beddor	20	4:00	50-mile winner
3	Frank Beddor	58	4:00	50-mile winner
3	Steve Beddor	21	4:00	
3	Irwin Berman	55	4:42	
3	Lloyd Brodniak	38	2:49	
3	Craig Chambers	34	2:47	50-mile, 6:07; 100-mile, 21:14; Ironman Triathlon, 12:27

Years on Diet	Name	Age	Marathon Time	Other Events
6	Robert De Castella	25	2:08:18	Winner of 4/9/83 Rotterdam, Holland, Marathon, defeating Alberto Salazar
	Rolet De Castella	59	2:58	
10	Noel Johnson	83	4:50	
2	Nick Karem	39	3:45	
2	Mr. & Mrs. Kocher	40, 35	4:00	
3	Allan Korolowicz	29		100-mile
2	Ridge La Mar	34	3:30	
1	Scott Molina	22	2:24	Ironman Triathlon, 9:40
5	Roger Nichols	35	3:00	
4	Hilda Richardson	67	6:10	
3	Debbie Robison	28	5:00	
3	Grace Robison	47	5:00	
3	Monroe Rosenthal	35	2:45	Ironman Triathlon, 12:08
2	R. T. Ryan	47	3:15	
1	John Scheff	30	3:00	Ironman Triathlon, 11:36
7	David Scott	28	sub 3:00	Ironman Triathlon, 9:08
3	Gina Serafin	44	5:03	
3	Tony Serafin	21	3:58	
2000	Tarahumara Indians			200 miles, 48:00
6	Ed Wehan	39	2:37	50-mile, 5:53; 100-mile, 18:48

By now I hope you will see how thoroughly nutritious and safe the Pritikin diet is, even for people who tax their bodies to the limit. If you have any lingering doubts as to whether it is wise to forgo high-fat-and-protein diets, the following chapter should put your mind to rest.

10
CHAPTER

Run and Die
on the
American Diet

Goodloe Byron, 49 years old, U.S. Congressman from Maryland, had run 6 Boston Marathons, with a best time of 3:28:40, and had finished a 50-miler. He was 5 feet 7 inches tall and weighed 130 pounds, had run almost every day for several years for at least ½ hour, and had not smoked for 25 years. Then why, toward the end of an easy 15-mile training run, did he drop dead?

Byron had read extensively about health and running, and was intrigued by Dr. Tom Bassler's flat statement that anyone who runs a marathon in under 4 hours and is a nonsmoker has absolute immunity from heart disease.

Strongly influenced by the belief in the immunity of marathon runners to heart disease, he ignored his physician's warnings about his gradually closing coronary arteries, as shown in successive treadmill tests from 1974 to 1978. Dr. Robert Flynn, Byron's personal physician, said the last test, in January 1978, indicated severe abnormality and was positive for heart disease. "I advised him to stop running completely until further tests could be done with Dr. Sam Fox [head of the Cardiology Exercise Project of Georgetown University]."

Byron continued to run, and though he made four appointments with Dr. Fox in the next 10 months, he canceled them because of his Congressional work load. His cholesterol level in 1974 was 305 mg/dl, and in 1978, the year of his death, had declined to 228 mg/dl. A safe cholesterol level would have been below 160 mg/dl.

But Byron ignored his diet and his doctors; he believed that running made him immune to heart disease. And so he died of heart disease on October 12, 1978.

Dr. Manuel G. Jimenez, who did the autopsy, said the coronary arteries were filled with cholesterol, "extensive and diffuse, involving both coronary arteries and main branches. The coronaries were narrowed to only pinprick openings. Congressman Byron's coronary arteries were worse than most I've autopsied."

After receiving the autopsy report, Dr. Bassler said the death had not been caused by heart disease. "He probably wasn't eating one of the six foods that [Bassler recommends] marathoners eat: yeast, yogurt, peanuts, beer, wheat germ and vitamin C."

Dr. Jimenez politely commented that Bassler's conclusions were *not* supported by the evidence: ". . . for me, it was plainly coronary insufficiency due to atherosclerosis."

The information about Byron's untimely death comes from a study of sudden death in marathon runners on the regular American diet that was conducted by B. F. Waller and W. C. Roberts, pathologists at the National Institutes of Health. In the same study, they reported on 4 other runners besides Byron. All were free of any evidence of heart disease before they started running, and all died while running. The lowest cholesterol level was 228 mg/dl, and all had coronary arteries severely narrowed or closed with cholesterol deposits. Waller and Roberts evaluated Bassler's much-publicized statement that marathoners were immune to heart disease, and on the basis of their evidence, they stated "that Bassler's thesis that marathon running provides 'immunity to atherosclerosis' is incorrect." Their conclusion was: "Thus, coronary heart disease appears to be the major killer of conditioned runners aged 40 years and over who die while running."

New Zealander Dennis Stephenson had reason to wish

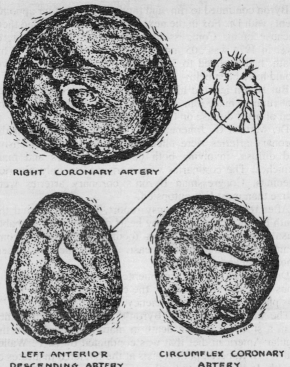

RIGHT CORONARY ARTERY

LEFT ANTERIOR
DESCENDING ARTERY

CIRCUMFLEX CORONARY
ARTERY

CROSS SECTIONS OF CONGRESSMAN BYRON'S
ARTERIES SHOWING EXTENSIVE CLOSURE
(Drawn from photographs provided by William C. Ruberts, M.D., Natl. Insts. of Health)

Bassler were right. Despite a lifetime of running in which he held records for 100-mile runs and 24-hour endurance races, he still suffered from heart disease. He died the day after his last marathon. In his early 50s, he was very fit, but toward the end, he had had the same warning signs as Byron: pains in the chest and arm (usually the left arm) and feelings of fatigue in his last marathon.

His autopsy revealed the same coronary cholesterol closures Byron had. If only he had followed a low-cholesterol diet, like his Australian neighbor Rolet de Castella.

In his early 50s, Rolet was fortunate to have survived his first heart attack, but years of running had not spared him from heart disease. After a year of incapacitating angina despite the best medical care, he went on the Pritikin diet. Within weeks his pain disappeared. Rolet cautiously resumed his running, and now, 5 years later, has run 16 marathons, including a sub-3-hour. Not bad for a man of 59, with a damaged heart and previously cholesterol-filled arteries. Rolet learned that running does not prevent heart disease, but proper diet, even after a heart attack, can return you to an active, vigorous life.

It is unfortunate that runners who develop heart disease by eating too much cholesterol and fat are not aware that the symptoms can be reversed. Ron Clarke, former holder of many world running records, at age 45 underwent coronary bypass surgery for his cholesterol-filled arteries. If Clarke had followed Rolet de Castella's diet, the chances are 80 percent that he would never have had bypass surgery.

In 1976–77, 64 people came to the Pritikin Centers instead of having bypass surgery, and have now been followed for 5 years. More than 80 percent never had to have their bypass surgery; 80 percent had angina when they came, but after 5 years, only 30 percent had angina; our deaths in 5 years for heart disease average only 0.6 percent per year, the lowest ever reported in medical journals for any type of treatment for heart patients like these.

You may not be aware too that of all those who undergo coronary bypass surgery, 10–20 percent suffer complete blockage of all their bypasses within the first year. On a high-cholesterol diet, bypasses can close ten times as fast as did the original arteries. It is crucial to go on a low-fat, low-cholesterol diet after bypass surgery.

Jim Shettler's sudden death shocked the running community. Jim had trained like a marathoner since the age of 15. Lean at 6 feet 1 inch and 150 pounds, he had a slow pulse and low blood pressure. He was a nonsmoker and had competed for 25 years in 3000-meter to 10-mile runs. He had run many marathons. On a day in 1976, at age 42, he ran for 3 hours over hilly terrain in preparation for his next marathon. The following day, in Oakland, California, he died.

The autopsy was very clear: a main left artery was almost entirely closed with cholesterol deposits. There was little question that this blockage had created a fatal arrhythmia (irregular heartbeat) and sudden death.

If there were any truth in Bassler's statements that 1) marathon runners cannot develop heart disease and 2) if you have heart disease, 10,000 miles of training runs will clean the cholesterol from your arteries, Jim would have been alive. Cholesterol cannot be "burned out" by running or any other exercise. Cholesterol cannot be used for calories of fuel. So to advise runners that because they are active they do not have to watch their cholesterol intake closely is deceptive and dangerous, and I urge you to get your cholesterol under control.

Dr. John Vogel reported on a case identical to Jim Shettler's (*Adv. Cardiol.* Vol. 26, Karger, Basel, 1979, pp. 121–124). A 64-year-old male marathon runner woke one night just one month after his last marathon with a strange sensation in his chest. He went to a hospital's emergency room, where he developed ventricular fibrillation—an irregular heartbeat in which the rate increases up to 300 beats per minute and the heart stops pumping blood. It means death is imminent. Fortunately, he was revived with emergency measures. An angiogram, or X-ray of his coronary arteries, showed cholesterol deposits narrowing a main left artery by 90 percent. He had immediate bypass surgery, and with the improved blood flow, the arrhythmia disappeared.

The surgeons noted that his right coronary artery was 30-percent closed, but felt the condition wasn't advanced enough to bypass. To protect himself, the patient put himself on many supplements, vitamins E and C, lecithin, brewer's yeast, wheat germ, and so on. He carefully followed Bassler's recommendations and drank beer regularly, and especially after marathons.

Two years later, his treadmill test became abnormal. Another angiogram revealed that the right coronary artery, which had taken 64 years to close 30 percent, had in 2 years closed 100 percent. In that 2-year period, he had run a sub-4-hour marathon.

In 1978, 2 years later, he was running 10–15 miles each day, in preparation for a marathon a month away, when again he went into arrhythmia. He got to the hospital too late, and never regained consciousness. The autopsy revealed that an unbypassed left artery had completely closed, producing a fatal heart attack. This man's dietary supplement program was no protection against the rapid artery closure that finally killed him.

The evidence tells me that this man's dietary supplement program had a great deal to do with the rapid artery closure that finally killed him, since it was the only real change in his lifestyle.

Dr. Thomas Pickering of Cornell University has studied arrhythmias (abnormal heart rhythms) and finds that they occur more frequently during exercise; this, he suggests, could be the principal cause of runners' deaths. He said that a person is at increased risk of arrhythmia death if he runs, and at little risk if he doesn't.

Irwin Baker found that to be true: his arrhythmia almost killed him (page 48). When he had been on the Pritikin diet for only 6 weeks, his arrhythmia had disappeared and he could stop his medication and start running. That was 6 years ago, and he has run many marathons and ultramarathons since then. Arrhythmia and sudden death in runners could be more closely attributed to the wrong diet.

In 1982, Dr. George Sheehan reported a study that sounded the death knell for Bassler's theory of the invincible runner. "DISHEARTENING NEWS" was the headline, and Sheehan wrote, "Men who have taken up running to prevent a heart attack may find it all a waste of time. A five-year study done at Methodist Hospital in Houston reports that a large proportion of men, aged 40 to 60, who were long-distance runners developed evidence of coronary heart disease."

The 41 subjects in the study had been marathon runners for at least 2 years before the study began. At the beginning of the investigation, 5 men had positive (abnormal) stress tests; by the end of the third year, 13 had developed positive tests; by the 5-year mark, 18 recorded positive stress tests.

None of the men had chest pains yet, or other heart-related symptoms, at the end of the 5-year study.

When those runners who tested abnormal were checked with the normal runners, there was no difference in average:

1. Miles run per year (1400);
2. Age (48 years);
3. Cholesterol (192 mg/dl);
4. Bruce treadmill time (12 minutes).

A short time later, three of the abnormal group worsened. One died following a heart attack, another was required to undergo coronary bypass surgery, and the third was confirmed to have heart disease.

Heart disease gradually evolved in all of these men, and in time most of them could show an abnormal stress test, followed by heart attack, angina, and death. Running itself cannot prevent these tragedies.

Rarely is there an opportunity to watch as the arteries of a healthy runner gradually close through the years. Dr. Jeffrey Handler reported the case of a highly trained marathon runner, a 48-year-old Marine, who after a 1-month period of chest pain checked into the Naval Regional Medical Center in San Diego for evaluation. This man had competed in athletic events since childhood and had begun a vigorous running program 8 years before. He was running 50–60 miles a week at an 8-minute/mile pace, and before a marathon increased to more than 70 miles per week. Not only had he completed 7 marathons, but he had also done 10K runs and 52-mile ultramarathons. Usually he finished in the top 10 percent of his age group.

The angiogram revealed a 99-percent closure of one of his main left arteries with cholesterol deposits, the same as in Jim Shettler's case and with Dr. Vogel's patient.

How could this Marine, in superfit condition, a non-smoker, and whose cholesterol level was only 185 mg/dl despite the fact that he was on the high-fat and high-cholesterol Marine diet, develop heart disease? Dr. Handler comments: "This patient remains the best described example of the failure of a vigorous running program to prevent the progression of coronary atherosclerosis.

"Unfortunately, statements regarding the protective value of running have been made in the medical literature and have been widely circulated among runners. These assertions are not only inaccurate, but potentially dangerous. They foster the tempting illusion of invincibility in the runner.''

The Marine's blood cholesterol of 185 mg/dl did not prevent cholesterol plaque from closing his arteries. He was perhaps unaware that eating dairy products can keep total cholesterol low while still allowing cholesterol deposits in the artery walls to form the cholesterol boils that eventually prevent blood from reaching part of the heart muscle.

The Masai, an East African nomadic cattle-herding tribe, exemplify this phenomenon. Milk is the staple of their diet, and the average Masai drinks 3 to 5 quarts a day. During the dry season, when the supply of water, milk, and other food is low, the Masai drink fresh cow's blood, and eat plenty of meat. Yet they do have low total cholesterol levels (135 mg/dl), and it was formerly believed that the Masai were safe from coronary heart disease in spite of their high-cholesterol, high-fat diet.

However, 10 years ago, the hearts and aortae of 50 Masai men, most of whom had been killed in accidents, were collected for autopsy (*Am. J. Epid*. 95:26, 1972). Measurement of the aortae showed extensive atherosclerosis, and the coronary arteries showed thickening equal to that of elderly American males. The blood cholesterol of the Masai is indicative neither of the amount of fat in their diet (66 percent of the 3000 calories they consume—50 percent higher than American); of their cholesterol intake (600 mg—same as Americans); nor of the degree of atherosclerosis. Why? Because the large quantity of milk they drink artificially lowers the amount of cholesterol found in their blood. Studies suggest that a factor in milk lowers blood cholesterol levels (*Am. J. Clin. Nutr.*, 1974, 27: 464–69). While there is a positive correlation between the amount of cholesterol in the blood and the incidence of cardiovascular disease, low cholesterol levels influenced by the consumption of dairy products are misleading and cannot guarantee freedom from disease now or in the future.

Sudden death from ventricular fibrillation is probably the main cause of runners' deaths. In 1958, Dr. Claude Beck of the Cleveland Clinic had studied fibrillation and concluded that it could not occur unless one or more areas of the three coronary arteries and their branches were substantially closed. During periods of little activity, the amount of blood required by the heart is so small that even if one artery is 90-percent closed, the heart looks healthy and pink. But when you exercise vigorously, the heart requires more blood, so if you have an artery closed by 90 percent, the part of the heart nourished by the closed artery turns blue.

This uneven, or checkerboard, distribution of oxygenated blood produces uneven electrical currents, and when the difference in blood flow becomes too great—the faster the heartrate, the more uneven it will be—ventricular fibrillation is almost inevitable, and almost inevitably fatal.

Dr. Meyer Friedman, cardiologist at Mount Zion Hospital in San Francisco, supports this concept. "The greatest danger," he says, "is the immediate occurrence of arrhythmia, a ventricular fibrillation of the heart—and that's instant death. *That can only affect the people who have serious coronary-artery disease* [my emphasis]. But only 50 percent of the people who died instantaneously during exercise were aware of the fact they had serious coronary disease. In fact, a study at Johns Hopkins found that 28 percent of heart attack victims had seen a physician within two weeks prior to their deaths [Baltimore study]. At autopsy, of course, we find their blood vessels are pretty badly occluded" (*The Jogger*, June 1979).

Some have thought that sheer exhaustion and collapse can precipitate the irregular rhythms of ventricular fibrillation. In the 1968 Olympic Games in Mexico City, the high altitude caused hundreds of participants to collapse. The oxygen deprivation created loss of sight, migraine headaches, nausea and vomiting, blue lips, drop in systolic blood pressure to 60 mm mercury, rapid heartbeat, and other symptoms; but none of the athletes died or developed heart problems. If your heart is free of significant coronary-artery closure, exhaustion does not result in injury.

Too many people die when they exercise more vigorously than usual, as when they shovel snow; play tennis, golf, or other sports; or run marathons. Sadly, the running death of Jim Shettler, 42, winner of the National AAU Masters 25K run, heads a steady procession of others who ran for their health but died of their diets. We remember:

- JIM DOOLEY—37, who directed the expansion of the Anaheim stadium for the Los Angeles Rams, died running near his home.
- ROBERT CLARKE—49, physiologist, died during his daily run.
- COL. GILES HALL—50, USAF Director of Health Professions Recruiting for the Air Force, a daily jogger for 20 years, died while jogging.
- DR. ROBERT SUMMERS—54, longtime Administrator of the Miami Heart Institute, died while jogging.
- DR. EDWARD LAUTH—46, who instituted a jogging program for the American Heart Institute, died while running.
- DR. DAVID DOROFF—49, psychologist, completed an 18-mile training run for the New York Marathon, had a normal reading in a stress test conducted by his cardiologist, and then dropped dead in the doctor's office. Two of his three coronary arteries were 90 percent closed, and the third, 60 percent.
- DUANE ARMSTRONG—59, a 5-year member of the Seniors Track Club (California), died while jogging.
- RON HOLMES—37, a member of the Seniors Track Club, died during the Napa Valley Blossom Time Run. His recent physical had been perfect.
- DR. STEPHEN W. ROYCE, JR.—51, marathon runner and member of the Seniors Track Club, died in his sleep.
- RICHARD PEEK—58, marathon runner, died after a 12-mile run.
- RUSS HARGREAVES—67, a retired recreation-department supervisor, died while running.
- DODGE PARKER—29, player coach of the Orange County (California) Stars of the International Volleyball Association, died of a heart attack.
- BILL ENGLISH—19, football player, died of a heart attack.
- CHUCK HUGHES—28, Detroit Lions receiver, died of a heart attack.
- JOSEPH MALLON—20, suffered a heart attack while jog-

ging on his college campus. His life was saved by instant emergency measures.

In 1971, before exercise deaths became a subject of national interest, Dr. Ernst Jokl published a monograph on more than 100 cases of sudden death during exercise. Dr. Jokl writes: "The group studied by us is distinguished by the fact that the cardiac diseases had proceeded without symptoms and without impairment of physical fitness. Several of the victims had been outstanding athletes. Among the postmortem findings, coronary atherosclerosis and degenerative changes of the myocardium [heart muscle] were the most frequent. . . .

"Even the most strenuous exercise will not cause death in subjects with normal hearts."

Like to run? Don't move to Rhode Island. Dr. Paul Thompson reported data from that state from 1975 to 1980. For each sedentary man 30 to 64 years of age who experienced sudden death, there were 7 joggers. Seven jogging sudden deaths to one sedentary sudden death! Dr. Thompson writes: "Exercise contributes to sudden death"—and I add: only on the American diet.

If you like to run, great!—your body will benefit immeasurably from the exercise. But please, get your diet under control too. By now you know that the Pritikin Program of proper diet and exercise can pave the way to a long, healthy, vital life. What becomes abundantly clear, however, is that the diet and exercise are integral parts of the program, and neither should be undertaken to the exclusion of the other. Now here's how you begin.

PART THREE

THE
28-DAY
PROGRAM

11

CHAPTER

Revving
Yourself Up!

You are now undoubtedly convinced that people who commit themselves to the Pritikin life of healthful eating and regular exercise are "winners"—whether in a marathon or in conquering the "blahs" or even in saying goodbye to the need for medication, sickbed, or wheelchair. You probably think, "If they can go so far to improve health and fitness, so can I." And indeed you can. The decision to try this program is a momentous first step toward a lifetime of high energy, normalized weight loss, reduced risk of fatal diseases, and a wonderful feeling of success.

Your 28-day commitment will be one of the most important choices you make in your life. So many people who come to the Pritikin residential centers tell me this decision is the best thing they have ever done for themselves (except for marrying their spouse, they will add, if he or she is in earshot). In just 4 weeks, you too can expect substantially improved health and fitness and newfound vitality, and you will look better too. Many diet-related symptoms, such as headaches, chronic fatigue, and constipation, may have completely disappeared. Most of you will be so enthusiastic that you will "sign on" for life as a Pritikin Program follower.

Your 28-day stint is a kind of journey or adventure—not to new lands, but to new inner experiences. As with any journey, some planning is essential so that each day you experience success and feel you are advancing toward your goals. If you understand the program and its rationale as described in this book, you have made a successful beginning. It helps, too, to be specific about your personal health and fitness goals. Make a list of what you hope to achieve during the initial 28 days of the program. Having your goals on paper will help keep you motivated because you will be able to see precisely how much closer you are to your goals each day. Your goals, of course, are for you alone. In this program you compete only with yourself. To help you establish your goals and keep track of your successes, use the chart on page 118.

MEETING THE 28-DAY DIETARY CHALLENGE

While you have made the commitment to begin the program, very possibly you have some anxiety about your ability to adhere to the diet for 28 days; perhaps even some concern about whether you will like the food. Will you enjoy a diet that by usual American standards appears Spartan? How will you manage without cheeses, hamburgers, omelettes, ice cream, or other favorite foods you will have to forgo on the Pritikin diet? The new diet will be easier to adjust to than you think. Fortunately, preferences are mainly a matter of conditioning, as you will realize if you consider the unusual varieties of foods and eating habits of people from all over the world. It should help you to know that many former gourmets (including myself!) who've converted to the Pritikin diet tell us they enjoy their food now more than ever, and that they would never consider returning to their former diets. Most of them did miss the old tastes for a while— steaks and chops, rich sauces, fried foods; but their new diet now tastes great to them and they feel terrific. What could be better?

All kinds of people have adopted the Pritikin diet quite happily. Some operated restaurants featuring the most elegant cuisine; others were gourmet chefs, professional or amateur; but most were just ordinary folk who loved good eating, and some lived to eat. What a shock to discover that the rich diet they thought so essential to their enjoyment of life turned out to be so expendable, and that their new diet is heaped with eating pleasure! Some of these talented people have created new and delectable Pritikin diet recipes, a number of which appear in this book.

From among the hundreds of testimonials we've received about the tastiness of Pritikin vs. "regular" food, I think the letter from Rita Green, a registered nurse, says it best. "I thought it would be impossible to give up cheese, desserts, McDonald's hamburgers, etc.," she writes, "but what I have found is that there are so many wonderful foods that ARE allowed that I don't even miss the old foods, and the great part is that I can now eat as much as I want. . . . I never used to cook much before. Now I find that I take such care about what I eat and I have a ball trying all the recipes in your book and making up a few of my own. . . . I don't even feel tempted to go back to the way I used to eat. One thing this program provides which is so much better than all the other diets I have tried . . . is FLEXIBILITY. I really do feel like I'm cheating when I eat bread. That's not diet food. I have always thought that potatoes, fruits, bread, bananas, desserts, etc. had no place on a weight reduction diet."

She also wrote that by nature she is inclined to be a bit lazy and self-indulgent when it comes to food and exercise, had been 25–30 pounds overweight since she was a teenager, and had never before been able to stick to a diet. Now she has lost 30 pounds without feeling deprived. As a nurse, she was motivated, too, by the many sick people she saw. As she wrote: "I know very few people over 60 years old not on Lasix, potassium supplements, Digoxin, Aldomet, etc., and having to deal with their side effects and not actually feeling any better, anyway. I plan to stick to the Pritikin Program and don't expect to have to be sick like the old people I nurse."

It won't be long before you too are able to make that

magic connection between a mode of eating and a sense of well-being that will motivate you to stay with the program for life. When you achieve that awareness, you too will find it easy to pass on taboo foods forever.

In the meantime, don't forget that you're on a special new journey and it will take time to be comfortable with the new cuisine, as well as new rituals and customs. Now a word or two about backsliding. It has happened to *all* of us, so don't punish yourself too harshly. Don't give up because you ate a brownie in the 4th day of the program. If you do slip and eat unwisely, don't let it give you the excuse to do it again. Get right back on the program! The most important factor in determining your success in achieving your 28-day health and fitness goals is your overall degree of dietary compliance. While a little deviation or cheating on occasion is not going to be too consequential, departing too much and too often from the Pritikin diet standards will seriously compromise your results.

It would be ideal if everyone who embarked on the 28-day program were able to follow the suggested 28-day diet plan with little or no modification. If you are lucky, you will be able to do this. But life is complicated, so you will need to anticipate what may interfere with or distract you from the program. Most people will occasionally be confronted with meals not on the diet plan. It could be a company banquet, a friend's wedding, or Thanksgiving dinner at your aunt's. Here are some useful suggestions on how to cope in these situations.

- Eat a good-sized snack, almost a complete meal, before you arrive so that you are not very hungry. You can then pick and choose from the meal the items that are on the Pritikin diet.
- Try to arrange in advance with your hostess or the person in charge to have something appropriate for you to eat.
- After you arrive, ask a waiter or your hostess to help you by providing your salad without dressing, a second helping of the fresh fruit cup, additional plain bread, and so on.

Restaurant dining can be your nemesis, but you can also eat out Pritikin style and have a thoroughly enjoyable time. Insofar as you are able, try to minimize eating out during the initial 28-day period; but here are a few suggestions for times when you do eat out.

● Select a restaurant most likely to meet your needs. Suggest to your friend the restaurant with the excellent salad bar instead of the bistro that serves omelettes and pastries.

● If you do find yourself at the bistro after all, you can still lunch on a nice big fresh salad, sourdough bread, and a small bowl of fresh fruit.

● Don't be shy about asking the waiter or waitress to have the kitchen make minor modifications in serving some of the foods. Specify a *dry* baked potato (to avoid having it arrive doused with sour cream); *unbuttered* vegetables; salad *dry* but accompanied with a slice of lemon; a piece of fish broiled without butter (split the piece with your table partner, since it will be very likely too large for Pritikin-size limits), and so on.

The daily coffee break at the office needn't be your downfall either.

● When the coffee and doughnuts tempt you, dash to your desk for the Pritikin-style snacks you brought from home and avert a mini-crisis.

● Use the extra time to exercise. Walk around the office, or if possible, go outside for a short brisk jaunt. Whenever you feel the urge to eat unhealthful foods, move—not to the candy counter, but to the corridor or outside for a brief walk.

The key to success in all these special eating-out situations is to anticipate the problems you will confront and work around them in a manner that enables you to adhere as closely as possible to the Pritikin diet.

How well you meet these dietary challenges at home and away from home will be reflected in the checklist on page 124. If you need to improve, the chart will help you spot the source of your problem.

ESTABLISHING YOUR 28-DAY HEALTH AND FITNESS GOALS

1. Weight

Do you want to lose a little weight, a lot of weight, stay at your present weight, or even gain weight? The Pritikin diet used properly is ideal for any of these purposes.

Losing Weight on the Pritikin Diet

If you need to reduce as little as 2–3 pounds, or as much as 100, the Pritikin diet is the most healthful way to get it off and keep it off. And because a diet high in complex carbohydrates has much more bulk, it is consequently much more filling than a conventional diet of even more calories. You won't be hungry even if you decide you need to restrict caloric intake for a while. Suggestions for low-calorie meals are in Chapter 16, in the sections on the dinner menus, dinner salads, luncheons, snacks, and beverages, and in the 28 menu plans for dinner.

Even on the regular unrestricted-calorie diet plan most people will lose weight at a slow, steady rate unless they make a conscious effort to eat more of the *higher*-calorie Pritikin diet foods. Such a weight loss occurs for several reasons: reduced salt intake will result in some water loss; a high-complex-carbohydrate diet is inherently less caloric than the conventional high-fat diet most Americans consume—a gram of carbohydrate has only 4 calories, compared with 9 calories in a gram of fat; and most people who begin the Pritikin diet start eating lots of raw-vegetable salads, low-calorie soups, and other low-calorie vegetable combinations, with the result that there is a reduction in their total caloric intake even if they aren't consciously trying to restrict calories. A word of caution here: if you are already lean and should not lose weight, you will have to restrict your consumption of the lower-calorie foods on the Pritikin diet, like salads and soups. This is discussed in more detail in the section called "Gaining Weight or Maintaining Weight" on page 112.

On the unrestricted-calorie plan, most people will lose ½ pound to a pound or more per week until they reach their optimal weight. So if you have only a little weight to lose, or are not even in a hurry to lose it, or if you don't want to deprive yourself—even a little—then by all means, just follow the regular unrestricted-calorie plan on the 28-day calendar. But if you want to take off weight quickly, some deliberate caloric restriction will help you to do so. With some calorie counting, in the 28-day period, women should be able to lose from 6 to 15 pounds and men from 8 to 25 pounds.

If you follow the suggestions in Chapter 16 for restricting calories, you will be eating the same basic diet, except that some foods have been omitted and some portion sizes reduced. You will eat approximately 1200 calories per day. At this level, most women and some men can function without discomfort and are able to be physically active. If you want to follow a calorie-restricted diet but need an intake somewhere *between* 1200 calories and the regular unrestricted-calorie plan, you simply adjust your caloric intake upward. Caloric values are provided for all foods on the menus. Some people may wish to follow the 1200-calorie menus on some days, and on other days opt for something in between the 1200-calorie and the regular menus. If you are feeling a little tired, you may need to increase your caloric intake slightly, or to eat more often. You should suit your own preferences and requirements from day to day.

Some Factors Affecting Rate of Weight Loss

The amount of exercise you do will certainly affect how quickly you lose weight. If walking is to be your form of exercise, figure 400 calories expended in one brisk hour's walk covering 4 miles. Joggers will be expending 600 to 900 calories in the same time. To lose a pound of fat, you must burn and not replace 3,500 calories; therefore you will need to burn at least 2000 calories per week through exercise for physical activity to be a significant factor in your rate of weight loss.

The ratio of muscle cells to fat cells in your body composition is another factor to consider. Muscle cells and fat cells have different metabolic rates. Muscle cells burn more energy than fat cells, so muscular people, and men in general, lose weight faster than women and less muscular people.

Also, your rate of weight loss will depend on how overweight you are at present. Even on the same diet, people who are very much overweight tend to lose faster than people who are just a little heavy.

If you have been on a high-protein diet up to now, that too will affect your weight loss, because the high-protein diet has forced too much water from your tissues. When you go on the high-complex-carbohydrate Pritikin diet, your tissues will regain normal water content, so there will be a period when you will seem not to be losing weight. In fact, your weight loss is simply being masked briefly by the water gain.

Gaining Weight or Maintaining Weight

If you *don't* want to lose weight or if you have only a little to lose, and a week or two into the program find yourself slipping below your optimal weight in a steady, continuous drop, you will need to make *two dietary modifications:* 1) increase portion sizes and servings of grains and grain foods, such as bread, cereal, rice, and other grains; and 2) limit your intake of low-calorie dishes, such as raw mixed-vegetable salads and almost all soups. (Even higher-calorie soups tend to have lots of filling bulk for their caloric value.) You can continue to use the regular unrestricted-calorie menus, but double your morning cereal portions, eat bread or bowlfuls of rice or other grains between meals for snacks, and have second and third helpings of grain dishes. On the other hand, limit salads to one small salad per day, and avoid soup other than in small amounts as a base for scoopfuls of rice or other grains or pasta.

> These words of caution are not to be taken lightly. It's easy to avoid losing too much weight, but once the weight loss has occurred, it is hard work for some people to gain it back on the Pritikin diet.

Now turn to the chart of 28-Day Health and Fitness Goals —if weight loss is one of your goals on the program—and fill out the section on weight. First indicate your present weight ("Present Level"), then make a guesstimate as to what you will weigh after the 28-day program ("28-Day Goal"). After the 28-day program is completed, you can enter your actual weight ("28-Day Accomplishment"). When making your guesstimate, take into consideration whether you will be on the regular diet or restricting your calories, and if so, by how much. Consider also the amount of exercise you expect to be doing, and any other factors that seem relevant.

2. Cholesterol Level

Your cholesterol level can be determined by a blood test and is now generally acknowledged to be the single most reliable indicator of arterial health, aside from a surgical technique called angiography, in which a catheter is inserted into the artery to assess artery blockage. The health of your arteries—that is, their freedom from blockage by cholesterol—is the key to your overall health and resistance to heart disease.

Blockage of the coronary arteries that feed the heart muscle is the cause of heart disease, the number-one killer in our country (52 percent of all deaths) and in other countries on an "affluent nation" diet. But you don't have to be middle-aged or older for artery blockage to affect your functioning. Blockage of the small arteries leading to the ears impairs our hearing, and although we do not realize it in most cases, we can no longer perceive certain frequencies.

When blood, and the oxygen it carries, is unable to reach *any* of the body tissues in sufficient amounts because of artery blockage, problems result. Visual impairment, joint pain, loss of mental acuity all develop when cholesterol deposits in arteries prevent adequate blood flow.

What Should My Cholesterol Level Be?

Unfortunately, healthy blood cholesterol levels are not possible on the conventional American diet, owing to the inordinate amounts of cholesterol present in the typical diet. What most physicians call "normal" cholesterol levels are in fact average cholesterol levels for any given age group in our population, and do not indicate freedom from artery disease. In populations in which degenerative diseases do not exist, cholesterol levels don't exceed 160 mg/dl at any time of life, but in our society it is considered "normal" for

113

blood cholesterol levels to increase with age. American medical scientists who are abreast of the epidemiological studies and other research are beginning to advocate cholesterol levels not exceeding 100 mg/dl plus your age, with a maximum of 150–160 mg/dl.

While cholesterol levels are usually an accurate reflection of arterial health, in about 15 percent of cases the values obtained in the cholesterol tests will be deceptively low. False readings occur in individuals who use large quantities of polyunsaturated fats or dairy products. These foods artificially lower the level of cholesterol and can cause it to be deposited in the tissues.

Now is the time to find out what your cholesterol level is. It's the one laboratory test I urged you to take before starting the 28-day program, because: 1) you should know your cholesterol level (it's more important than knowing your bank balance!) and 2) I would like you to experience at first hand the dramatic drop in cholesterol level possible on the Pritikin diet. The Pritikin diet—among all popular diets, including the American Heart Association diet—is the only one capable of substantially reducing cholesterol levels. At the same time, it's a good idea to have your triglycerides (blood fats) measured. Triglycerides are also significant in determining your degree of risk for coronary heart disease. They too will drop quickly and impressively on your new program.

In 28 days, your cholesterol level will drop 10–50 percent, depending upon its present elevation. At levels of 300 or higher, drops of 40–50 percent may occur; the average drop is 26 percent. If you already know your cholesterol level, or as soon as you have been tested, turn to the chart on 28-Day Health and Fitness Goals and fill out the section on Cholesterol Level, entering your present level and 28-day goal in the proper spaces.

3. Blood Pressure

As many as 75 million Americans are afflicted with high blood pressure; even children are becoming hypertensive in large numbers. To control high blood pressure, official medical agencies say that hypertensives must go on medication and stay on it for the rest of their lives. In many cases, however, you may not have to take this medication, which can have serious side effects, including impotence in men, gout, and diabetes.

If your blood pressure is higher than it should be, you can expect it to drop by as much as 15 percent after 28 days on the Pritikin diet and exercise program. This may seem suspect to you until you understand the mechanism. Fat causes red blood cells to bunch up in clumps (agglutinate); the cells stick together as though they had adhesive on their surfaces. In such clumps, they are unable to pass through the smaller vessels of the circulatory system and actually act like little corks to block circulation at thousands of locations. As in any hydraulic system when part of the system is blocked, pressure of the fluid flowing in the system becomes elevated. Now, on the Pritikin diet, with fats in the bloodstream substantially reduced, the blood cells become "unclumped", the circulatory system therefore expands, and pressure drops accordingly.

In addition, on the typical American diet, high in total fat, the body produces excess thromboxane A-2, a prostaglandin (a hormonelike substance). This prostaglandin makes cells sticky and contracts arteries, raising blood pressure.

Because the Pritikin diet is low in total fat and contains primarily polyunsaturated fats, more of the prostaglandin called prostacylin is synthesized. This prostaglandin inhibits cell stickiness and dilates arteries, both of which result in lower blood pressure.

When you have your cholesterol-level test, ask to have your blood pressure measured as well. Using the chart on page 118, indicate what your present blood pressure is and what you expect it to be in 28 days. Even if your blood pressure is in the acceptable range, you can still expect an improvement. Our data show that on the Pritikin diet, normal individuals can expect a 6-percent drop in systolic pressure and a 7-percent drop in diastolic pressure. At the end of 28 days, you can record *your* improvements.

4. Increased Endurance and Fitness

As you progress into the 28-day program, you'll notice improved endurance and fitness in many ways. The hill that had you puffing last week doesn't seem as taxing when you climb it now; and you have increased the total distance of your walk or run appreciably without strain. A low resting pulse rate is a good indication that you are physically fit. Your resting heart rate will probably be lower after 28 days of being on the program—another sign you're more fit than you were before you began. To measure your improvement, we would like to have you give yourself a Step Test, both before you start the 28-day program and then again at the end of the four weeks. The Step Test gives you an accurate measurement of your resting pulse rate and the speed of recovery to a resting heart rate after vigorous activity.

For the test, find a stool that is about 10 inches high. You'll also need a watch or clock with a second hand. Start by taking your pulse. Sit on the stool and count your pulse for 60 seconds by gently placing your index and middle fingers over the large neck artery (carotid) or over the artery at the base of your wrist below the thumb. Turn to the 28-Day Health and Fitness Goals chart on page 118. Under the "Endurance and Fitness" section, record your pulse in the space for Resting Heart Rate in the Present Level column.

You are now ready to begin the test. From a standing position, step up onto the stool with one foot, then the other; then step down again one foot at a time. Repeat this procedure over and over at a steady rate as fast as you comfortably can for as long as 5 minutes. Each time you step onto the stool and then back to the ground counts as one time. If possible, maintain a rate of 30 times per minute for 5 minutes, but don't push yourself excessively.

As soon as you stop, sit down on the stool. After one minute, take your pulse for 30 seconds. Multiply this number by 2 to obtain your pulse rate per minute. Record your one-minute postexercise pulse rate in the space in the chart allotted for it. Also record the duration of the Step Test and the rate of the Step Test in their respective spaces.

You are now ready to make your guesstimate as to how

much improvement you may make in these figures at the end of 28 days. The average improvement leads to a 5-percent drop in resting heart rate and a 10-percent drop in recovery heart rate. At the end of 28 days, when you take the Step Test again, I am confident you'll be very impressed with your results!

5. Decreased Fatigue

You will also notice improvement in increased stamina and alertness during the day. If you normally experience drowsiness, decreased attention span, and physical tiredness in the afternoon hours, you'll begin to notice changes. Several different factors are at work here, but principal among them is the decrease in the amount of fat in your bloodstream. When tiny arteries and capillaries become blocked by the fat from high-fat meals, your brain and muscles become oxygen-deprived. The already high fat level in your blood gets still another dose of fat as you digest your hamburger or quiche, and you begin to nod off when you need to be at your brightest.

Low blood sugar, which can compound the problem of reduced mental alertness, can also be remedied on the Pritikin diet. Complex carbohydrates are broken down S-L-O-W-L-Y and released into the bloodstream *a little at a time,* so that at no time is there a deficiency of blood glucose to the brain and other cells. Blood glucose is the only fuel that can be used by the brain, and it is important that glucose be available to your brain at all times. Often when people feel fatigued they will eat a candy bar or other product high in sugar, a simple carbohydrate. Your body digests simple carbohydrates almost instantly, and glucose enters the bloodstream in a rush, all at once. Such large amounts of sugar in the bloodstream trigger an overcompensating response, and the body begins to work overtime to rid the blood of the excess glucose. As a result, there is an even greater drop in blood sugar a little later, and you will feel more tired than ever. A high-protein diet will not overcome the problem of low blood sugar; it almost guarantees, in fact, that the problem will continue. The many horrors of a high-

YOUR 28-DAY HEALTH AND FITNESS GOALS

HEALTH AND FITNESS AREA	PRESENT LEVEL	28-DAY GOAL	28-DAY ACCOMPLISHMENT	AVERAGE 28-DAY IMPROVEMENT
Weight (if reduction is desired)*	wt in lb	wt in lb	wt in lb	Loss of 2–4 lb (mostly water) on unrestricted-calorie diet; loss of 6–15 lb (women) and 8–25 lb (men) on restricted-calorie diet
Cholesterol Level (in mg/dl) (Should not exceed a total of 100 plus your age with a maximum of 160 mg/dl)	_____ mg/dl	_____ mg/dl	_____ mg/dl	10–50% drop, depending upon amount of elevation
Triglyceride Level (in mg/dl) (Should be less than 120 mg/dl)	_____ mg/dl	_____ mg/dl	_____ mg/dl	10–50% drop; may occasionally rise for a month or two and then drop
Blood Pressure (Should not exceed 135/85 at any age) Systolic (upper figure)/ Diastolic (lower figure)	_____ systolic _____ diastolic	_____ systolic _____ diastolic	_____ systolic _____ diastolic	Up to 15% drops; in normal individuals, drop of 6% in systolic and 7% in diastolic rates

* If you plan to lose more than 10 pounds, you may wish to check first with your physician to determine what your ideal weight should be on the basis of your bone structure and other factors; you may also wish to consult Chapter 5 of my book *The Pritikin Permanent Weight-Loss Manual* (Grosset & Dunlap, 1981), which deals with this subject in detail.

Endurance and Fitness (Step Test)				
Resting Heart Rate (per minute)	___ per min	___ per min	___ per min	5% drop in Resting Heart Rate
Duration of Step Test (no. of minutes)	___ minutes	___ minutes	___ minutes	___ minutes
Rate of Step Test (steps per minute)	___ steps/min	___ steps/min	___ steps/min	___ steps/min.
Recovery Heart Rate (Start counting 1 minute after step test; count for 30 seconds, multiply by 2, and record in "per minute" space)	___ per min	___ per min	___ per min	10% drop in Recovery Heart Rate
Afternoon Alertness* (On scale of 0–100%: 0% = very fatigued; 100% = very alert, no fatigue)	Day 1: ___ Day 2: ___ Day 3: ___	___ % Day 1 ___ % Day 2 ___ % Day 3	___ % Day 1 ___ % Day 2 ___ % Day 3	A 10–50% increase in alertness ___ % Day 26 ___ % Day 27 ___ % Day 28

* You will probably have some muscle fatigue as a result of your new exercise program; don't confuse this fatigue with brain fatigue that reduces your alertness.

119

protein diet are discussed in more depth in Chapter 6 on pages 53–56.

Besides eating less fat and more complex carbohydrates, you'll be further combating problems of afternoon fatigue through your exercise program. If you haven't been exercising at all or very much up to now, you'll probably experience some muscle fatigue after you start your exercise program that may last from 2 to 6 weeks. That kind of fatigue is normal and simply tells you your body is adjusting to conditioning. Muscle fatigue is not to be confused with *brain fatigue,* which causes you to be lethargic and sleepy by midday.

To make an approximate measurement of brain fatigue as it affects afternoon alertness, make an evaluation for 3 days before starting the 28-day program, rating yourself on a scale of 0 percent—very fatigued—to 100 percent—very alert. The evaluation should reflect your condition each day for the 3-day test from approximately 2 to 6 P.M. Enter the figures in percentage values on the 28-Day Health and Fitness Goals chart on page 118 for "Afternoon Alertness," "Present Level." Then make your guesstimate of improvement expected in afternoon level of alertness as evaluated at or near the end of the 28-day period. While this test is entirely subjective, it still yields worthwhile information for you in this area.

Of course, it is important that you have adequate sleep at night during the testing periods, and during the 28-day period in general, to maximize your gains. Being well rested will enable you to exercise more efficiently too, although you may find that on the Pritikin diet and exercise program you need *less* sleep to feel refreshed in the morning. You may also find that you will sleep more soundly because of the tranquilizing effects of exercise and improved health.

I have singled out five major areas in which you may expect marked improvements in the 28-day period on the program: 1) weight normalization without hunger; 2) reduction in blood cholesterol level; 3) reduction in blood pressure; 4) increased endurance and fitness as measured by reduced resting heart rate and recovery heart rate; and 5) decreased fatigue. But there will be other benefits that will further contribute to your sense of well-being, both physical and emotional. For example, you will notice that you have become more regular in your bowel habits; and you will feel an emotional high from having exercised initiative in changing your lifestyle and then successfully implementing your decision. In addition, there will be emotional benefits from *feeling better* physically. So expect to enjoy your relationships more; to feel less irritable; to take pleasure in looking better in your clothes (and out of them); and to enjoy your day-to-day activities, work and play, far more than you ever have.

PEOPLE CAN BE HELPFUL

Your family, friends, co-workers, and other associates can be great assets in helping you to adhere to the 28-day program. At best, they will offer you encouragement, reinforcement, and companionship—or at the very least, neutrality and noninterference.

You will need to give some thought to setting the right tone with the people closest to you as to your commitment to the 28-day program. If you are in earnest about your commitment and let the important people in your life know, you will already have taken the first big step in gaining their understanding and support. When you discuss your commitment with them, you have acknowledged to yourself and to them your intent to make some significant lifestyle changes. In so doing, you firm up your own resolve and you increase the awareness of the people who will be at your side as you begin the program.

STARTING THE PROGRAM WITH A COMPANION

The ideal way to start the 28-day program is to do it with a companion—either your spouse or a friend. You will reinforce each other, and have much more fun in the process. Hopefully, you can share in the preparing of meals, making them less work and more enjoyable. The advantages are tremendous.

If you are not living with someone who wants to join you,

perhaps a close friend or co-worker will have an interest. You could exercise together and share a few meals. Even if you cannot find someone who can be with you for meals and exercises, just having someone you know start the program simultaneously with you can be a great boon. You can check with each other, and share laughs and helpful hints. You can even plan to celebrate together when you reach that important 28th day.

SETTING THE SCENE AT HOME AND AWAY FROM HOME

Family members at home may surprise you by expressing an interest in going on the program with you. The program is suitable for entire families, and you will find more detail on this in Chapter 14 under "Special Situations." If your family is uninterested or uncooperative, don't be discouraged. Read selections to them from Chapter 1 and tell them about the "winners" described in Chapter 9, in an attempt to gain their backing in your efforts to be a winner too. But if they fail to respond to your reasoning, don't alienate them with missionary tactics. Let the example of your improvement during the 28-day program be your message. Whether or not they are enthusiastic about your venture, you still have to live together. Think through your needs, the logistics of meal preparation, and how others may have to adjust to your new schedule—for example, you may be exercising when you would previously have been available. Work out a *modus vivendi* that will enable you to carry out your program requirements with as little upheaval as possible.

You may also need to work out some understandings with others as well. The friend who is used to going out with you to restaurants you will no longer frequent may be a bit miffed, and perhaps the neighbor with whom you sat around in your kitchen enjoying coffee and pastries will feel abandoned when you now use the time for your exercise period. Sociability and food are very much intertwined in our lives, and when we want to change such patterns others may feel quite threatened. Be sensitive to their reactions, and let friends or co-workers understand that you value them and their association, but you must do what is required to follow through on your decision.

Tell them, too, that you need and welcome their support and encouragement. And remember that even in going about the program in a quiet way, you can be a tremendous inspiration to others.

Now your final task before starting the program is to establish where you are today. Use the checklist on page 124, and then as the days pass, you will have a report card of your progress.

RATE YOURSELF ON

Compliance: Place X in the day's box if you didn't exercise when

Week	1							2				
Day	1	2	3	4	5	6	7	8	9	10	11	12
Exercise												
Smoking, all substances												
Diet: Egg yolks												
High-fat dairy: cheese, ice cream, butter, whole milk												
Margarine, oils												
Nuts, peanut butter, seeds												
Fish, fowl, meat more than 3–4 oz/day												
Organ meats: liver, kidney, etc.												
Alcohol: more than 1 drink/day												

Feeling of Well-Being: Rate yourself on a scale of 1 to 10:
1 = Terrible; 10 = No problem.

Afternoon drowsiness												
Evening drowsiness												
Constipation												
Uncontrolled eating, binges, etc.												
Insomnia												
Depression												

THIS CHECKLIST

you were supposed to, smoked, or ate the foods listed.

				3						4					
13	14	15	16	17	18	19	20	21	22	23	24	25	26	27	28

12
CHAPTER

What to Expect Each Week— and by the End of 28 Days

NO SURPRISES! WHAT TO EXPECT IN WEEK 1

On day 1 of your new life, you will give up some habits, and learn some new ones. Let's start with the ones you're giving up.

1. Coffee, Tea, Chocolate, Cola Drinks

All of them contain caffeine or caffeinelike substances called methylxanthines, which a number of physicians believe might cause fibrocystic breast disease. Dr. John P. Minton of Ohio State University treats women with fibrocystic breast disease by eliminating coffee, tea, chocolate, and cola drinks from their diets. Most of his patients recover in a few months. The breasts lose their tenderness, swelling, and discomfort, and the cysts gradually disappear.

The day after you eliminate this foursome from your diet, you may have a minor headache and a feeling of uneasiness. If you were a heavy consumer, your headache may intensify on the third and fourth days, but on the fifth and sixth days it will gradually disappear.

Most people can tolerate the discomfort, but if it gets too much, take headache tablets, especially before bed, so that you can get a good night's sleep.

On the second day after eliminating methylxanthines you will feel a new calmness. Your heart will beat more slowly, and you'll be less uptight about things. If you're accustomed to the pick-me-up of caffeine, on the second day you may feel tired in the morning, especially if your habit is to get by on very little sleep.

For the first week, it's important to increase your hours of sleep. Go to bed 1 hour earlier the first night. If you are tired when you wake up, get to bed 1½ or 2 hours earlier the second night. This will help overcome the fatigue associated with any longtime sleep deprivation you may have had from being a heavy caffeine user. The extra sleep that first week will also be helpful for your new exercise program.

2. Alcohol

Alcohol is a sensitive subject. If you can abstain for 28 days, fine! If you must have some, then limit yourself to 1 beer, glass of wine, or cocktail 4 times a week. Alcohol is a rich source of empty calories, and it raises the level of fats or triglycerides in the blood. Alcohol should be especially limited by people just starting the program because it makes it more difficult to resist eating unhealthful foods or smoking.

3. Smoking: Cigarettes, Cigars, Pipes

On a high-carbohydrate diet, you can stop smoking without having to worry about weight gain. In fact, this diet permits you to lose weight at the same time as you stop smoking, and to really fill your stomach so that you won't feel hungry.

The diet is ideal for giving up smoking, because the chemistry of your blood and your body tissues will change so that the urge to smoke is greatly reduced, and in a week or so 90 percent of the urge will be gone.

I suggest that you stop smoking at once, and when you have the urge to smoke, drink a glass of water slowly instead. By the time you finish drinking, the urge will probably be gone. It lasts for only a minute. By the third day, 50 percent of the urge will be gone, and by the end of the first week, you'll be surprised at how easy it was, even if you smoked three packs a day.

After not smoking for a while you'll notice less fatigue during the day, and this will continue to improve. Soon, not only will your energy level be higher, but your sight, hearing, and ability to concentrate and remember will improve remarkably.

Remember, on the Pritikin diet, giving up smoking is essentially a 1-week problem.

4. Calorie-dense, Fiber-poor Foods

For those who have not experienced a high-carbohydrate diet, the end results of a diet of this type can be very surprising:

  a. Eat all you like and not gain weight? Yes!
  b. Eat all you like and lose weight? Yes!

Giving up calorie-dense fatty foods such as pastries, fat spreads, and cheeses, will enable you to lose weight without feeling hungry, because you can eat large quantities of high-fiber foods. You can also expect to be free from problems of constipation for life.

If you have a tendency toward ulcers, hiatus hernia, spastic colon, or ulcerative colitis, you probably have been told to avoid roughage. In fact, the soft, fiber- or roughage-free diet is the most probable *cause* of these colon disorders, and unfortunately, it is mistakenly used as the treatment. Instead, cook *all* your vegetables for the first week. After that, slowly introduce raw vegetables, and if you develop any discomfort, back off and slowly start again.

Exercise

If you have not had a regular exercise pattern, you'll start with whatever level of *walking* is comfortable. Don't overdo! Your joints, muscles, tendons are not conditioned, and too much can cause swelling, pain, tearing, and unhappiness.

As you gradually exercise, you may experience some stiffness the next morning as you get up. This is very normal, and will take from 1 to 3 weeks to disappear, depending upon your age. Extra sleep the first week is a marvelous repairer of tired, unconditioned muscles.

If you have an exercise program, this conditioning problem doesn't apply to you unless you intend to considerably increase your exercise time.

By the end of Week 1, you should notice the following:

1. If you gave up coffee, tea, cola, and chocolate—
Calmer, more restful sleep; less daytime fatigue; heartburn and headaches gone.

2. If you gave up smoking—
A feeling of being more alive; all your senses more alert; 90 percent of the smoking urge gone; and you are now kissable.

3. If you gave up alcohol—
You're more alert and more relaxed at the same time.

4. If you gave up calorie-dense foods—
You have more energy, and you're starting to lose a little weight; constipation disappears.

5. If this is your first regular exercise program—
Most of your joint stiffness and muscle fatigue should be gone. Your endurance will be at least 50 percent greater than on Day 1.

6. Other changes—
Warm glow of feeling better. You may still require some extra sleep. Your food volume intake will be 25 percent greater because of bulkier foods that have less calories.

If you are of normal weight or up to 10 pounds heavier than you would like to be, stay on the normal full-calorie diet. Excess fat will gradually disappear, and most people come down to their lean muscle mass in a month or two.

It's not necessary to go on the weight-reduction guidelines unless you are more than 10 pounds overweight. Stay on the weight-reduction guidelines until you are 5 to 10 pounds more than you would like to be, and then shift to the normal-calorie diet. You will drift down to your normal weight in a month or two.

High-protein dieters who switch to this diet may gain from 1 to 5 pounds the first week.

Don't panic! It's only the water that your dehydrated tissues need so desperately. In an effort to dilute the poisonous end products of a high-protein diet, the body gives up more water than it should and now will replace that water and become healthy again.

Within the first week, high-protein dieters will experience a dramatic shift from constant fatigue to a feeling of being alive all through the day.

WEEK 2

The worst is over. Withdrawal headaches, aches, pains, stiffness of joints and muscles are largely behind you.

If weight loss is your goal, the amount you lose in the second week will be representative of how much you will lose steadily as the weeks progress, until you reach your optimal weight.

Examine your feet carefully for blisters, red spots, tender areas. Make sure your shoes are large enough, since your feet may be swelling slightly from the increased exercise. Feel the tips of your toes: if they are tender, you may require longer shoes.

By Week 2, you should be aware that your stamina is increasing, and that you're feeling better and more alive generally.

Sleep. Stay with the increased rest for the next few days, and then gradually reduce your hours of sleep on the basis of your needs. If you're getting up at 5 A.M. and feel completely rested but would like to sleep until 6 A.M., go to bed 1 hour later at night.

Exercise. Don't overdo, or proceed too fast!

After 1 week you may feel so much better that you'll want to walk 20 miles, or run for an hour. Resist the temptation. Increase your activity according to schedule for Week 2, so as not to risk an injury.

Food. By this time, you're almost accustomed to eating without salt, sugar, and fat. If you have discovered a favorite day's menu, repeat it as often as you like.

Try to get into the habit of cooking double quantities of food so that you'll have leftovers and save preparation time.

Friends. Be sure to tell your friends how well you are doing. They will be proud of you and want to cooperate. But avoid friends who say, "Just this once." If you succumb, you may never make it to 28 days. Be firm. Planning is essential so that you stay closely on your new diet.

WEEK 3

Halfway mark!
By this time, you'll notice several changes.

Fatigue. Now you won't feel like dozing after lunch or in the early afternoon. You'll enjoy your new vitality, and you'll even want to walk (15–20 minutes) during your lunch break.

Exercise. Who'd have guessed you'd have so much energy! You'll do your exercise without much effort and feel refreshed, not tired, when you are finished. *Don't* overdo, no matter how well you feel. You'll live a long time. Give your muscles and joints time for conditioning.

Weight. If you were trying to lose weight, you will now notice that your clothes are looser. But don't see your tailor yet; wait for the full 28 days.

Food. By this time, you should be an expert on food preparation and dining out. Your taste buds should now start to appreciate the whole grains and the good taste of natural foods. Devote the extra time you've saved by using leftovers to your exercise.

Sleep. With all this new effort, you will now find that your sleep requirement is less. Some people report sleeping ½ hour to 1½ hours less per night. Everyone is different, but if, when you awaken, you do not feel the need to go back to sleep, you have had enough sleep.

Alertness. You will notice a new feeling of being alive in both body and mind. You will have faster reactions, better memory and concentration, absence of fatigue, and an urge to be active.

WEEK 4

Almost there. Although this is the last week of the introduction to the Pritikin Program, by now you will see it as a beginning to a whole new way of life.

Friends will notice the changes that are happening in you. Several may even follow your example. Now would be the time to develop new friends, as well: people who enjoy being active—running, hiking, folk dancing, and so on. And perhaps you can teach them your new food habits.

Exercise. At the end of this week you will do your second endurance step test. The only way to be sure of your progress is to measure it. You'll be proud of your increased stamina. By this time, exercise should be an integral part of your daily schedule. In another month or so, you should reach your permanent endurance goals.

Alertness. Get ready to gauge your alertness on Days 26, 27, and 28. You will be pleasantly surprised by comparing them with Days 1, 2, and 3.

Final testing. Make an appointment to have your blood cholesterol tested and your blood pressure taken. Record these on your progress card.

Food. You should be experienced enough now to invite friends to help celebrate your 28th day. Make it a party; have fun, and give yourself credit for how far you've come.

What next? In the first 28 days, you will have improved your fitness and health by about 60 percent of what is possible for you. To attain 100 percent of your potential improvement may take from 6 months (if you are younger than 35) to 3 years (if you are older than 65). The best part is that as you get older, you feel younger!

GOALS YOU SHOULD HAVE ACHIEVED AT THE END OF 28 DAYS

Congratulations on completing your first month on the Pritikin Program! By this time you should be feeling the results of your new lifestyle. You should—
- Have more energy
- Be able to walk farther and faster
- Have lost several of your unwanted pounds (and possibly inches) if you were overweight
- Look more alert
- Be able to concentrate longer without feeling tired
- Be spending less money on food
- Be able to run, rather than drag yourself, up a flight of stairs

We have provided a scorecard so you can record all your successes. If you wish to send the card to us, we would be happy to evaluate your progress, pinpoint the areas in which you can improve further, and tell you how to go about it.

Of course, your health and level of fitness will continue to improve, so we have provided scorecards for your 6-month and 1-year checkups.

PROGRESS CARD—28 DAYS

We will be happy to evaluate your progress if you fill out this page, fold it along the dotted lines on the reverse side, and send it to us. Please include a self-addressed stamped envelope.

Name_____Date_____

Age_____Sex_____Height_____Ideal weight_____

Address_____

Phone_____Date started program_____

HEALTH AND FITNESS		Day 1	Day 28
Weight	pounds		
Cholesterol level	mg/dl		
Blood pressure	Example: 120/70		
Endurance and fitness (Step Test)			
Resting heart rate	per minute		
Duration of test	minutes		
Rate of test	steps/ minute		
Recovery heart rate (Start counting 1 minute after step test, count for 30 seconds, multiply by 2, and record in "per min." space)	per minute		
Afternoon alertness (On a scale of 0–100%: 0% = very fatigued; 100% = very alert, no fatigue)			
Other:			

Name _____

Address _____

City & State _____

Zip _____

HEALTH GOALS
P. O. Box 5335
Santa Barbara, CA 93108

Under

PROGRESS CARD—SIX MONTHS

We will be happy to evaluate your progress if you fill out this page, fold it along the dotted lines on the reverse side, and send it to us. *Please include a self-addressed stamped envelope.*

Name_____ Date_____

Age_____Sex_____Height_____ Ideal weight_____

Address_____

Phone_____Date started program_____

HEALTH AND FITNESS		Before (copy from Day 1)	Day 28 (copy from previous progress card)	After 6 months
Weight	pounds			
Cholesterol level	mg/dl			
Blood pressure	Example: 120/70			
Endurance and fitness (Step Test)				
Resting heart rate	per minute			
Duration of test	minutes			
Rate of test	steps/ minute			
Recovery heart rate (Start counting 1 minute after step test, count for 30 seconds, multiply by 2, and record in "per min." space)	per minute			
Afternoon alertness (On a scale of 0–100%: 0% = very fatigued; 100% = very alert, no fatigue)				
Other:				

Name _____

Address _____

City & State _____

Zip _____

Place
stamp
here

HEALTH GOALS
P. O. Box 5335
Santa Barbara, CA 93108

Under

PROGRESS CARD—ONE YEAR

We will be happy to evaluate your progress if you fill out this page, fold it along the dotted lines on the reverse side, and send it to us. *Please include a self-addressed stamped envelope.*

Name_____ Date_____

Age_____Sex_____Height_____Ideal weight_____

Address_____

Phone_____ Date started program_____

HEALTH AND FITNESS		Before (copy from Day 1)	Day 28 (copy from previous progress card)	After 6 mos (copy from previous progress card)	After 1 year
Weight	pounds				
Cholesterol level	mg/dl				
Blood pressure	Example: 120/70				
Endurance and fitness (Step Test)					
Resting heart rate	per minute				
Duration of test	minutes				
Rate of test	steps/ minute				
Recovery heart rate (Start counting 1 minute after step test, count for 30 seconds, multiply by 2, and record in "per min." space)	per minute				
Afternoon alertness (On a scale of 0–100%: 0% = very fatigued; 100% = very alert, no fatigue)					
Other					

Name _____

Address _____

City & State _____

Zip _____

HEALTH GOALS
P. O. Box 5335
Santa Barbara, CA 93108

13
CHAPTER

Planning
Your
Exercise Program

You will now be "revved up" and eager to get on with your program. And great things lie ahead, because whether you are a marathon runner or are just now embarking on a regular exercise regimen, the combined exercise and diet program will soon have your circulatory system operating at its very optimal and you will be feeling terrific.

By now you understand that although exercising is healthful, it can kill you IF you are on a diet high in cholesterol and half of your calories come from fat.

Exercise protects against heart disease by putting a demand on the heart, to which the body gradually adapts. Adaptation involves strengthening of the heart muscle, reduced tendency to clot formation, an increase in blood volume, and most important, an increase in the size of the vessels supplying the heart.

However, the majority of adult men and many women who for years have been eating the typical fatty American diet and leading the typical sedentary American life will already have moderately to severely narrowed heart vessels owing to too little activity and to dietary-induced cholesterol growths protruding into the vessels. If these artery-diseased people suddenly take to the track, the heart muscle, because of insufficient blood from the narrowed coronary arteries, will have difficulty pumping the blood through the 70,000 miles of blood vessels in the body fast enough to meet the oxygen demand of the working muscles, especially the legs and the heart. This is the danger. Creating a need for a little more oxygen puts a small stress on the cardiovascular system and promotes healthful adaptations. But strenuous physical activity by people cardiovascularly unfit can create such a shortage of oxygen that the heart is unable to function properly, and sudden death can result.

It's important to remember the significant role of both exercise *and* diet in the Pritikin Program. If you are able to adopt only one part of the program, it should be the dietary part. But combining diet and exercise will ensure the most improvement in your condition.

You will observe that once you begin your exercise program you have more stamina than before. Endurance studies comparing a high-fat diet and a high-carbohydrate diet show that the subjects on the high-carbohydrate diet were able to exercise more than three times as long as when they were on the high-fat diet. Does that mean you should eat before exercising—and if so, how much? Since the long muscles of the legs or arms and the stomach muscles may be in competition for blood supply if you exercise following a large meal, I suggest you wait to eat a meal until after you exercise. People with heart disease ought to eat only lightly before exercising. Almost everyone is able to eat a snack, such as fruit, before exercising with no ill consequences; and some people, myself included, have no problem whatsoever with strenuous exercise even after a large meal—but many others do. You'll need to experiment to find out what's best for you.

TYPE OF EXERCISE

Aerobic exercise refers to rhythmic, repetitive activities involving the large voluntary muscles of the legs or arms. It is strenuous enough to cause sufficient elevation of the heart and respiratory rates, but not so strenuous that it cannot be sustained for a sufficient length of time. You won't derive the aerobic benefits if you stop to window-shop or admire the flowers during your run. You have to keep going so you're breathing a little harder and your heart beats a little faster continuously for 15–30 minutes, depending on the type of exercise. For it to be beneficial, your body must make a great enough demand for oxygen over a long enough period of time. Gradually your system will adapt so that an increased supply of oxygen is brought to the cells. For maximum benefit, you should do aerobic exercise 4 times a week or more. For most people, the best aerobic exercises are jogging or brisk and sustained walking. Many other types of exercise are fun, and provide additional benefits, but it is still important to do 4 hours of walking or 2 hours of jogging per week. If you like, you can substitute some other form of exercise for walking or jogging if you are sure it keeps your pulse at your target heart rate (see page 144) for at least 20 minutes.

Swimming is an excellent exercise if you sustain the effort by doing continuous laps. Tennis and racquetball may qualify if they are performed continuously for a long enough period of time at a sufficiently high level of exertion. Outdoor bicycling usually does not qualify because the exertion required is uneven. You may work hard going up a hill but then coast downhill. I advise most people to embark on a program of either brisk walking or jogging as the simplest, best, and most readily available forms of exercise for helping to achieve their fitness and health goals.

Serious joggers or people with a good walking regimen have probably already worked out logistical problems involved in a regular exercise program, but may wish to work out a more intensive regimen than their present one.

PLANNING YOUR INDIVIDUAL EXERCISE PROGRAM

Will you be walking? Jogging? Or a combination of the two? Where will you be exercising? And when?

People who have not been exercising regularly for the past several months would do best to begin with a walking program. Plan to start your walking at a pace that is just comfortable. It will take a while for your muscles and joints to adapt to vigorous and prolonged exercise without sustaining injury. Until your muscles gain strength, they will limit the amount of exercise in which you are able to engage. Then you can sustain sufficient elevation of your heart rate for a long enough period of time to be beneficial to your heart.

If your muscles are up to it, you should exert yourself until you can feel your heart beating harder and you are breathing more heavily without being short of breath. The best way to judge if you're exerting yourself too much is to take the breath test: if you are too short of breath to talk, hum, or sing to yourself, you should slow down. However, if you don't exert yourself enough, you won't derive the desired benefits.

For those of you who enjoy testing and measuring, you can see if you're working hard enough by calculating your target heart rate. Simply subtract your age from 220, which will give you an estimate of your maximum heart rate per minute. If you haven't had a regular exercise program, multiply this number by 0.7, or if you have been exercising, by 0.75. If you smoke or are 20 pounds or more overweight, multiply by 0.65. This is your target heart rate per minute. Divide by 6 to obtain your target rate for 10 seconds. Interrupt your exercise and take your pulse for 10 seconds (see page 116) and see if you're on target.

Example:

	220	
	-48	(age)
	172	(estimated maximum heart rate)
	$\times 0.7$	(factor for sedentary, nonobese nonsmoker)
	120.4	(target heart rate/minute)
$\div 6 =$		
	20.0	(target rate for 10 seconds)

HOW TO DRESS FOR EXERCISE

Many people who want to lose weight overdress in the mistaken notion that if they sweat they will lose more weight. But you will gain back weight loss due to sweating as soon as you drink your next glassful of water. Overdressing to promote sweating during strenuous exercise serves no useful purpose, and can lead to dangerous heat exhaustion.

Dress in comfortable clothes and avoid becoming overheated. If you're chilly when you start out, wear layers of clothing that can be shed as you warm up. More calories are burned when your skin is cool.

You can simply tie the arms of your sweater around your waist, or you may want to carry a backpack for the layers of clothing shed as you get warmer. Carrying a backpack—or any weight, for that matter—will also increase the number of calories you burn during exercise, and if you're carrying enough weight, it can substantially improve your aerobic physical fitness. But I don't recommend that beginners add weight for several months.

Proper shoes are of the utmost importance. Tennis shoes or sneakers are not good for either walking or jogging because they do not cushion your weight adequately or give proper support. Buy good jogging shoes for either walking or jogging. Look for excellent fit and comfort, good arch support, rounded heel for shock absorption, light weight, flexibility, and cushioned sole. Pinch the toe to check cushioning.

Proper shoes will go a long way in preventing blisters and other foot and knee problems. Should a blister develop, simply purchase some moleskin from your pharmacy. Cut a small circular piece of the moleskin a little larger than your blister. Cut a hole in the circle the size of your blister and apply to your foot so that the blister peeks out of the hole. Change the dressing as necessary until the blister is gone.

Wear thick, absorbent socks. Try several brands until you find the one that's right for you. Make sure there is plenty of room for your toes, because your feet will swell slightly when you exercise.

WARM-UP AND COOL-DOWN

It's important to warm up before and cool down after your exercise sessions. "Warm-up" and "cool-down" sound like factory terminology. In truth, your body *is* very much like an industrial operation, and its equipment, which includes your heart and muscles, needs a warming-up period and a cooling-down period in order to run most efficiently and without mishap.

The warm-up period is simply a few minutes of slow exercise, such as walking at a moderate pace, at the beginning of the session to allow your heart rate to increase gradually. Warm-up also allows your blood vessels to dilate slowly until they have enlarged as much as possible to accommodate the increased blood flow from strenuous exercise. Most walkers automatically start at a slower pace, then gradually ease into brisker walking. You can either walk a few minutes as indicated in the Walking and Walk/Jog Progression charts, or spend a few minutes warming up by doing the optional warm-up exercises that follow.

The cool-down period has the opposite effect to the warm-up period; by gradually decreasing the intensity of exercise, you will put less strain on your heart. Also, fast walking or jogging causes lactic acid to be formed from the glucose in your system. Lactic acid can accumulate in the calf muscles, causing fatigue and cramping. If you walk for a while after the exercise session, it will help flush the lactic acid from your muscles and prevent soreness the following day. A warm bath will also help to relax your muscles, but always wait half an hour for your blood vessels to return to normal after exercise before taking a hot bath or shower or getting into a Jacuzzi or sauna. The heat will cause further dilation of the blood vessels, which puts a strain on the heart.

OPTIONAL WARM-UP EXERCISES

* These exercises should be done slowly and gently. *Do not bounce or force the stretch.*

LATERAL STRETCH

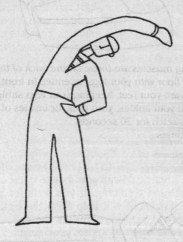

1. Standing tall, with shoulders relaxed, place left hand on hip.
2. Raise right arm and bend it over head.
3. Pushing hip in with left hand, reach as far as you can with your right arm and upper body.
4. Hold for 30 seconds.
5. Do the exercise in the opposite direction.
6. Repeat 3 times.

THE PRITIKIN PROMISE

HAMSTRING STRETCH

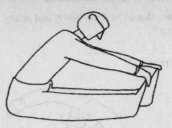

The hamstring muscles are those on the back of the thigh.
1. Sit on the floor with your legs extended in front of you.
2. Reach toward your feet, keeping your legs straight.
3. Grab on to your ankles, your toes, or insides of your feet.
4. Hold the stretch for 20 seconds.
5. Repeat 5 times.

LEG LIFT

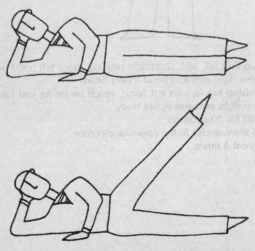

1. Lie on left side, left elbow bent, left hand supporting head, and right palm on floor in front of chest.

148

2. Slowly lift right leg, keeping knee straight and breathing out.
3. Slowly lower leg, breathing in.
4. Do exercise while lying on right side.
5. Repeat each side 8 times.

PUSH-UPS

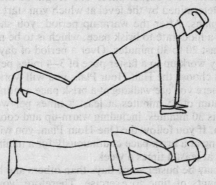

1. Begin with knees on floor and elbows straight.
2. Slowly bend elbows and lower your upper body close to the floor, keeping back straight.
3. Exhale, and push floor away by straightening arms.
4. Repeat 10–20 times.

After doing push-ups, stretching in either of the positions below will relax your muscles and feel good.

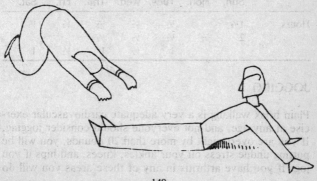

WALKING

If you've chosen walking as your form of exercise, follow one of the Walking Progression Plans starting on page 154. Before brisk walking, you should warm up by walking for a few minutes at a casual pace. The length of the warm-up will be determined by the level at which you start, as shown on the plans. After the warm-up period, you should have reached a moderate to brisk pace, which is to be maintained for at least 20 to 30 minutes. Over a period of days you will gradually work up to a faster pace of 3–4 miles per hour.

If you choose the Half-Hour Plan, you will work up to the point where you are walking at a brisk pace continuously for a minimum of 25 minutes at least 8 times per week. Each session is 30 minutes, including warm-up and cool-down, in duration. If you follow the One-Hour Plan, you will work up to walking at a brisk pace continuously for a minimum of 55 minutes at least 4 times a week.

You may be busier some days than others and have varying amounts of time to exercise. Therefore, you can mix hour-long and half-hour-long walks during the week. Just don't let more than 3 consecutive days lapse between sessions, and try not to let more than 1 day go by, especially until you're in better condition. Below is a chart showing examples of different combinations of duration and frequency that will enable you to meet the minimum requirements of 4 hours and 4 times a week.

	Sun.	Mon.	Tues.	Wed.	Thu.	Fri.	Sat.
Hours	1½		½	½	½	½	½
	2	½	½	½	½		
			1	½	1	½	1

JOGGING

Plain brisk walking is a very adequate cardiovascular exercise at any age, and not everyone should consider jogging. If you are overweight by more than 20 pounds, you will be putting undue stress on your ankles, knees, and hips if you jog. If you have arthritis in any of these areas you will do better not to jog; and if you have orthopedic problems that could be aggravated by jogging, such as an appreciable difference in leg length, an ankle injury that flares up easily, or a hip that has been broken, you would do better with walking or other sports. Would-be joggers who are over 35 or have high blood pressure or a cardiac problem should not begin a jogging program without first having their physician administer an EKG stress test to decide whether they are ready for jogging and to determine a safe but effective exercising heart rate.

If you're already jogging and have none of these problems, just continue to do so at least 4 times a week. If you haven't even been walking on a regular basis, but want to take up jogging, follow one of the Walking Progression Plans before starting to jog. If you can already walk briskly for an hour, have no health problems, and wish to jog, follow the Walk/Jog Progression Plan on page 155. Start your jogging at a slow speed of 5 to 6 miles per hour, as at first you'll be burning mostly glucose to provide your energy. Later your body will adapt and use more fat for energy during exercise. Until that time, if you jog too fast you might run out of steam. As your level of fitness improves, you can gradually increase the rate at which you jog to 6½–7½ miles per hour.

Many authorities advise joggers to make a conscious point of always beginning with 5 minutes of walking at a moderate pace followed by the stretching exercises below:

TO STRETCH CALVES:

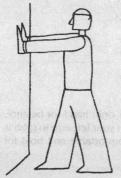
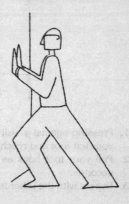

THE PRITIKIN PROMISE

1. Stand with your arms straight ahead of you and place your hands flat against the wall.
2. Move one foot directly forward and the other back so that the distance between them is about 10–12 inches.
3. Keeping your body straight and heels on the floor, bend your forward knee and your arms. This will bring your head close to your hands and stretch your straight back leg. Hold for 5 seconds.
4. Stretch each leg 5 times.

TO STRETCH THIGHS:

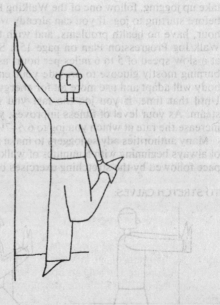

1. Pressing against a wall with your right hand for balance, lift your left foot and reach back with your left arm to grab it.
2. Pull your foot back as far as comfortable and hold for 30 seconds.
3. Repeat with the other foot.

TO STRETCH HAMSTRINGS AND LOWER BACK MUSCLES:

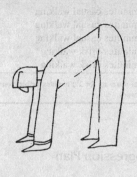 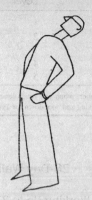

1. Stand with feet about 12 inches apart and drop your head forward. Lean forward at the waist as far as you can, keeping your back straight, and reach your hands toward the floor. If you are flexible, you will be able to place your palms on the floor. Hold for 30 seconds.
2. Return to erect position.
3. Place hands on hips, drop your head backward, and lean your upper body back as far as you can. Hold for 30 seconds.
4. Repeat the sequence, but lean forward, this time bending your back.
5. Do the sequence 6 times, alternating between straight back and bent back when bending forward.

Follow the Walk/Jog Progression Plan and gradually work up to a minimum of 20 minutes' continuous jogging. You will be exercising for half an hour a minimum of 4 times a week including the 5-minute warm-up and cool-down periods.

Exercise has tremendous physical and emotional effects. It's an important part of the Pritikin Program, and if you are as diligent about your exercise as you are about your diet, you will have made great gains in your level of fitness by the end of the month.

Day	Level	Walking sessions
1– 7	1	10 minutes casual walking
8–14	2	15 minutes casual walking
15–19	3	20 minutes casual walking
20–24	4	20 minutes brisk walking*
25–	5	25 minutes brisk walking

* Remember, when you reach level 4 you have to warm up for 2½ minutes before your brisk walking and cool down for 2½ minutes afterward.

28-Day Walking Progression Plan

Working Up to 2 Half-Hour Sessions per Day
Begin at any level that is comfortable for you and stay at that level for 1 week. If you haven't exercised in several years, it is best to start at Level 1. As you progress, you may shorten the time spent at any level if you feel ready to do so. You'll have to exercise 3 times a day for short but progressively longer periods and work up to 2 half-hour sessions a day. Walk at a casual pace for 2½ minutes prior to and after brisk walking sessions. This will allow you to warm up and cool down safely.

You are now walking one hour a day. Well done!

28-Day Walking Progression Plan

Working Up to 1 Hour-Long Session per Day
Begin at any level that is comfortable for you and stay at that level for 1 week. If you haven't exercised in several years, it is best to start at Level 1. As you progress, you may shorten the time spent at any level if you feel ready to do so. You'll have to exercise twice a week for shorter but progressively longer periods and work up to an hour-long

Times per Week	Example
24	4 times/day, 6 × in 7 days (days 1–7)
16	4 times/day, 4 × in 7 days (days 8–14)
12	3 times/day, 4 × in 5 days (days 15–19)
12	3 times/day, 4 × in 5 days (days 20–24)
8	2 times/day, 4 × per week (days 25–)

session. Walk at a casual pace for 2½ minutes prior to and after each session. This will allow you to warm up and cool down safely.

Day	Level	Walking Sessions	Frequency
1– 7	6	30 minutes brisk walking	7 times in 7 days (days 1–7)
8–14	7	35 minutes brisk walking	6 times in 7 days (days 8–14)
15–19	8	40 minutes brisk walking	4 times in 5 days (days 15–19)
20–24	9	50 minutes brisk walking	3 times in 5 days (days 20–24)
25–	10	55 minutes brisk walking	4 times per week (days 25–)

You are now walking 1 hour a day. Terrific!

28- to 40-day Walk/Jog Progression Plan

If you can walk briskly for an hour and your health permits, you can start jogging. Warm up by walking at a moderate pace and gradually increase to a brisk pace. After jogging, walk at a brisk pace and gradually decrease your speed in order to cool down slowly.

If you follow this suggested timetable, you will be jogging continuously for 15 minutes after 28 days. You can progress faster, but if it's more comfortable for you to remain at a given level for a longer period than indicated on the chart, you should do so until it's comfortable for you to progress to the next level.

THE PRITIKIN PROMISE

Day	Level	Routine	Duration	Frequency
1–7	11	Walk briskly Alternate: Jog 1 minute and walk 1 minute, 5 times Cool down	25 minutes 10 minutes 5 minutes	4 times in 7 days (days 1–7)
8–14	12	Walk briskly Alternate: Jog 2 minutes and walk 1 minute, 5 times Cool down	20 minutes 15 minutes 5 minutes	4 times in 7 days (days 8–14)
15–19	13	Walk briskly Alternate: Jog 3½ minutes and walk ½ minute, 5 times Cool down	10 minutes 20 minutes 5 minutes	3 times in 5 days (days 15–19)
20–24	14	Walk briskly Alternate: Jog 4½ minutes and walk ½ minute, 4 times Jog continuously Cool down	15 minutes 20 minutes 10 minutes 5 minutes	3 times in 5 days (days 20–24)
25–29	15	Walk briskly Alternate: Jog 4½ minutes and walk ½ minute, 3 times Jog continuously Cool down	5 minutes 15 minutes 15 minutes 5 minutes	3 times in 5 days (days 25–29)
30–35	16	Walk briskly Alternate: Jog 4½ minutes and walk ½ minute, 2 times Jog continuously Cool down	5 minutes 10 minutes 20 minutes 5 minutes	3 times in 5 days (days 30–35)
36–	17	Walk briskly Jog continuously Cool down	5 minutes 30 minutes 5 minutes	4 times per week (days 36–)

You are now exercising 40 minutes a day. Congratulations!

156

14
CHAPTER

Using the Diet During Pregnancy, Infancy, and Other Special Situations

Although you are probably convinced that the Pritikin Program makes sense for you, I realize that you may have questions about special situations: Is the diet good for infants and growing children? Can vegetarians go on the Pritikin diet? What about maintaining the program while traveling? While backpacking? What if my family won't cooperate? In this section we will deal with all of these questions and more.

THE PRITIKIN DIET FOR CHILDREN

If members of your family, including your children, are thinking about joining you in the 28-day program, you are probably wondering about the suitability of the diet for growing children, whether toddlers, gangling adolescents, or somewhere in between.

Protein Requirements of Children

The adverse effects of eating too much protein and the excessive amounts consumed by most Americans have been discussed on pages 53 to 56. But do children, with their fast rate of growth, do well on a diet (the Pritikin diet) in which protein is restricted to 13 percent?

If you keep in mind that infants fed exclusively on mother's milk (only 6 percent protein) who are in the fastest growth stage of the life cycle are able to *double their birth weight in six months*, it becomes obvious that the Pritikin diet, which contains more than twice the protein present in breast milk, suffices for any growth stage.

The protein mania has misled more than one generation of well-meaning parents who have been anxious to provide the very best nutrition for their children. Be assured your child—whatever his or her age—will have more than enough protein on the Pritikin diet.

You can read more about protein needs and the damage done by excess protein in Chapter 23, pages 454 to 470.

Other Nutritional Needs of Children

For growing children and adolescents, the basic diet plan as outlined in the 28-day calendar will guarantee all their nutritional needs. (A special section on infants' nutritional needs follows.)

However, because they are growing, children and adolescents will require relatively more calories and more of some nutrients, on a body-weight basis, than adults. They can have larger servings of higher-calorie foods such as whole grains and whole-grain bread and pasta; starchier vegetables such as white and sweet potatoes, winter squash, and peas; or hearty bean-based soups or other bean dishes. Don't put young children on a low-calorie version of the Pritikin diet, with lots of salads and thin soups; the low-calorie diet may not be high enough in calories or certain nutrients for a growing child.

To ensure an adequate supply of vitamins and minerals, make sure your children have such green vegetables as broccoli, Brussels sprouts, kale, bok choy, and other leafy greens such as the darker varieties of lettuce and mustard, turnip, and collard greens. Spinach, beet greens, and Swiss chard should be limited because they are high in oxalates, which inhibit the absorption of calcium. Other good choices include carrots, winter squash, sweet potatoes, peas, asparagus, sprouts, cantaloupes, papayas, oranges, bananas, and other year-round or seasonal fruits and vegetables.

In addition to nutritious foods, children need regular exposure to sunlight in order to obtain vitamin D; exposure to outdoor sunlight causes the skin to manufacture this vitamin. Even half an hour per day of facial exposure is adequate.

Sometimes young children do not care for fancy dishes, or for casserole combinations. Often they are most receptive to simply prepared foods—plain baked or mashed potatoes, whole-grain cereals, lightly steamed vegetables, and so on. Many children enjoy a bowl of hot brown rice with cinnamon, skim milk, and a small amount of sliced banana or diced apple. For younger children, try steamed or baked vegetables such as potatoes, carrots, broccoli, cauliflower, or winter squash, cut in large pieces that can be eaten with the fingers. Children usually love thick, hearty soups, with brown rice, barley, split peas, beans, potatoes, or whole-wheat pasta. Children's snacks could include fresh fruit, whole-grain crackers or bagels, air-popped popcorn, or oven-baked corn tortilla chips.

If you are wondering about cholesterol-laden foods and their effect on children, you should be aware that children's arteries start to be blocked by cholesterol deposits in the same way as adults'. The effect will show up first in functions that depend upon the circulation in the smallest arteries, such as those serving the hearing organs. In Wisconsin, where large amounts of cholesterol-rich dairy products are consumed, tests on hearing reveal losses in the higher frequencies (14,000–18,000 cycles per second) even as early as 15 years of age. By age 25, the loss of hearing in this range is substantial.

Buildup of arterial cholesterol plaque in children starts early in life and is cumulative. Do everything you can to obtain your children's cooperation, and give them the benefit of clean arteries and the superior health and functioning possible with an uncompromised circulatory system. Limit their intake of high-cholesterol foods, using the same Pritikin guidelines you will use for yourself.

Nutrition for Infants

How early in life can children begin the Pritikin diet? Infants under 6 months of age should be breast-fed and given no other foods. Starting solid foods too early seems to promote many lifelong allergies. The intestinal tract in early infancy is not ready to accept nourishment other than mother's milk. (Many babies on formula experience stomach upset.) After 6 months of age, cereals, fruits, and vegetables can gradually be introduced into the infant's diet. Usually, babies over 1 year can join the rest of the family on the Pritikin diet.

Make sure your baby tolerates a food well before adding a new one. Avoid giving babies foods containing salt, sugar, or excessive amounts of spices. Read labels, and do not buy commercially processed foods that contain large amounts of these substances or chemical additives. Now is the best time to prevent your child from developing a taste for inferior foods.

You can make your own baby food quite easily using a blender. However, be aware that infants have delicate digestive systems and are sensitive to low levels of bacterial contamination that will not pose a problem for older children or adults. Therefore, cleanliness is mandatory when you're preparing and serving baby food, and it is best to prepare the infant's meal fresh before each feeding. If it is necessary to store baby food, take precautions to ensure that the food is not stored too long or under conditions conducive to the growth of bacteria.

The vitamin D requirements of infants can be met by a brief exposure to the outdoors. Fair-skinned babies will need 15 minutes a day; darker-skinned babies, slightly longer. Most babies have longer outings in their prams. As with older children, they needn't be naked—just exposing your baby's face is sufficient.

THE PRITIKIN DIET DURING PREGNANCY AND LACTATION

Pregnancy

The basic additional dietary requirement during pregnancy is a higher intake of calories. These supplemental calories should come from foods acceptable on the Pritikin diet—largely complex carbohydrates such as grain products, dried beans and peas (legumes), vegetables, and fruits.

During pregnancy there is an increased need for some nutrients such as folic acid and calcium. Pregnant women can meet this need by eating frequent servings of broccoli; Brussels sprouts; kale; collard, mustard, and turnip greens; bok choy; and darker varieties of lettuce. These vegetables should be eaten at least several times a week, preferably every day.

Many pregnant women are concerned with obtaining sufficient protein. If a woman is following the Pritikin diet, the additional calories she consumes while pregnant will provide ample protein for herself and the developing fetus. Moderate amounts of lean meat, fish, and chicken can be included in the diet if desired, but they are not necessary. Vegetarians can obtain adequate protein from grains and legumes.

It is especially important during pregnancy to obtain optimal amounts of all the nutrients. Note, however, that optimal means neither too little nor too much. Pregnant women who are following the Pritikin diet and who are basically healthy will be obtaining all the nutrients they need and should not take vitamin or mineral supplements unless advised to do so by their physician.

Women who are overweight should not attempt to lose weight during pregnancy unless they do so with the approval of and under the supervision of their physician. Otherwise, they could increase their risk of having a low-birth-weight baby, and such babies have lower survival rates.

The most important period of fetal development is the first three months of pregnancy. Often, however, women don't realize they are pregnant until several months have passed.

Therefore it would be best for women to adhere to healthful diets all the time.

Exercise is also important during pregnancy. In addition to the aerobic benefits provided by exercise, it has been found that women who maintain their level of physical fitness while pregnant have faster deliveries with fewer complications. We suggest that pregnant women consult their obstetricians for assistance in selecting an appropriate exercise program.

Nursing Mothers

The Pritikin diet is also excellent for lactating mothers. Once again, the basic additional dietary requirement is extra calories, in this case to maintain the mother's milk production. There is also a somewhat greater need for calcium and folic acid, which can be met by eating the foods mentioned in the discussion above on pregnancy. Nursing mothers on the Pritikin diet will receive adequate amounts of nutrients unless they are on a very-low-calorie version of the diet and are losing weight rapidly.

Although vitamin and mineral supplements are usually not needed by either nursing mothers or their babies when the mother is following a good diet, the advice of a pediatrician should be followed in this matter.

FAMILY COOPERATION

Some families are exemplary in their adherence as a family to the Pritikin diet. Dr. and Mrs. Alan (Jerry) Michels and their many children, ranging in age from teenagers to infants, have been on the program for four years. Young, attractive, and very much involved in work, family, church, and their California community, JoAnne and Jerry Michels opted for the Pritikin lifestyle because they were concerned with prevention (Jerry's father and stepfather had both died of heart disease) and because they weren't feeling as well as they would like. The Pritikin diet is also consistent with guidelines of the Mormon Church, in which the Michels family is active

They introduced the dietary changes to the children gradually in order to minimize balking, though some objections did—and do—exist. When the children were first served dry toast and bread without butter or margarine, says JoAnne, there were complaints until one of the children thought of dunking the bread in their milk and an enthusiastic dunking mania ensued. And since the Pritikin guidelines say sugar is better than fat in a trade-off, jam is sometimes served.

The change in eating style has had side benefits. Main meals, says JoAnne, are not such big deals anymore, because the children fix mini-meals for themselves all through the day. She adds, "Eating this way has cut our food budget by 30 percent."

Their day starts with hot whole-grain cereal, such as rolled oats eaten with cinnamon and bananas, or cold Grape-Nuts, or whole-wheat pancakes. Other grains are eaten at other meals along with lots of steamed vegetables, raw salads, hearty soups, and bread. For snacks, JoAnne favors a hot baked potato, processed in minutes in her microwave oven, or cut-up veggies.

JoAnne and Jerry think it's okay to cheat once in a while —perhaps even advisable—though they are committed to the diet as a permanent way of life for themselves and, hopefully, for their children. "Psychologically, it's not good to think you're on rations, that you're missing something," says JoAnne, in defense of the occasional cheat. But she also says her food tastes have changed and when she occasionally does cheat, it is disappointing. JoAnne says being on the Pritikin diet with her family has restructured their lives, and they are able to devote more time and attention to maintaining physical well-being, as well as to their family life.

Each family situation is unique. Perhaps yours will be another Michels family, but it could also happen that you will have less cooperation from your spouse or offspring.

Take a positive attitude toward your particular situation. If your family members have no interest at all, perhaps in time they will, particularly when they notice the benefits you have derived. Or perhaps they will make minor modifications from time to time, gradually evolving toward a more healthful dietary lifestyle. Every change in the right direction is helpful, and one good change may soon beget another.

INFORMATION FOR VEGETARIANS STARTING THE PRITIKIN DIET

Vegetarians, like parents with growing children, may wonder whether the Pritikin diet can provide them with all the needed nutrients. Lacto-ovo-vegetarians, who eat eggs, cheeses, and other milk products, may worry about their health if they give up egg yolks and high-fat milk products, since they will not be eating the 3½ oz of low-fat meat, poultry, or fish permitted per day on the Pritikin diet. Stricter vegetarians, called vegans, who eat no animal products in any form, wonder how the additional abstinence from the nonfat dairy products and egg whites permitted on the Pritikin diet, but not on theirs, will affect their health. They will now need to pass up foods they often eat in large quantities: nuts, oil-rich vegetables like avocados, and vegetable oils.

Let me assure you that the diet has been carefully, scientifically designed, and that even the strictest vegetarian who goes on the Pritikin diet can meet all nutritional requirements indefinitely, with the single exception of vitamin B_{12}. Vegans can fulfill their vitamin B_{12} requirement with a 1000-mg (microgram) tablet of vitamin B_{12} taken once a month. Lacto-ovo-vegetarians, who use milk products, can obtain all the vitamin B_{12} necessary by drinking ½ glass of milk per day. No other supplements should be necessary, ever.

In adapting the menu plan, if you are a vegetarian, you will find that most of the recipes are suitable as they are. In a few that call for chicken stock, you may substitute vegetable stock. Chicken-stew-type recipes can be made into interesting vegetable stews by replacement of the chicken with potatoes, carrots, squash, or another vegetable you like. In other cases, you may choose to substitute a vegetarian entrée from another day's menu for the entrée made with animal food, or to simply eliminate it without a replacement and, instead, double up on other parts of the meal, such as grain dishes.

PROBLEMS WITH INTESTINAL GAS (FLATULENCE)

Virtually everyone who goes on the Pritikin diet enjoys a burst of new vitality and sense of well-being, but some people do develop an unpleasant problem with intestinal gas. Usually, the problem is of a temporary nature, though it may persist for a few months. Intestinal gas, or flatulence, may be a by-product of the diet resulting from the change in intestinal flora that takes place when you go from a high-fat diet to one high in complex carbohydrates. This change is desirable, because the kind of bacteria that predominate in the intestinal tract of persons on a high-fat diet are associated with a high risk of colon cancer. Nevertheless, if you are one of those who are bothered with persistent flatulence, it can be a real nuisance.

Here are some suggestions for counteracting the problem:

1. Bran, beans, and peas—because they have the highest percentage of indigestibles—are responsible for 95 percent of the flatulence that occurs in susceptible people. Unless you need the bran to keep your bowels regular, you don't require it on the high-complex-carbohydrate Pritikin diet. Experiment with eating beans and peas, and bran if you think you need it, in small amounts; or eliminate them from your diet altogether for a while, and then reintroduce them gradually.

2. Lightly cooked vegetables are sometimes easier to digest initially than raw vegetables. Eat more cooked vegetables and only a few raw vegetables, then gradually switch to more raw vegetables.

3. Overeating can be a factor in flatulence problems, so avoid eating too much food at any one time. People who eat small amounts of food frequently throughout the day seem to have fewer digestive problems than people who eat large meals spaced relatively far apart.

4. Don't eat excessive amounts of vegetables in the cabbage family—broccoli, cabbage, cauliflower, Brussels sprouts

—as they contain sulfa compounds which can contribute to flatulence.

If you do develop a flatulence problem, it should resolve itself fairly quickly. Keep in mind that the temporary discomfort is outweighed many times by the benefits of your new dietary lifestyle.

FOLLOWING THE PRITIKIN DIET AWAY FROM HOME

The ultimate challenge is trying to follow the Pritikin diet if your work and social schedules are such that you must eat out much of the time, or if you are planning an extended trip. Or perhaps you like to go backpacking. The following suggestions should be helpful.

Workday Lunches—Brown-Bagging It

For most people, the meal most frequently eaten away from home is weekday lunch. Taking your lunch with you is the best way to stay on the Pritikin diet, packing leftovers from the previous night's dinner or other suitable food. It's done in the very best circles. Many a captain of industry, male or female, has been an inveterate brown-bagger. Lots of good brown-bag lunch suggestions are given in Chapter 16, pages 207 to 210.

Restaurant Eating

For many, however, lunch is going to be a restaurant meal, whether by necessity or by preference. If so, make a point of finding conveniently located restaurants that serve the most Pritikin-like food or are willing to make minor modifications for you. Many alumni from our Center programs have "trained" restaurateurs to provide them with Pritikin-style breakfasts, lunches, or dinners. Some of these restaurants are posh establishments in Washington, D.C., Manhattan, and other major cities. This approach might work for you.

Restaurants with good salad bars are often your best

choice for lunch. Even some of the fast-food restaurants are beginning to offer salad bars—which may provide a solution in a pinch. Watch out for salads already bathed in oily or creamy dressings. While none of the separate dressings are likely to be Pritikin-OK, you can flavor your salad with vinegar or a wedge of lemon, and sometimes you can find a salsa or other cooked-vegetable combination on the salad bar that looks oil-free and will make a good topping for your raw vegetables.

In restaurants where your food is brought to you, good communication with the person who takes your order is the key to your success in getting what you want. You may think you've been understood, only to find when your order arrives that the breast-of-turkey sandwich on sourdough bread that was supposed to be dry has both butter and mayonnaise on it. Or the fish that was to be broiled dry is glistening with butter, and the baked potato accompanying it has been doused with sour cream. So when you order, ask to have your order repeated to you, and explain that your special requests are of the utmost importance because you are on a special diet. If you are courteous but firm, you are likely to win these minor skirmishes.

In ordering restaurant dishes with poultry, fish, or other animal foods, it's important to keep in mind your 3½-oz-per-day limit for such foods. Take home a doggie bag with your leftovers, or split a large serving with a dining partner. If he or she is a Pritikin-type eater too, you can sometimes ask for one order of the fish or meat dish, and then order extra butter-free vegetables, plain mixed green salads, or baked potatoes to round out the meal.

Restaurants serving Chinese or Italian foods are often good choices. In Chinese restaurants, you can order steamed vegetables with diced breast of chicken and a couple of mounds of plain white rice. The Chinese, unfortunately, don't use brown rice, and the fried rice, which looks deceptively like brown rice, is merely white rice that has been fried and colored by soy sauce.

Since Chinese food is prepared to order, you should be able to get a good meal by asking that the vegetables and chicken be cooked in plain chicken broth or water, not cooked in oil. Specify that you don't want MSG (monosodium glutamate), a sodium flavoring agent that acts like salt and also causes allergic problems in some people. Nor do you want salt, soy sauce, or sugar to be used, but that you like lots of fresh ginger and garlic. You can add a *little* soy sauce when the dish arrives, if necessary, using the soy-sauce shaker at the table.

If communication with a barely bilingual waiter is a problem, you can whip out a reproduction of the instructions that appear on pages 169 to 174 for ordering Pritikin-style vegetables in six different languages, including Chinese.

Italian restaurants may offer spaghetti served with a tasty marinara sauce, and in some instances you may be able to order pizza with tomato sauce, bell pepper, onions, and other vegetables, but made without cheese, fatty sausage or meat balls, or salty anchovies.

Some restaurants in larger cities are now offering Pritikin-style meals and are advertising it. If you know of such a restaurant in your vicinity, you're in luck. But in any case, there's no need to fall off the Pritikin wagon if you are eating out.

Traveling on the Pritikin Diet

Travelers are faced with a variety of problems. They eat in airplanes, in motel rooms, and in restaurants, and sometimes they buy food in a market anywhere in the world to be eaten picnic style.

In American supermarkets or in exotic markets, you can often assemble in a single trip a few items that will last without refrigeration for one or more days and provide at least part of the menu for several meals. If you can take food with you, select assorted fruits, tomatoes, cucumbers, and even cabbage; the best bread or crackers you can find; and canned vegetable juices, when available, for several fine, impromptu mini-meals.

When traveling by car, packing some edibles in a Styrofoam picnic basket or icebox enables you to dine in style. Air travel, however, can be more inhibiting. When I travel by air, I order a special meal when I buy my ticket, but I also take along a loaf of my whole-wheat bread, several boxes of whole-grain rice crackers, and some fruit, including with special meals. Others, sad to say, tend to botch things up horrendously. However, when making your reservation, it's worth taking the time to place an advance order with the

---

**How to Order Your
Pritikin-Spanish Meal**
(*show this to your waiter*)

**SIN ACEITE, SIN SAL, Y SIN
AZÚCAR. ESPECIALMENTE SIN
"MSG." VEGETALES VARIADOS
AL VAPOR, POR FAVOR.
GRACIAS.**

No oil, no salt, no sugar. Especially
no MSG. Assorted steamed
vegetables, please.

Thank you.

---

bananas. When my meals in-flight turn out to be disappointing, as happens occasionally, I feast instead on banana sandwiches made from my food cache. Some airlines do well with special meals. Others, sad to say, tend to botch things up horrendously. However, when making your reservation, it's worth taking the time to place an advance order with the

---

How to Order Your
Pritikin-French Meal
(*show this to your waiter*)

**POINT D'HUILE, POINT DE SEL,
POINT DE SUCRE. SURTOUT
POINT DE MONOSODIUM-
GLUTAMATE. LÉGUMES
VARIÉS CUITES À LA VAPEUR,
S'IL VOUS PLAIT. MERCI
BEAUCOUP.**

No oil, no salt, no sugar. Especially
no MSG. Assorted steamed
vegetables, please.

Thank you.

---

airline commissary for a Pritikin-style meal. Ask for unbuttered vegetables, fish or chicken broiled or poached without oil or fat, and a boiled or baked potato, plain, with fresh

---

How to Order Your Pritikin-Chinese Meal
(show this to your waiter)

素菜什錦
請勿放油塩糖
尤其是味精
祇要清蒸
謝謝

No oil, no salt, no sugar. Especially no MSG. Assorted steamed vegetables, please.

Thank you.

171

fruit for dessert. You're gambling, but you may hit the jackpot.

Some of the foodstuffs that campers and backpackers use

How to Order Your
Pritikin-Italian Meal
(*show this to your waiter*)

SENZA OLIO, SENZA SALE,
SENZA ZUCCHERO.
SPECIALMENTE SENZA "MSG."
VERDURA MISTA A VAPORE,
PER FAVORE. GRAZIE.

No oil, no salt, no sugar. Especially
no MSG. Assorted steamed
vegetables, please.

Thank you.

(See the next section) may also be handy to carry in your suitcase when traveling. And when you're eating in foreign restaurants, the foreign-language instructions for Pritikin-

How to Order Your
Pritikin-German Meal
(*show this to your waiter*)

KEIN ÖL, SALZ, ODER ZUCKER.
BESONDERS KEIN GLUTAMAT.
EINE AUSWAHL DER
GEDÜNSTETEN GEMÜSE,
BITTE. DANKE.

No oil, no salt, no sugar. Especially
no MSG. Assorted steamed
vegetables, please.

Thank you.

style steamed vegetables may prove helpful. I suggest you photocopy the pages, then clip the sections apart and tuck them in your wallet for use at home and abroad.

How to Order Your
Pritikin-Israeli Meal
(*show this to your waiter*)

בלי שמן, בלי מלח, בלי
סוכר, בלי מ.ס.ג'. מיבחר
ירקות מבושלים. בבקשה.

תודה רבה.

No oil, no salt, no sugar. Especially
no MSG. Assorted steamed
vegetables, please.

Thank you.

Backpacking on the Pritikin Diet

Backpackers who follow the Pritikin diet report that they carry uncooked or lightly toasted rolled oats (both are edible without further processing), whole-wheat pita bread, toasted corn tortillas, and freeze-dried foods, such as bananas, apples, string beans, and carrots. Some recipes that are handy for backpackers, providing concentrated calories and nutrients, are *Granola* (page 353), *Garbanzo "Nuts"* (page 399), and *Camper's Chile* (page 370), which can be cooked on the trail in minutes to provide a hearty meal.

Entertaining and Being a Guest on the Pritikin Diet

By all means accept invitations to dine at people's homes and invite them to yours while you're on the Pritikin diet—your social life needn't take a backseat because of your new lifestyle. When you are invited out and think your host or hostess may be amenable to a few simple requests (e.g., not dressing your salad, setting aside a portion of the vegetable dish for you before adding the sauce, and so on), don't be shy about asking. It's common these days for people to have dietary restrictions, and you won't be regarded as an oddball. If you are not in a position to make special requests, eat a mini-meal before venturing out, as we suggested earlier. You are less susceptible to food seduction when you are not hungry and will then be able to choose small portions from the foods offered that are closest to Pritikin requirements. Double up on them if you wish to make up for bypassing taboo foods.

When it's your turn to entertain, use some of the menus and recipes on the 28-day calendar. Suggestions for entertaining with these menus appear on pages 214 to 215. You'll find suitable menus for dinners, lunches, and brunches for either sit-down or buffet service. When using the menus, you needn't apologize or explain to your guests; they'll enjoy the dishes thoroughly, though you may feel that for your guests you need to allow a larger serving per portion of the chicken, turkey, or fish entrées than is allotted by Pritikin standards. On the other hand, your guests may enjoy a *bona fide* Pritikin meal. They may, in fact, be so happy with it that they'll want to prepare one for you in return!

Whenever you dine out—whether at a restaurant, at a friend's home, or elsewhere—you can indeed stick to the Pritikin diet, if you have

1. the motivation;
2. enough forethought to anticipate the situation you will face;
3. a repertoire of solutions for varying situations; and
4. the ability to be politely but firmly assertive in dealing with the people who will be preparing, serving, or selling you food.

Hanging in, while dining out, can be satisfying.

SPECIAL ITEMS

This is the time to take stock of your kitchen equipment and
lay in a supply of basic foodstuffs you'll be using on the
program, so that once you begin you won't find yourself
without essential cookware or ingredients.

It would also be advantageous to spend a few hours making special items called for in some of the recipes (bread
crumbs made from a good whole-wheat bread, defatted
chicken stock, and the like) and to store them in your refrigerator or freezer ready for instant use.

PRITIKIN-STYLE COOKING EQUIPMENT YOU'LL NEED

Unless you are a beginning cook, you will probably have
most of the items you'll require, such as good knives and a
chopping board, stainless-steel skillets and pots of various
sizes equipped with good-fitting lids, a colander, and oven
casseroles with covers. Some of the recipes call for the use
of an electric blender, and many people enjoy using a food
processor, especially for cutting up large quantities of vege-

tables. If you don't have either, the blender would be the more important acquisition. Crushing garlic in a garlic press is faster than mincing with a knife, so you may want one if you don't have one now. A hot-air corn popper is a good investment, too, for making that fun-to-eat low-calorie snack.

For Pritikin-style cooking, you'll also require nonstick baking pans and a nonstick skillet or crêpe pan so you won't have to use oil. Another must is a collapsible stainless-steel steamer basket that fits into a saucepan or large pot, for steaming vegetables.

If you like a particular recipe and it freezes well, you may want to double or triple it for freezing or for lunches. For such freezer and refrigerator storage you'll need a good supply of plastic containers in various sizes with tight-fitting lids. Heavy aluminum-foil disposable baking dishes in which you can store, freeze, and reheat will also prove useful, as will heavy seal-top plastic bags, which are also great space savers in the refrigerator or freezer, since they conform to the shape of the food placed in them.

SPECIAL INGREDIENTS AND FOODS FOR PRITIKIN-STYLE COOKING AND EATING

Most of the foods you'll shop for are familiar items, especially if you have been conscious of nutrition in the past and have tried to use whole foods rather than refined foods. In that case, you'll know where to find whole-grain products, such as breads and crackers, cereals, and pasta, and whole grains such as brown rice or cracked wheat. If most of this is new to you, allow yourself a little extra time for your first "Pritikin" shopping trip. If you don't find what you need on the regular supermarket shelves or in the supermarket health-food section, by all means ask the store manager for these items, or shop in health- and natural-food stores. On the Pritikin diet you'll have to take the additional precaution of making sure that the whole-grain products you select—especially breads, crackers, and pasta—are free of butter or oil of any kind, or egg yolks. Pritikin bread is in many markets now, either in the regular bread section or in the freezer. If you can't find it or another good-quality whole-grain bread without added oils or other fats, select products in which oil or fat is the last or almost-last item in the list of ingredients, since ingredients are given by weight in descending order. Better yet, calculate the percentage of fat in the product, as shown in the examples on page 181. Except for the allowed 3½–4 oz per day of poultry, fish, or lean meat (or soybean-product substitute), the upper limit for acceptable fat content for any food on the Pritikin diet is 15 percent of the total calories of that food.

But even for health buffs now converted to the Pritikin diet and familiar with all kinds of whole-grain products—including interesting specialty breads, like pita bread, sprouted-wheat bread, chapatis, and corn tortillas—there may be some unfamiliar foods or ingredients used in the recipes, especially among the dairy foods. Sapsago cheese is one. Though not essential to any recipe, it contributes a cheesy flavor when grated into casseroles or other dishes.

Other dairy products may include foods you have been using, such as milk, buttermilk, cottage cheese, yogurt, and canned evaporated milk, but the Pritikin diet permits *only* the use of nonfat or skim-milk versions of these foods. The terms are more or less synonymous, but skim-milk products may be slightly higher in fat content, up to 1 percent by weight. The dairy foods you consume should be nonfat or under 1 percent by weight. Products that are as high as 2 percent fat by weight, like low-fat cottage cheese, really may be almost 30 percent fat by calories—twice the fat content permitted on the Pritikin diet. Because of the high water content of milk and other dairy products, fat content by weight can appear to be low, but this is deceptive.

You should be able to find most of the dairy products you'll need with acceptably low fat content. If you can't find a suitable yogurt, it's easy enough to make your own; see page 409. In different parts of the country, skim-milk cottage cheese appears in various guises—sometimes as a dry-curd product, other times in a pressed brick, and still other times in a form that resembles regular or low-fat cottage cheese. If you can't find anything but low-fat cottage cheese, put it in a strainer and rinse it under cold running water until the rinse water runs clear. Much of the creaming mixture should wash off, reducing the fat content of the product.

Acceptable buttermilk is often available, but if you can't find a product low enough in fat content, simply strain off the visible fat particles—though you will not be able to remove the larger quantity that has been homogenized. (We use the term "skimmed buttermilk" to refer to buttermilk that has had its fat content reduced this way.) For some uses, such as baking, you can substitute nonfat milk that has been soured with lemon juice (½ lemon per cup milk) for skimmed buttermilk, with fair to good results.

In some of our recipes for salad dressings, you will notice that pectin appears as an ingredient. We like the way it gives body to the dressings and makes the greens glisten. You may be familiar with pectin, which derives from fruit and is used as a thickener in the making of jams and jellies. Apples are particularly rich in pectin, and there is even some indication that eating several apples a day may help in lowering blood cholesterol levels. You'll find pectin in most supermarkets near the jams and jellies.

Other thickeners used in sauces and other recipes are arrowroot and cornstarch. You may not be familiar with arrowroot as a thickener. While it does not reheat as well as cornstarch, in some applications, such as certain sauces, it is more desirable because of the clarity it provides. You'll find arrowroot in the spice section where you shop.

HOW TO CALCULATE FAT CONTENT OF ANY PRODUCT

Total fat intake on your diet should not exceed 10 percent of total calories. You can achieve this by limiting intake of animal foods, such as poultry, fish, or lean meat, to 1½ lb per week (approximately 3½ oz per day), and not eating any other foods in which fat content is greater than 15 percent of total calories. A large part of your diet—vegetables, fruits, and grains—is substantially below 10 percent fat in calories and helps to keep the average down to acceptable levels.

You determine the fat content of a product this way: if the

fat content per serving is given in grams and the calories per serving are also given, simply multiply the number of grams of fat by 9 (the approximate number of calories in a gram of fat), then divide that figure by the number of calories per serving. Move the decimal point two places to the right and you have the percentage of calories from fat for that product. The same method would be used if grams of fat are given per 100 grams, rather than per serving. Here are some examples:

Knudsen's buttermilk	Deming's canned salmon
120 calories per cup serving	170 calories per ½ cup serving
4 g fat per cup serving	9 g fat per ½ cup serving
4 × 9 = 36 calories fat (approx.)	9 × 9 = 81 calories fat (approx.)
$^{36}/_{120}$ = .30 = 30% fat (approx.)	$^{81}/_{170}$ = .48 = 48% fat (approx.)

Besides being aware of the fat content in the foods you buy, you should also be on the lookout for sodium, often present in commercial products like bouillon cubes and seasoning combinations under names you may not recognize as sources of salt: monosodium glutamate, hydrolyzed yeast, sea salt, or garlic and onion salt. Our bodies need a little sodium, but excessive amounts are bad for everyone, especially if you have a tendency to hypertension. The healthy adult requires little more sodium than an infant—approximately 58 mg per day. You receive more than enough sodium from natural foods and the water you drink. In our recipes, when a slight saltiness seems important even with the most imaginative seasoning, we have specified a little soy sauce, which is also a sodium source. A teaspoon of soy sauce contains 440 mg of sodium, as compared with about 2200 mg for a teaspoon of salt. (A teaspoon of salt weighs about 5 gm and is approximately 40 percent sodium.) It is better still to use the salt-reduced milder soy sauce available at most supermarkets. Condiments such as capers and mustard with high salt content, and other high-salt-content foods, should be restricted too; use salt-reduced brands when available; and if your doctor has ordered you to limit your sodium intake, it would be wise to choose canned vegetable products, such as tomato sauce and juice, whole tomatoes, and so on, that are available without added sodium. Four gm of salt, or about 1600 mg of sodium, should be the maximum daily intake for healthy people, and those with hypertension should strive for even lower levels.

In the Pritikin diet scale of priorities, the worst offenders are cholesterol in excess of 100 mg per day, and fat in excess of 10 percent of total calories. Cholesterol and fat are therefore the substances you'll be tracking most closely on a daily basis. Moderate salt intake is less dangerous for healthy people, although too much salt will cause the tissues to hold a great deal of excess water, which burdens the cardiovascular system. For persons with elevated blood pressure, however, fat *and* salt must be avoided. We recommend they use salt-free canned goods and omit soy sauce in the Pritikin recipes.

Sugar is less detrimental to your health than fat and cholesterol, but this should not be interpreted as a license to go out and eat sweets every day. Cutting down on refined sugars is high on the list of Pritikin priorities. None of our recipes use refined sugar in any form, including brown or raw sugar, nor do they use molasses, honey, or fructose. Our preferred sweeteners are either apple juice or grape juice. Be aware, however, that these are sugars too. As a result, we do not recommend fruit juice as a beverage and use it only as a recipe sweetener. Dried fruits, which are especially high in natural sugars, are also limited, and never eaten as a snack. In addition, *read labels* when you shop. Many canned vegetables, such as corn, peas, tomatoes, and beets, have a great deal of added sugar, which may be described on the label as "dextrose" or "corn sweeteners." Avoid them.

LAYING IN A FOOD SUPPLY FOR THE 28-DAY DIET

If you have room to store a good supply of nonperishables such as grains, dried beans, spices, canned goods, and freezer items, you'll be that much ahead. A complete *Shopping List* for these foods appears on pages 188 to 190.

If you can, keep a good stock of Pritikin-OK frozen foods useful for meals and snacks—corn on the cob, lima beans, vegetable combinations without sauces, and fruits without sugar. It would also be convenient to have on hand frozen fish and poultry to use with some of the recipes, including items like packaged chicken breasts, both with and without the bone, and turkey breast slices, now available in many supermarkets. When you select them, choose packages containing small breasts or slices, so that you are able to keep cholesterol intake per serving within bounds. (Chicken breast halves, unskinned, should weigh no more than 7–8 oz each; boned chicken breast halves, unskinned, should weigh about 5 oz each. The edible chicken on such market purchases will be about 4 oz per half breast.)

Since you are starting a new kind of cooking which derives much food flavor from the judicious use of herbs and spices, now is a good time to replenish your spice supply with fresh spices to replace those that have been in your cupboard for ages. Old spices lose their potency. It's a good idea to label your new spice purchases with the date of purchase.

Perishables, such as dairy foods, fish and poultry (though these can be frozen), fresh fruits, and vegetables have to be purchased more frequently, of course. Most of the produce items called for in the recipes and menus are probably familiar to you; but if not, we'd like to acquaint you with just a few of our favorites that you may not now be using. These include romaine lettuce, bok choy, cilantro, and chiles. Bok choy and romaine lettuce are outstanding greens for their nutritional value, as well as their palatability, and deserve a prominent place in your diet alongside other healthful greens such as collards, kale, turnip greens, and mustard greens. We prefer to use spinach or Swiss chard sparingly because of their high oxalic acid content, which interferes with mineral absorption.

Romaine lettuce. Head lettuces, like iceberg lettuce, are sometimes especially desirable because of their crisp texture and have for this reason been specified in one or two of our recipes, but in general, the superior nutritional qualities of romaine and other dark green lettuces, as well as their fine flavor, make them better choices for the salad bowl. In addition, romaine lettuce is excellent cooked and is used extensively in this manner in French and other European cookery. Instead of throwing away the outer leaves of romaine lettuce not suitable for your salad, why not steam some of them? See our recipe for *Romaine Succotash* (pages 258 to 259).

Bok choy, a type of Chinese cabbage, may already be somewhat familiar to you as an ingredient in Oriental dishes. Try it as a vegetable dish; you'll be delighted with its light, delicate flavor and crisp texture. See our recipes on page 305. You can also use the hearts of bok choy raw in salads, or blanched, as the Chinese do. Bok choy may be found in the market under other names, such as Chinese chard or Chinese mustard. (Don't confuse it with another Chinese cabbage called pe-tsai, or celery cabbage. Ask your grocer to show you which is which.)

Cilantro, also called coriander and Chinese or Mexican parsley, is a favorite herb in the cuisine of Latin American and Asian peoples. Although it is a member of the parsley family, its flavor is very unlike that of the parsley with which we are familiar. Cilantro is used in several of our ethnic recipes, where it is a valued ingredient both for its distinctive flavor and for its nutritional qualities. The seed of the plant (coriander seed) is also an important spice.

Chiles (also spelled chili, chilli, or chillie!). These peppers are cousins of the ordinary bell pepper, and while some are mild, other varieties range from hot to inferno! For our purposes, two of the more readily available chiles suffice. For recipes in which a mild chile flavor is desired, we call for "green chile"—known in the complicated chile nomenclature (there are endless varieties) as the California or Anaheim green chile. It is available in many markets in either fresh or dried form, as well as in cans. Fresh green chiles are bright shiny green; they vary from 5 to 8 in in length and about 1½ to 2 in in diameter at the top, tapering to a point. In dried form, they are a dark red. When fresh chiles are canned, they turn soft and mossy green in color. To use the whole canned chiles, slit open the side of each chile and remove the seeds and pith, which are *very* hot. Then use as is, or dice. Or, buy the ready-diced canned green chiles. While Mexican cooks peel fresh green chiles before using them, we have not found it necessary to do so for our recipes.

When a hot chile flavor is desired, we have specified the little jalapeño chile—darker green than the California green chile and only about 2½ in long and about 1 in in diameter at the stem end. Many markets carry the fresh form, but if they are not available where you live, use the canned or bottled jalapeños, sometimes labeled "hot peppers" with the word "jalapeño" underneath.

You need to take some precautions in working with the chiles, especially the hot ones. The juice, seeds, membranes, and stems are the hottest parts and should be removed. Mince fine, since a little goes a long way. But most important, to avoid any possibility of skin irritation, don't touch any part of your face, and especially your eyes, until you have washed your hands well after working with chiles.

Trying vegetables, and fruits, too, that you have not used in the past is part of the adventure of your new diet. You can do your gastronomic traveling right at home on the 28-day diet, enjoying wonderful-tasting and unusual fruits— new varieties of melons, delicious little kiwis, papayas, the new seedless red grapes, persimmons, or fresh figs. The possibilities for your evening fruit cup are endless.

ADVANCE FOOD PREPARATIONS

Most Pritikin cooks like to prepare a few staple ingredients or foods ahead of time. You may find these suggestions helpful.

Salad Dressings. Although a few commercial salad dressings may be acceptable, most contain oil, sugar, and lots of salt and chemical additives. Although many people are content to eat a large salad plain with just a wedge of lemon or a sprinkling of good vinegar, some of us prefer a dressing on our salads. The dairy free salad dressings will keep in the refrigerator for at least 4 weeks. See the recipes starting on page 402.

Chicken and Vegetable Stock. Many recipes call for chicken or vegetable stock. In most cases, vegetable stock will do as well, but sometimes chicken stock is really preferable. It's easy to make your own. Fill a stockpot with chicken backs and necks and a few vegetables (onion, carrot, celery tops and stalks, etc.), bay leaf, parsley, and garlic; cover with water; and boil gently for 1 to 2 hours. If you bone your own chicken breasts, be sure to save the bones for the stockpot. Strain and place the stock in the refrigerator overnight. Remove the congealed fat carefully with a slotted spoon; then strain through cheesecloth or Handi Wipes. Pour 1-cup portions into heavy plastic seal-top bags for freezing, or freeze in ice-cube trays for smaller stock portions.

You can store vegetable stock in the same way, using either liquid left over from steaming vegetables or a stock you prepare from scratch by cooking a variety of vegetables from the vegetable drawer of your refrigerator with lots of garlic and a bay leaf in a big pot of water. Use celery stalks; large onions, quartered; leeks, cut in half; a few carrots; and well-washed vegetable scraps (bell pepper tops, onion skins, celery tops, etc.). Broccoli, cauliflower, green beans, mushrooms, zucchini, green onions, and cilantro are also good candidates for the stockpot. This is a good way to use up vegetables that are just slightly past their prime.

Bread Crumbs. You will need fine bread crumbs for making piecrusts or for breading. Use whole-grain wheat bread without oil, and grind in an electric blender or food processor. You can store the crumbs in jars with tight covers or in heavy plastic seal-top bags in the freezer for months.

Yogurt. Yogurt is used in a number of the Pritikin recipes and is also convenient to have on hand for combining with fresh or frozen fruit for snacks and desserts. If nonfat yogurt, or yogurt with fat content not exceeding 1 percent fat by weight, is not available in your area, consider making your own with our easy recipe (page 409).

Mock Sour Cream. This staple in Pritikin cookery, made in a blender from skim-milk cottage cheese and skim milk or skimmed buttermilk, and used like sour cream, is another item Pritikin dieters like to have on hand. It keeps well refrigerated for several days or can be frozen. The recipe appears on page 408.

Sapsago Cheese. A few recipes, such as Pritikin pizza (page 293), call for grated Sapsago cheese, and many people like to sprinkle the grated cheese over spaghetti or tacos. To have it refrigerator-ready for such uses, grind small chunks of the cheese in a blender until they are well pulverized and powdery-fine, then store in a small covered jar or in a heavy plastic seal-top bag in the refrigerator.

Other Useful Advance Food Preparations. In our food-development kitchen, we have found that certain procedures speed recipe work. Fresh *garlic cloves* are peeled and stored in the refrigerator in a heavy-duty plastic seal-top bag, ready for use. Fresh unpeeled *ginger root* is cut into pieces and stored in a plastic bag in the freezer ready for use when grated fresh ginger is required. *Onions* too, when frozen, keep their flavor, grate easily, and are less apt to make you "tearful." We cut a peeled onion in half and store it in a plastic bag in the freezer. *Parsley* is washed, drained, and minced fine or cut into small sprigs and placed in a small aluminum-foil pan, uncovered, in the refrigerator, and permitted to air-dry. When sufficiently dry, it is transferred to a covered jar and placed on our spice shelf, or used right from the refrigerator pan. When we find *fresh dill* or other hard-to-find fresh herbs in the market, we buy a bunch, clean and trim it, and store it in the freezer in a seal-top plastic bag. It's great to be able to snip a bit when needed.

Now that you're ready, here's your shopping list.

28-Day Pritikin Diet Shopping List of Nonperishable Items

(includes recipe ingredients and daily diet needs)

GRAINS AND GRAIN PRODUCTS

Cracked-wheat cereal

Rolled oats, regular

Whole-wheat pasta, without egg yolk or soy flour (spaghetti; linguine; elbow macaroni; spiral and flat noodles)

Corn noodles (wheat-free corn pasta)

Cornmeal, yellow, whole- or coarse-grained

Brown rice, long-grain (short-grain if preferred)

Barley, whole

Bulgur wheat, medium- or coarse-grained

Buckwheat, whole groats

Bran, unprocessed miller's

Millet, hulled

Couscous, parboiled dry

Wild rice

Four-grain cereal (wheat, oats, rye, and barley)

Corn for popping

Flour, wheat (whole-wheat pastry; whole-wheat regular)

Flour, potato

Crackers* (whole-grain rye, wheat, or rice, without added oil, fats, or sugars)

Other whole-grain breakfast cereals that are acceptable, for cooking or to be eaten as dry cereals, if desired

LEGUMES

Beans, dried (pinto; red; black; navy; garbanzo; kidney)

Lentils, dried

Split peas, yellow

CANNED GOODS

Evaporated skim milk

Tomato products* (juice and V-8; sauce; paste; whole and Italian plum; diced in juice; and crushed in puree)

Beans, without sugar or additives, if substitute for home-cooked dried beans is desired (See list under "legumes")

Chiles, green (whole, diced, and salsa)

Pimientos, whole and sliced

Artichoke hearts, water-packed

Beets, sliced, in water

Water chestnuts

Pumpkin

Fish, shellfish (tuna, water-packed; pink salmon; whole clams)

Pineapple, unsweetened, canned in own juices (crushed; chunks; and small-size juice)

Applesauce, unsweetened

Apricots, whole, water- or juice-packed

188

Peaches, whole, water- or juice-packed; baby-food peaches

MISCELLANEOUS STAPLES

Nonfat dry milk (powdered)
Cornstarch
Arrowroot
Active dry yeast
Baking powder (choose brand free of aluminum compounds)
Baking soda
Carob powder, unsweetened
Unflavored gelatin
Pectin (for making some salad dressings and cooked fruit recipes)
Tapioca, small pearl, quick-cooking
Agar (for making nonfat yogurt)
Matzo meal

FREEZER FOODS

Fruit-juice concentrates (apple, orange, pineapple), unsweetened
Fruits, unsweetened (cherries; blueberries, cranberries, and other berries; other fruits)
Vegetables, plain (corn kernels and corn-on-the-cob; green beans, French-cut and regular cut; lima beans; asparagus spears; peas; peas and carrots; any other desired)
Breads, acceptable (whole-wheat, rye, or sourdough; specialty breads such as corn tortillas, whole-wheat tortillas or chapatis, Bible bread, sprouted-grain bread, whole-wheat pita bread, whole-wheat English muffins, etc.)
Chicken (breast halves; boneless breast halves; and bones, necks, and backs for making chicken stock)
Turkey breast (whole and packaged slices)
Beef, very lean, ground (for *Bolognese Sauce*, if desired)
Fish and shellfish (salmon steaks, halibut, sole, bass, cod, red snapper, or other lean firm-fleshed white fish; and lobster chunks)

FLAVORINGS AND CONDIMENTS

White grape juice, bottled
Vinegars (rice, cider, red wine, tarragon, herb-flavored wine vinegars)
Soy sauce* or tamari
Mustards* (French's prepared; Dijon)
Capers
Pepperoncini (peppers in wine vinegar)
Sapsago cheese
Tabasco (hot pepper sauce)
Hot sauce
Picante sauce
Angostura bitters (for flavoring mineral-water beverages)
Postum (for some dessert recipes)
Date sugar (health-store item; for some dessert recipes)
Flavor extracts (pure vanilla, almond, lemon, orange, banana)
Wines, dry, white and red, for cooking (sherry, Burgundy,

Chablis, etc.); rum and
brandy, for use in some
desserts

DRIED FRUITS, HERBS, AND SPICES

Fruits for cooking and baking—
(currants, raisins, and dates)
Allspice, ground and whole
Anise, ground and seed
Basil leaves
Bay leaves
Caraway seeds
Cardamom, ground
Cayenne pepper
Celery seed, ground and whole
Chile powder, mild and regular
Chile con carne seasoning
Chives, freeze-dried
Cinnamon, ground (and sticks,
if desired)
Cloves, ground and whole
Coriander, ground
Cumin, ground
Curry powder
Dill seed
Dillweed
Fennel seeds, ground and
whole

Garam masala (Indian spice)
Garlic powder; dried minced
garlic
Ginger, ground
Italian seasoning
Marjoram leaves
Mexican seasoning (Schilling's)
Mint leaves
Mustard, dry; Chinese-style hot
mustard
Mustard seeds, black
Nutmeg, ground
Onion powder; dried minced
onions
Oregano leaves
Paprika
Pickling spices
Poppyseed
Pumpkin-pie spice
Poultry seasoning
Red pepper, hot dried crushed
Rosemary
Saffron
Sage, ground and leaf
Savory
Sesame seeds
Tarragon leaves
Thyme, ground and leaf
Turmeric

---

* Low-sodium brands are available and are desirable for those need-
ing to limit sodium intake as much as possible.

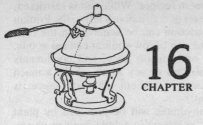

16
CHAPTER

How to Use the
Menu Plans and Recipes,
with Suggestions
for the 28-Day Diet

In this chapter, you'll find all the information you need to use the 28-day program of menus and recipes in Part IV (the 28 dinner menus and recipe selections for breakfast, lunch, and snacks). Also provided in this chapter are some general suggestions for mealtime planning, a sample 3-day menu plan, and specific information about the cooking methods used in the recipes.

NUTRITIONAL GUIDELINES AND DIET PLANNING

Our meal plans ensure a nutritionally adequate diet while safeguarding against excesses of fat and cholesterol. Protein intake is also deliberately restricted to safe levels. Carbohydrates form the mainstay of the diet (about 80 percent of total calories), and those favored are unrefined grains and other high-complex-carbohydrate foods, providing maximum fiber and other nutritional benefits. Simple carbohydrates are kept to a bare minimum and are found in the diet mostly in the form of whole fruit or in small amounts of fruit juice used as a sweetener in recipes. While salt is restricted, fine adjustment of the level of restriction is left to the Pritikin dieter. Further salt restriction can be achieved in the recipes, for example, by the use of low-sodium canned goods, such as tomato sauce and tomato juice, and condiments such as salt-reduced mustard or soy sauce. (Salt, a much more concentrated source of sodium than soy sauce, is never a recipe ingredient.)

Your complex carbohydrates will be provided by plant foods unprocessed or "as grown"—whole-grain products, such as pasta; tubers (like potatoes or sweet potatoes); vegetables; legumes (beans and peas); and fruits. We have purposely excluded high-fat plant foods, such as nuts and seeds (except for small seeds, used in small amounts, whole or ground, as seasoning, such as sesame, cumin, fennel, and so on); olives; avocados; and expressed oils, such as corn oil or soy oil or margarine made from plant oils.

You could be very healthy on a strict vegetarian diet if you took care to include as well minute amounts of some unusual plant foods, such as miso or tempeh—fermented foods used in Asian cultures—to provide you with the necessary vitamin B_{12}. Strict vegetarians can also take vitamin B_{12} supplements made especially for them from plant sources. But animal foods, selected carefully and eaten in prudent amounts, can be a good source of nutrients as well. The problem occurs, as we have stressed, when you eat the wrong kind of animal products, or *too much* of the right kind. Some animal foods, such as egg yolks, organ meats, and fatty meats, are too high in cholesterol or fat and have no place on your diet. Low-fat, low-cholesterol animal foods, however, such as light meat of chicken or turkey, most fish (except certain fatty varieties), and lean meat are safe to eat in limited amounts, but total intake should not exceed about 24 oz per week (or 3½ oz per day, on an average). The body can safely process that amount because the cholesterol contained in 3½ oz of low-cholesterol animal food sources is just about the amount that the body eliminates each day in the feces.

Whole dairy foods are excessively high in fat and cholesterol. Removing the fat fraction in the skimming process also removes most of the cholesterol associated with the fat.

But the high protein content remains the same and could be a problem if you eat too much of nonfat dairy products.

Recommended Intake of High-Protein Foods

High-protein foods, like skim milk and skim-milk products and beans and peas (legumes), can bring your total protein intake to unsafe levels, even when animal muscle foods (fish, fowl, shellfish, and meat) are limited. To avoid this, follow these guidelines:

Beans and Peas

Restrict intake to 1 meal per day on days when you are not eating fish, fowl, shellfish, and meat; on other days, avoid them.

Dairy Foods

Restrict intake to 1 glass (8 oz) of skim milk or equivalent in other skim-milk products on days when you are eating fish, fowl, shellfish, and meat; on other days, you may increase your intake to 2 glasses (16 oz) of skim milk or equivalents in other skim-milk products.

Because protein intake can build up surprisingly quickly when dairy foods and legumes are consumed together with even limited amounts of animal muscle foods, it might also be wise to limit your total intake of fish, fowl, shellfish, and meat to about 16 oz per week, even though 24 oz per week is permitted in most cases. You can control this by eating no meat, fish, or poultry for 3 days each week.

You will see how to make dietary exchanges of skim milk and various skim-milk products in the Pritikin Guidelines chart, following, and in the Table of Foods to Use and to Avoid (pages 196 to 199).*

Both these charts will help you understand the general principles underlying the Pritikin diet. While the 28 dinner

---

* If you would like a brochure with the rules and the *Table of Foods to Use and to Avoid,* please write to me at P.O. Box 5335, Santa Barbara, CA 93108.

menus will give you detailed suggestions for your evening meals, you will often need to make independent choices for other meals and snacks. Most people follow our recommended breakfasts of a whole-grain cereal and fruit, whole-grain bread or toast, and a little skim milk, a meal high in complex carbohydrate and safely within protein limits. At lunchtime and snacktime you will likely find choices more difficult at first. Watch out for those high-protein dishes. Too much skim-milk cheese, too many bean dishes, too much yogurt—all can be poor choices, especially on days when you are having fish, poultry, or other animal foods for dinner. Your success in the 28-day program depends on your making the right food choices. So take some time to familiarize yourself with the rules and the table, and refer to them frequently. Please be aware that both are based on the Pritikin maintenance diet, not the therapeutic diet used at the Pritikin Centers which makes further restrictions for people with specific illnesses.

PRITIKIN GUIDELINES

Adhere carefully to the Do's and Don't's of the Table of Foods to Use and to Avoid and to the following rules:

1. Eat two or more kinds of whole grain daily (wheat, oats, brown rice, barley, buckwheat, etc.) in the form of cereals, side dishes, pasta, bread, etc.
2. Eat two or more servings of raw-vegetable salad and two or more servings of raw or cooked green or yellow vegetables daily. Potatoes may be eaten every day.
3. Eat one piece of citrus fruit and up to 3 or 4 fresh-fruit servings daily.
4. Do not use sugar or honey of any kind. When sweeteners are necessary, use pureed fresh fruit or fruit juices.
5. Limit protein intake from animal sources† as follows: Up to 24 ounces (raw weight) per week of low-fat, low-

---

† Vegans, eating no animal protein at all, may require a supplement of Vitamin B_{12} once every several weeks.

cholesterol meat, fish, shellfish, or fowl, with a maximum of 4 oz (raw weight) per day.

Up to 16 ounces (2 glasses) skim milk on vegetarian days and up to 8 oz (1 glass) per day when full daily allotment of fish, fowl, or meat is eaten. ‡

6. On vegetarian days, 8 oz of cooked beans or peas may be substituted for meat, fish, or poultry. Avoid on other days except for small amounts in salads.

7. If you have constipation problems, add some unprocessed wheat-bran flakes (starting with 1 tablespoon daily) to your cereal, soup, or other foods.

8. Eat 3 full meals daily. Don't go hungry between meals; snacks are encouraged. For snacks, eat fruit (not exceeding daily fruit allotment), vegetables, and raw salad, or whole-grain bread or crackers that are free of oil, fat, added wheat germ, or sweeteners.

9. Flavor with herbs and spices, instead of salt. Keep salt intake minimal.

10. If you need to lose weight, increase vegetables and decrease grains. If you need to gain weight, decrease vegetables and increase grains.

THE 28-DAY DINNER MENUS

Twenty-eight completely different dinner menu plans are provided, many with alternative entrée selections, so that you will have many choices. Use only those menu plans and entrées which you like and find convenient to prepare. You may wish to use only half a dozen, or you may want to try them all. Some are elaborate enough to be used for a dinner party or other occasion when you wish to entertain. You will find specific suggestions for such special occasions later in this chapter. Other menus are quite simple, sometimes

---

‡ Substitutions may be made for the milk, as follows: 8 oz milk = 8 oz buttermilk, 6 oz nonfat yogurt, 5 tablespoons nonfat dry milk, 4 ounces evaporated skim milk, or 2 oz skim-milk cottage cheese. Since cottage cheese is not as good a source of calcium as the other dairy foods, no more than 2 oz cottage cheese per day is recommended.

Table of Foods to Use and to

CATEGORY	FOODS TO USE
FATS, OILS	None.
SUGARS	None.
POULTRY, FISH, SHELLFISH, MEAT, AND SOYBEANS	Chicken, turkey, Cornish game hen, game birds (white meat preferred; remove skin before cooking). Lean fish, lobster, squid, and other shellfish. Lean meat. Soybeans and tofu (soybean curd).
EGGS	Egg whites.
DAIRY FOODS	Nonfat (skim) milk, nonfat buttermilk (up to 1% fat by weight). (8 oz = 1 serving)
	Nonfat yogurt. (6 oz = 1 serving)
	Nonfat (skim) dry milk. (5T = 1 serving)
	Evaporated skim milk. (4 oz = 1 serving)
	100% skim-milk cheese, primarily uncreamed cottage cheese such as hoop cheese or dry curd cottage cheese, or cheeses up to 1% fat by weight. (2 oz = 1 serving)
	Sapsago (Green) cheese.
BEANS, PEAS	All beans and peas (except soybeans).
NUTS, SEEDS	Chestnuts.

QUANTITY PERMITTED	FOODS TO AVOID
	All fats and oils, including butter, margarine, shortening, lard, meat fat, all oils, lecithin (as in vegetable spray).
	All extracted sugars, including syrups, molasses, fructose, dextrose, sucrose, and honey.
Limit acceptable poultry, fish, and meat to 3 to 4 oz per day, maximum 1½ lb per week.	Fatty poultry such as duck, goose.
	Fatty fish such as sardines, fish canned in oil, mackerel.
Lobster, oysters, clams, scallops, or squid; 3½ oz/day (replaces entire daily allotment of poultry, fish or meat).[1]	Fatty meats such as marbled steaks and pork.
Shrimp or crab, 1¾ oz/day (replaces entire daily allotment of poultry, fish, or meat).[1]	Processed meats such as frankfurters and luncheon meats.
Soybeans and tofu: 3½ oz/day (replaces entire daily allotment of poultry, fish or meat).	Organ meats: liver, kidneys, hearts, sweetbreads.
	Smoked, charbroiled, or barbecued foods.
7/week max. (Raw: 2/week max.)	Egg yolks. Fish eggs, such as caviar, shad roe.
	Cream, half-and-half, whole milk, and low-fat milk or products containing or made from them, such as sour cream, lowfat yogurt.
	Nondairy substitutes such as creamers, whipped toppings.
2 servings/day (on vegetarian days); 1 serving/day (on other days)	Cheeses containing over 1% fat by weight.
1–2 oz/week max.	
Limit to 8 oz cooked beans on days when fish, poultry, or meat is not eaten. Avoid on other days except for small amounts in salads, or other dishes.	Soybeans and tofu (soybean curd) unless substituted: 3½ oz soybeans or tofu = the poultry, fish, or meat allotment.
Not limited.	All nuts (except chestnuts). All seeds (except in small quantities for seasoning as with spices).

Our revised recommendations are based on a conservative interpretation of the newest data concerning cholesterol and other possibly atherogenic sterols in shellfish.

CATEGORY	FOODS TO USE
VEGETABLES	All vegetables except avocados and olives.
FRUITS[2]	All fresh fruits.
	Unsweetened cooked, canned, pureed, or frozen fruit.
	Dried fruit.
	Unsweetened fruit juices.
	Frozen concentrates, unsweetened.
GRAINS	All whole or lightly milled grains: rice, barley, buckwheat, millet, etc.
	Breads, cereals, crackers, pasta, tortillas, baked goods, and other grain products without added fats, oils, sugars, or egg yolks.
SALT	Salt.[3]
CONDIMENTS, SALAD DRESSINGS, SAUCES, GRAVIES, AND SPREADS	Wines for cooking. Natural flavoring extracts. Products without fats, oils, sugars, or egg yolks.
DESSERTS OR SNACKS	Dessert and snack items without fats, oils, sugars, or egg yolks.
BEVERAGES[4]	Mineral water, carbonated water.
	Nonfat (skim) milk or nonfat buttermilk.
	Unsweetened fruit juices.
	Vegetable juices.
	Red bush or chamomile tea preferred.

[2] If triglycerides are above 125 mg%, eat only fresh fruit in the permitted amount.

Avoid on the Maintenance Diet

QUANTITY PERMITTED	FOODS TO AVOID
Limit vegetables high in oxalic acid such as spinach, beet leaves, rhubarb, and Swiss chard.	Avocados.
	Olives.
5 servings/day max.	Cooked, canned, or frozen fruit with added sugars.
24 oz/week max.	
1 oz/day max.	Jams, jellies, fruit butters, fruit syrups with added sugars.
4 oz/day max. (28 oz/week). ...or...	Fruit juices with added sugars.
1 oz/day max. (7 oz/week).	
Unlimited.	Extracted wheat germ.
Limit refined grains and grain products (i.e., with bran and germ removed) such as white flour, white rice, white pasta, etc.	Grain products made with added fats, oils, sugars, or egg yolks.
	Bleached white flour; soy flour.
Limit salt intake to 3–4 gms/day by eliminating table salt and restricting use of high salt or sodium (Na) foods such as soy sauce, pickles, most condiments, prepared sauces, dressings, canned vegetables, and MSG (monosodium glutamate).	Salt from all sources in excess of permitted amount.
Dry white wine preferable. Moderate use.	Products containing fats, oils, sugars, or egg yolks such as: mayonnaise, prepared sandwich spreads, prepared gravies and sauces and most seasoning mixes, salad dressings, catsups, pickle relish, chutney.
Plain gelatin (unflavored): 1 oz per week max.	Desserts and snack items containing fats, oils, sugars, or egg yolks such as: most bakery goods, package gelatin desserts and puddings, candy, chocolate, and gum.
Limit varieties with added sodium.	Alcoholic beverages.
See restrictions under DAIRY FOODS above.	Beverages with caffeine such as coffee, tea, cola drinks, cocoa.
See restrictions under FRUITS above.	
Not limited.	Decaffeinated coffee.
2 cups per day.	Beverages with added sweeteners such as soft drinks.
	Diet and other soft drinks with artificial sweetener.

Normal salt (sodium) needs are provided by food in their natural state and additional intake should be kept to a minimum.
Recommendations on herb tea (other than those given) and coffee substitutes are under study.

built around a soup entrée, supplemented with vegetables and salad. Look over the 28 dinner menus to see which suit you best. "Timesavers," "Leftover Suggestions," and "Weight-Loss Suggestions" appear with each menu. Almost all the recipes in this book are new ones, so even if you are familiar with Pritikin recipes, you'll find lots of new and exciting dishes.

If you want to use all 28 menu plans, you will find that the sequence in which they are arranged gives you lots of variety from day to day. However, if this is not important to you, and if you were to use just one of the dinner-menu plans over and over again, you would still be well nourished as long as you also followed our breakfast and lunch suggestions.

If you are not attempting to restrict calories, your portion sizes may be as large as you like for most of the vegetable and grain dishes on the menu, but those containing dairy products or legumes, fish, poultry, shellfish, or meat need to be regulated by the rules concerning desirable limits for intake of cholesterol-bearing or high-protein foods (See rules and *Table of Foods to Use and to Avoid*, pages 196–199). A serving size of any recipe containing fish, poultry, shellfish, or meat will usually be no more than 3½ to 4 oz of the animal food, the maximum permitted per day by Pritikin guidelines. Similarly, a serving size of any dish containing dairy foods will not exceed the allowable daily limits for skim milk or its equivalents in other skim-milk products. At the bottom of each recipe containing cholesterol-bearing or dairy foods you will find information as to the amount contained per serving of poultry, fish, or meat, or (if present in significant quantity) of dairy foods.

You may eat suitable breads with all your meals in any quantity, unless you are trying to lose weight. If you want to lose weight, omit bread, and follow the recommendations for dieters on each menu, as well as all the general recommendations in this book.

You need to remember that if dinner leftovers contain poultry, fish, shellfish, or meat and are eaten for lunch, you may have used up your daily quota accordingly. Also keep in mind that large servings of dried beans and peas (legumes) should be eaten only once a day and only on days when animal foods are not eaten. If you have had a full serving of legumes or animal foods for lunch, you should choose a vegetarian dinner menu that does not feature legumes as a prominent ingredient in any dish.

VEGETARIAN DINNERS

Many of the dinner menus feature interesting vegetarian menus for use on days when you have had serving-size portions of animal food or legumes for lunch or simply prefer a vegetarian meal. These are as follows: Menu 1, page 230 (spaghetti with whole-wheat pasta); 2, page 236 (vegetable curry and rice); 8, page 264 ("fried" rice); 11, page 275 (vegetable stew); 12, page 278 (eggplant-tomato stew and Spanish rice); 15, page 290 (potato gnocchi or Pritikin pizza); 20, page 313 (cabbage rolls with potato-grain filling); and 24, page 333 (polenta with Italian sauce and vegetables, or tamale pie). There are also several other vegetarian dinner menus which feature legumes: menu 5, page 250 (Mexican red beans or black beans and corn bread); 18, page 306 (Boston baked beans and sweet potato bread); 19, page 310 (vegetable-barley soup and chef's salad with beans); and 27, page 345 (*Pasta e Fagioli*—pasta and beans). In addition, menu 12 offers an alternative legume entrée (spicy Mexican lentils), and menu 8 offers an alternative entrée using a small amount of beans (bulgur wheat with chick-peas and vegetables).

DINNER SALADS

In a few cases we recommend a particular salad when it will substantially enhance your dinner menu; but on most nights simply toss together greens and other raw vegetables as you like. We suggest that the backbone of your tossed green salad be dark green lettuce, such as romaine or butter lettuce, with a little iceberg or other crisphead lettuce added for color and texture, if you wish. Add other raw vegetables and ingredients of your choice—radishes, cucumbers, green onions, sprouts, tomatoes, just a few cooked garbanzo or kidney beans, or croutons you make by oven-toasting cubes of a good whole-grain bread sprinkled with a little garlic powder, if desired. Several excellent salad dressings appear, starting on page 402. Or you may prefer your salad plain, with a little vinegar, or with just a squeeze of lemon.

One good-sized green salad daily is sufficient unless you enjoy a luncheon salad as well, or you want to lose weight. If you want to lose a few pounds or more, you should eat a large green salad at lunch as well as at dinner. The salads will provide low-calorie bulk that will satisfy some of your hunger.

DESSERTS

Though no particular desserts have been specified for each of the 28 dinners, most people enjoy something sweet to end the meal. Pritikin desserts are quite delectable (See pages 410 to 433), but on most days your dessert choice should be fresh fruit—a whole piece of fruit, berries, half a grapefruit, half a melon, or melon with a lemon or lime slice. Or when you feel more festive, make a fruit cup of whatever fruits are in season. A special fruit mixture can also enhance the character of the meal. For instance, add fresh mango or papaya chunks to a fruit cup when you're serving menus 2 and 8, which have an Indian theme. Or for menus 4 and 10, which include Chinese recipes, a delightful ending to the meal would be marinated tangerine, tangelo, or mandarin orange segments (page 412).

For a simple hot dessert to end a meal, particularly if the meal has been made in the oven, why not bake sweet potatoes or yams at the same time, to be eaten as the final course? A baked apple or wine-sautéed bananas in berry sauce are also easy-to-do meal endings. (See recipes, page 411.)

Yogurt makes a fine base for a simple but satisfying smooth and flavorful dessert with the addition of fresh, frozen, or canned fruit. Top nonfat yogurt with fresh sliced peaches, strawberries, or blueberries, or with frozen cherries and sliced bananas; or add applesauce, raisins, and cinnamon. Or make *Lime Yogurt Sauce* (page 433) to top fresh-fruit chunks.

While simple fruit or fruit-and-yogurt desserts should suffice for most of your dinners, there may be times when something more seems to be called for. One of our pie, cake, pudding, and cookie recipes will be just the thing for special occasions.

BREAKFASTS AND LUNCHES FOR THE 28 DAYS

Of course you will be concerned about eating tasty, filling, and nutritious breakfasts, lunches, and snacks on the 28-day program. The suggestions that follow, together with the guidelines to the Pritikin diet and the *Table of Foods to Use and to Avoid,* provide the framework for you to plan your meals and snacks around the basic 28-day dinner menu plan. It also provides the basis for sound meal-planning advice when you're not following a strict menu program.

Breakfasts

Breakfast preferences vary greatly, but the easiest, most popular Pritikin breakfast is a bowl of hot cereal with a sprinkling of cinnamon, slices of banana or other fresh fruit, and a little skim milk, if desired. Once you get into the swing of preparing a cereal each morning as you go about your other early-morning activities, you'll find it really isn't time-consuming. Whole-grain bread, toasted, if you wish, can accompany the meal. Begin or end your breakfast with a citrus fruit—a whole orange or half a grapefruit—or berries in season, melon, or other seasonal fruits. At least one of your daily fruits should be citrus—and it should, of course, be the whole fruit, not juice.

If you are not in the habit of eating a hot cooked cereal in the morning, at least give it a try. You might find that you really enjoy it. Whole cooked cereals are very satisfying and have great staying power, keeping you from being hungry for many hours. But if you just don't like hot cereal, or don't have time to cook it in the morning, you can also have other whole-grain foods suitable for breakfast, such as additional bread or toast, *Apple-Oat Bran Muffins* (recipe page 357), Pritikin English muffins (now being sold at many supermarkets), pancakes, or a cold cereal such as our *Granola* recipe (page 353), or a commercial whole-grain unadulterated variety. Or you could make easy *Apple-Oat Crunch* (page 354), using uncooked raw oatmeal as a base. Most people are surprised that rolled oats are good uncooked, although in that form they actually have been partially cooked and can be eaten out of hand, almost like peanuts, if desired.

You could make two loaves of *Oatmeal Bread* (pages 356 to 357) to give you almost a one-week supply of a delicious bread that would be about the equivalent of eating a bowl of oatmeal each morning. Recipes for other breakfast foods, including two kinds of pancakes and French toast, are also found in Chapter 18: Breakfast Fare.

Sweet spreads for bread, toast, muffins, pancakes, or *Oatmeal Bread* could be as simple as a little mashed banana sprinkled with cinnamon; a few spoonfuls of applesauce sprinkled with a little nutmeg; or sliced fruit, such as pears or bananas. Or you could use *Apple Butter* (page 396) or the unusual *Fruit-Eggplant Spread* (page 362); or piquant *Apple-Mustard Spread,* discussed in the section on fruit-based sandwiches on page 209. For a special treat for French toast or pancakes, make *Hot Berry Sauce* (page 364). Or you can prepare *Blueberry Jam* (page 361) or *Apple Syrup* (page 363).

For a special breakfast beverage, make a *Hot Apple Toddy* or *Hot Carob* (Pritikin hot chocolate), as shown on page 392. A blended frozen-fruit-and-milk shake can be a nice breakfast treat, too, but be aware that these recipes use a large quantity of milk or milk equivalents, partially depleting your allotment for dairy foods for the rest of the day.

Luncheons

Your daily breakfast menu is quite likely to be fairly consistent during the 28-day program, and will usually be composed mainly of cereal, bread, and fruit. But your lunch can vary greatly from day to day, and you need to be very mindful of the rules regarding dairy foods, legumes, and animal foods.

Luncheon meals eaten at home and those packed to take to work or school present different logistical problems, so we will discuss them separately.

Luncheon at Home

Home luncheons may vary from a quick bite on the run to a more relaxed repast at which, possibly, you are entertaining guests. At home you have access to your stove and oven, so you can heat a bowl of soup, bake a white or sweet potato, boil an ear of corn, or reheat leftovers from dinner. Building lunch around a soup is very desirable. Many people like to cook their favorite soups in large quantities and store serving-size amounts in space-conserving seal-top bags. In the morning, you just remove a bag from the freezer to defrost in time for lunch. If you don't have soup in the refrigerator or freezer, you can make *Creamy Corn Soup* (recipe page 371) or *Leftover Vegetable Cream Soup* in minutes. Convert leftover cooked vegetables, such as asparagus, broccoli, cauliflower, or peas, to a cream soup by combining about ½ cup each of cooked vegetables and nonfat milk, with a little evaporated skim milk (to add a creamier taste) in a blender and pureeing, then seasoning to taste with spices, such as marjoram, rosemary, thyme, or other seasonings of choice.

You can round out your soup lunch with some good bread; a tossed green salad, if desired; and perhaps a baked potato. Calorie-trimmers should include a *large* salad, omit the bread and potato, and opt for lower-calorie soups. Soups, in general, are wonderful for calorie-watchers. The soup-salad combination is the best lunch for those wanting to shed some pounds, because both tend to be very filling for the number of calories they contain, especially when the soup has lots of broth and vegetables and not too much of grains or beans.

When you want a change from a baked potato, if you have some leftover potatoes, baked or cooked, you can make delicious "French Fries," (See page 372) or *Potato Cakes* (page 372).

Leftover cooked pasta, stored in the freezer (and thawed)

or in the refrigerator, can be a great help in concocting a fast but filling lunch. Just combine the pasta with leftover sauces and/or vegetables, then reheat in the oven. Pasta salads (See pages 376 and 378) made with leftover pasta are also delicious, quick, and easy luncheon dishes. Leftover rice can be utilized in similar ways, and rice, pasta, and potatoes make soups more substantial.

When you are starting lunch from scratch without the benefit of leftovers, try a baked sweet potato, boiled or steamed fresh or frozen corn on the cob, steamed artichoke or cabbage wedge or broccoli, steamed frozen corn kernels, or other fresh or frozen vegetables of your choice. If you're not counting calories, have some whole-grain bread along with your vegetables. Lower-calorie vegetables, such as artichoke, cabbage, broccoli, or greens, would be good choices for calorie-watchers who want an additional dish to supplement a soup-salad lunch. The chart that follows shows caloric values for common vegetables per 8-oz cup.

Add a little zest to a cooked vegetable, baked potato, or bread with *Salsa*, a spicy Mexican tomato-chile relish; *Mock Sour Cream*, our very satisfactory version of sour cream; *Mustard-Yogurt Topping*; or nonfat yogurt that you can purchase or make. Recipes for these toppings are on pages 407 to 408.

Caloric Values for Vegetables

Food Item	Calories in 8-ounce Cup	Food Item	Calories in 8-ounce Cup
Lettuce, Boston and Bibb (varieties of butter lettuce)	8	Turnip greens	29
		Green beans	31
		Mustard greens	32
Lettuce, romaine	10	Bell peppers, green, raw	33
Cucumbers, raw	16	Asparagus	36
Mushrooms, raw	20	Broccoli	40
Celery, raw	20	Spinach	41
Cabbage	24	Tomatoes, raw	45
Bok choy	24	Carrots, raw	46
Cauliflower	28	Bell peppers, red, raw	47
Squash, summer	29		

Caloric Values for Vegetables

Food Item	Calories in 8-ounce Cup	Food Item	Calories in 8-ounce Cup
Beets	54	Potatoes, white,	
Brussels sprouts	56	boiled in skin	118
Collard greens	63	Corn	137
Artichokes*	—	Potatoes, sweet, boiled	
Squash, winter	93	in skin (depending on	
Peas, frozen	109	variety)	±291

* The caloric value of artichokes varies widely, but they are a low-calorie food.

When you are not in the mood for soup, potatoes, or vegetables, and don't have leftover rice or pasta, but still want something hot, fast, and filling for lunch, what to do? Backpackers and campers enjoy *Camper's Chile* (page 370), which utilizes pantry-shelf items—fast-cooking bulgur wheat, pasta, tomato paste, and spices. If you keep packaged corn tortillas on hand and have leftover cooked beans and lentils from our bean and lentil recipes (pages 251, 252, 278), or even plain cooked pintos or other beans, you can make delicious tacos or tostadas in minutes. Recipes for these are on pages 250 and 251. Calorie-watchers who want to limit their use of high-calorie beans can substitute leftover *Eggplant-Tomato Stew* (page 279), which makes a wonderful filling for tacos.

In addition to the dishes mentioned above, the section on lunches provides lots of other recipes for occasions when you can enjoy a more leisurely midday meal. See also suggestions on entertaining (pages 213 to 215) for menu ideas you can adapt for special lunches.

We have not forgotten about those who prefer a sandwich over anything else, even when at home. Read on.

Lunches Away from Home

If you pack a lunch to be eaten at work or at school, your midday meal can be as delicious and filling as if you were to eat at home. If you are going to be eating in a restaurant or at someone else's home, please read or reread the discussion on pages 166 to 176 in Chapter 14.

If you can carry a thermos jar or bottle or don't mind eating at room temperature foods usually eaten hot, you can take leftovers of all kinds packed in insulated containers or plain plastic containers with good lids. You can carry soups, salads, rice, beans, casserole dishes, and anything that won't melt or spoil by the time you eat it. The rice dishes, such as *Spanish Rice* (recipe page 280), *Confetti Rice* (recipe page 304), *"Fried" Rice* (recipe page 265), *Snow Pea and Rice Salad* (recipe page 249), and others, or the *bulgur wheat* recipe (page 265), are particularly good lunch-box items. They are filling and tasty, provide you with good nutrition, and are simple to pack.

Potatoes offer other lunch-box possibilities. Cold baked yams or sweet potatoes can be packed as is and eaten out of their own shells with a plastic spoon. Leftover baked or cooked potatoes can be sliced and mixed with a little salad dressing for a simple potato salad. *Buttermilk-Mustard Dressing* (recipe page 406), *Mustard-Yogurt Topping* (recipe page 407), or *Vinaigrette Dressing* (recipe page 403) would be good dressing choices. Complete your improvised potato salad by chopping in some celery, green pepper, and green onion and adding dried spices such as dillweed or celery seed to taste. Your salad could be even more interesting with the addition of a tablespoon or two of our wonderful *Pickle Relish* (recipe page 388), great with many kinds of salads. If you like pickles, have a look at our recipe for *Pickled Cucumbers* (recipe page 389). Imagine, delicious pickles without a grain of salt! A slice or two of pickle enhances most lunches, particularly sandwich lunches.

Sandwiches. The sandwich *aficionado* needn't fret because peanut butter, lunch meats, and American cheese are no longer options. The Pritikin diet offers intriguing possibilities, but don't neglect your base: a delicious, nutritious bread. Select a good-quality whole-grain bread, such as Pritikin wheat or rye, whole-grain pita bread, oil-free whole-grain sourdough or chapatis when you can find them, sprouted-whole-grain bread (a dense, dark, delectable whole-grain bread made from sprouted wheat or rye berries, carried in some health- and natural-food stores), or other suitable breads, including whole-wheat bagels and Mexican "bread"—corn tortillas.

Now that you have your bread, what do you do with it? Some good sandwich suggestions follow, but when using sandwich spreads made with skim-milk cheese or yogurt, or beans, keep in mind the rules regarding dairy foods and legumes, so that you do not exceed your allotments.

● Slice thinly red onions, tomatoes, and pepperoncinis (pickled peppers in vinegar). Add lettuce and sprouts and place between two slices of bread that have been spread with a little *Mustard-Yogurt Topping* (page 406).

● Cooked beans, mashed, mixed with a little nonfat yogurt and a few seasonings as shown in the recipe on page 375, make a tasty spread.

● Slice hard-cooked egg whites (yes, you have discarded the yolks) and spread the bread with *Mustard-Yogurt Topping*, described above. Stuff the sandwich with some sprouts or other veggies, and enjoy.

● Fruit cooked with eggplant and pureed makes a marvelous, surprising sandwich spread. The eggplant provides a bland, smooth base and the fruit flavor is all you taste. *Fruit-Eggplant Spreads* (page 362).

● Slice a banana thinly lengthwise onto bread topped with a little hoop cheese or skim-milk cottage cheese, with or without *Apple Butter* (page 397).

● Try simple but delicious *Apple-Mustard Spread* teamed with a thinly sliced banana on warm toasted whole-wheat bread, or use it as a topping on crackers. Combine a peeled, medium-grated apple with about a teaspoon of Dijon mustard. The vinegar in the mustard keeps the apple from turning brown, so you can make up a quantity and keep it in a tightly covered container in the refrigerator for several days.

● Tuna-fish salad is a favorite sandwich filling for many, and we offer two good recipes (pages 385 to 387). Or try some of the cheese spread and vegetable pâté recipes on pages 373 to 375, adding lettuce, cucumber, and other vegetables to the sandwich, as you like. A particular favorite is *Salmon Pâté* (recipe page 374). Spread it on lightly toasted whole-wheat or rye bread; then layer lettuce, sliced tomato, and cucumber over the pâté.

● A "lox and bagel sandwich" (without the lox!) can be

surprisingly delicious. Place a fairly thin layer of pressed or spreadable skim-milk cottage cheese (such as hoop cheese or 1-percent-by-weight cottage cheese) mixed with some chopped chives or scallions over a split and warmed whole-wheat bagel. Good alternative spreads are the *Salmon Pâté*, mentioned above, or *Pimiento Cheese* spread (recipe page 374). Top your choice of spread with a thin slice of tomato and red onion, and eat open-face or covered with the other half-bagel.

● Some of the entrées make very good sandwich fillings. *Turkey Loaf* (recipe page 269) is the Pritikin diet answer to sandwich meat, has excellent flavor, freezes well, and contains only a little turkey ($\frac{1}{12}$th serving of the loaf has $\frac{3}{4}$ oz turkey. That is plenty for a sandwich and uses less than $\frac{1}{2}$ your day's animal-food allotment). Thinly sliced cooked breast of turkey or chicken is a fine sandwich filling, especially on days when you will be having a vegetarian dinner. A recipe for roasting turkey breast appears on page 318. Prepare the turkey breast for a dinner, then slice and freeze the rest, ready for sandwiches.

Accompany your sandwich with celery and carrot sticks or a salad, if you wish, and fresh fruit or even a baked apple. For extra munching, consider packing some air-popped popcorn, a little bag of Pritikin *Granola* (recipe page 353), or some of the snack items you will find later in this chapter, such as homemade tortilla or potato chips, or roasted garbanzo beans, which are eaten like nuts. Additional munchies, such as plain rye or rice crackers, provide healthful calories that will help to fill you up. Whatever you take, be sure you have given yourself enough to eat and a little extra for a midafternoon snack (to insulate yourself from food seduction in the wicked outside world!) and include a suitable beverage—small cans of salt-free tomato juice would be a good choice.

SNACKS AND BEVERAGES FOR THE 28 DAYS

Snacks

To round out your diet, you'll need to know more about Pritikin-approved snacks and beverages. For instance, an unusual feature of the Pritikin diet is that we *encourage* snacking. Present-day custom to the contrary, we humans do not function best on "3 squares a day." The body machinery runs most efficiently when we eat more than 3 times a day. You may want to have part of your breakfast meal midmorning, as we do at the Center, where cereal starts the day and a citrus fruit is served about an hour and a half later. Still later in the morning, we provide both raw and cooked vegetables, crackers, and bread. If you would like to eat this way, and are able to, you can snack on bread, crackers, raw or cooked vegetables, and some fruits on and off all day. You will have to observe the guidelines on fruits, though, as too much, especially cooked, canned, frozen, or dried fruit, can elevate triglycerides in your blood.

Later in the day or in the evening, you might find other kinds of snack foods appealing—air-popped popcorn or oven-toasted corn tortillas heated until crisp, then broken into wedges. Or if you are more ambitious, you could try *Potato Chips* (recipe page 399), *Garbanzo "Nuts"* (recipe page 399), or Pritikin *Granola* (recipe page 353), which makes an excellent snack food as well as breakfast food.

The sandwich spreads in the *Luncheon Dishes* section make great snacks with bread or crackers; or thin them to dip consistency, as directed in the spread recipes, for use with toasted corn tortillas or raw vegetables. *Salsa,* the zesty Mexican tomato-chile relish (page 407), and *Onion Dip* (page 398) are also good dips.

When you want a snack that is a mini-meal, *Quick Pita-Bread Pizzas* (page 295) might be just the thing. You can simplify preparation by using just one vegetable, perhaps the onions, or substituting whole-wheat English muffins for the pita bread.

You'll find exciting snack recipes in the section on *Beverages and Snacks;* but be on the lookout too for recipes with good snack potential in the breakfast, luncheon-food, and dessert recipe sections.

Snacking is fine for those who want to lose weight too. In fact, it's recommended. It is important to avoid getting too hungry, and those attempting to lose weight are advised to carry with them to work, on walks, and at other times when away from home plastic bags filled with raw vegetables for munching. If you are trying to lose weight, go easy on grain snacks, such as bread and *Granola*, and emphasize the raw vegetables. *Green Bean Guacamole* (recipe page 281) or *Salsa* are good low-calorie dips for your raw vegetables. Air-popped popcorn is a fun, satisfying treat containing fewer calories than almost any other snack.

BEVERAGES

While we don't discourage drinking liquids on the Pritikin diet, neither do we emphasize it. Oftentimes, we drink out of habit, or because of thirst developing from a diet containing too much sodium. On our salt-restricted diet, your thirst should abate, since a large part of the diet consists of vegetables and fruits (which are largely water). In addition, you will be eating foods cooked with water, so you will actually get ample water from your food. There is little need for most of us to drink water or other beverages, but habit, tradition, and enjoyment are compelling factors, and many of us want a beverage a few times during the day. Dieters will find that drinking fluids before or during meals creates a sense of fullness, so they are well advised to use water or other acceptable low-calorie beverages for that purpose. On the other hand, if keeping your weight up is a problem, I suggest you abstain from mealtime beverages.

Most beverages people drink, even if they are nonalcoholic, are not conducive to optimal health. If you are a milk drinker, even if you restrict yourself to skim milk, you will still consume too much protein if you drink more than 2 glasses a day. Since you will be having milk or milk products in other forms, in your foods, it would be better to drink water. In fact, if you don't particularly crave skim milk in the morning over your cereal, it might be a good idea to "save" the milk for later in the day. Then you can have skim milk or skim-milk products (yogurt, etc.) with your lunch, dinner, or snacks.

If you have been drinking coffee, tea, or caffeinated soft drinks, it is time to kick the habit. Caffeine is addictive, and you may have some withdrawal symptoms—headache, fatigue, or lethargy—which can last for several days. If you are unable to give up caffeine completely, perhaps you can cut down to one cup a day. But if you eliminate caffeine from your diet, you'll be one important step closer to better health. In addition, beverages containing caffeine further undermine dieters by stimulating the appetite. Even decaffeinated coffee, which retains caffeols, is an appetite stimulant.

Fruit juice, especially the ritual morning glass of orange juice, has become a mainstay of the American diet. But you are far better off eating the whole fruit than drinking the juiced version. When you juice fruit, you lose much of the fiber content and get considerably more sugar, since it takes several fruits to make up a glass of fruit juice.

Of available beverages, the best choices in the experience of thousands of Pritikin dieters are herb teas or beverages made with roasted grains, such as Postum or Roastaroma. At the Centers, we serve red bush *(Rooibosch)* and chamomile teas, and many people seem to like just plain hot water and lemon.

When you want a cold drink other than water, choose carbonated mineral water (watch for high sodium content in some brands), and serve with a slice of lime or with other fruit. (See page 396, *Mineral-Water "Mixed Drinks."*) A few drops of Angostura bitters in a glass of carbonated mineral water makes a "mixed drink" that is interesting. Choosing such a drink in lieu of an alcoholic beverage has become rather chic in this new health-minded age.

For special treats, though, two outstanding hot beverage snacks are *Hot Apple Toddy* and *Hot Carob* (page 392). A delicious cold treat which tastes much like a milkshake is the Pritikin *Smoothie* (page 393).

THROW A GRADUATION PARTY FOR YOURSELF— OR HOW TO ENTERTAIN PRITIKIN STYLE

At the end of the 28 days, wouldn't it be fun to have a graduation party? If you and one or more of your friends started the program together, perhaps you can co-host the party, sharing preparations for the feast. Hopefully, you will regard it as a graduation party *and* a commencement to a permanent new and healthy lifestyle. Whether or not you decide on a spectacular finish to the 28 days, you'll see the potential for fabulous entertaining using recipes from this book. The combination of delicious and unusual dishes will have your mouth watering!

Dinner-Party Buffets with an Ethnic Theme

● Italian (using recipes from menus 1, 9, 15, and 24). *Garbanzo Minestrone Soup*; *Caponata* and tossed green salad with *Italian Dressing* (page 406); *Turkey Balls in Tomato Sauce* or in *Bolognese Sauce* over whole-wheat spaghetti; *Polenta with Italian Sauce and Vegetables* or *Potato Gnocchi in Tomato Sauce*. Dessert: *Fruit Meringue* (page 413).

● Mexican (using recipes from menus, 5, 12, and 26). *Green Bean Guacamole* with raw-vegetable relishes and corn chips (recipe, page 398); *Chicken or Turkey Tacos*, oven-warmed corn tortillas, and assorted taco toppings—for do-it-yourself tacos; *Mexican Black Beans* or *Mexican Red Beans* and *Corn Bread*; *Gazpacho Mold*. Dessert: *Creamy Tapioca Pudding* (page 415).

● Middle East (using recipes from menus 2, 8, and 11). *Chilled Cucumber Soup* or tossed green salad with *Cucumber-Yogurt Dressing* (page 406). *Moroccan Chicken-Vegetable Stew* served with couscous; *Baked Eggplant with Yogurt* and pita-bread wedges. Dessert: *Carob "Cream" Pie* (page 422).

● Indian (using recipes from menus 2 and 16). *Sri Lanka Chicken Curry* and *Vegetable Curry I* with *Fruit Chutney* and *Mint Chutney*; hot brown rice; *Tomato-Cucumber Indian Relish*. Dessert: fruit cup with mango slices.

Sit-Down Dinner Parties

● Chinese meal (using recipes from menus 4 and 10). *Tofu-and-Snow Pea Soup*; *Lobster Szechuan Style* and/or *Jade Empress Chicken*; *Rice with Chinese Vegetables*. Dessert: *Marinated Mandarin Oranges* (page 412).

● Holiday meal (using recipes from menus 3 and 21). *Onion Dip* (page 398) and raw vegetable relishes; *Roast Breast of Turkey* and *Onion Gravy*; *Mashed Potatoes*;

Baked Winter Squash with Raisin Sauce or *Sweet Potato-Orange Meringue Pudding*; steamed Brussels sprouts; *Cranberry-Apple Compote* or *Cranberry-Apple Mold*. Dessert: *Pumpkin Chiffon Pie* (page 426).

Summertime Entertaining

• Elegant picnic (using recipes from menus 7, 18, 22, and 23). *Breaded Cinnamon Chicken* or *Mustard-Breaded Chicken*; *Fruited Rice Salad* (page 382) or *Potato Salad* (page 379); choice of *Caraway Slaw*, tossed green salad with *Sweet-Sour Vinaigrette Dressing* (page 404) or *Chilled Marinated Vegetables*. Dessert: *Cereal-Raisin Cookies* (page 430).

• Summer luncheon (using recipes from menus 4 and 23). *Orange-Carrot Soup* or *Cold Curried Zucchini Soup*; *Chicken Salad–Stuffed Tomato* (page 380) with *Fruit-Glazed Noodle Pudding* (page 418) or *Chinese Sesame-Chicken Salad* with *Snow Pea and Rice Salad*. Dessert: *Fruited "Chocolate" Cake* (page 427) or melon wedges with lime slices.

Casual Entertaining

• Sunday night supper (using recipes from menus 18 and 25). *Creamy Fish Chowder* or *Boston Baked Beans*; *Sweet Potato Bread*; hot corn-on-the-cob; deluxe tossed green salad (use artichoke hearts, sliced red onion, garbanzo or kidney beans—with the chowder, only—and other interesting ingredients) and *French Dressing* (page 403). Dessert: *Apple-Raisin Pie* or *Crumb-Topped Fruit Pie* (page 421).

• Brunch. *Millet-Applesauce Enchiladas* (page 367) or *Noodle Kugel* (page 417) and fruit salad; *Tuna–Green Pea Salad* (page 386) in tomato cups; oven-warmed whole-wheat bagels with choice of *Pimiento Cheese* (page 374) and *Salmon Pâté* (page 374), and vegetable platter with lettuce leaves, sliced tomatoes, sliced red onion, and pepperoncinis (for making "lox-and-bagel-sandwiches-without-the-lox"); *Molded Fresh Cucumber-Mint Salad* (page 327); *Pumpkin Bread* (page 308).

	DAY I
Breakfast	Half grapefruit *Cooked Rolled Oats** with sliced banana, nonfat milk, and sprinkling of cinnamon Whole-wheat toast
Lunch	*Vegetable-Barley Soup* Baked sweet potato Pita bread stuffed with *Eggplant Relish*, lettuce, and sliced tomato Carrot and celery sticks Apple
Dinner†	*Chicken and Potatoes in Mushroom-Tomato Sauce* Tossed green salad with *Italian Dressing* Cantaloupe with lime slice
Snacks During Day	Pear; Rye-Krisp crackers; Corn tortillas and *Salsa*; Air-popped popcorn; *Smoothie*

* Recipes for all italicized dishes are in book. See recipe index.
† Day I dinner = Dinner Menu 6; Day II dinner = Dinner Menu 25; Day III dinner = Dinner Menu 12

Menu Plans

DAY II	DAY III
Orange slices *Oat-Wheat-Rice Pancakes* with sliced banana and *Blueberry Topping*	Half grapefruit *Cooked Cracked Wheat* with sliced banana, nonfat milk, and sprinkling of cinnamon Whole-wheat toast
Tabbouli *Carrot Relish* Whole-wheat bread Fresh pineapple	*Corkscrew-Pasta Salad* on lettuce with garnish of canned artichoke hearts and beets Whole-wheat bread Fresh pear
Cioppino Hot corn-on-the-cob Steamed artichoke with *Mustard-Yogurt Topping* Baked Potato with *Salsa* Tossed green salad with *French Dressing* Fresh strawberries with nonfat yogurt	*Spicy Mexican Lentils* served with corn tortillas (taco style), with garnish of shredded lettuce, diced tomatoes, chopped green onions, shredded carrots, and Sapsago cheese *Spanish Rice* *Green Bean Guacamole* *Fruit Meringue*
Banana; Grapes; Rye-Krisp crackers; Whole-wheat bread and *Apple Butter*	Peach; Banana; Cantaloupe; Carrot and celery sticks; Rye- Krisp crackers; Air-popped popcorn

IMPORTANT POINTS ABOUT THE RECIPES

A few general instructions concerning ingredients and procedures:

Ingredients

• When the size of a vegetable or fruit is not indicated in the ingredient list, assume it to be medium size; when small or large size is to be used, we have specified.

• Recipes using chicken breast halves always call for small halves to keep cholesterol intake within guidelines. A half chicken breast, with skin, should weigh no more than 7–8 oz; a boned half chicken breast, with skin, should weigh about 5 oz. The edible chicken on such market purchases will be about 4 oz per half breast.

• If you wish to reduce sodium content further, choose sodium-reduced or no-salt-added ingredients whenever possible in canned goods, condiments, etc. In addition, you can rinse and drain capers, pepperoncinis, and other ingredients to wash off some of the added salt.

• Frozen apple-juice concentrate is the ingredient most often used to provide sweetening in recipes. It should be measured out in the thawed state. It's convenient and practical to keep a can in the refrigerator, defrosted, for use whenever needed.

• Stock (the liquid in which vegetables, chicken, fish, etc., has been cooked) is called for in many soup and entrée recipes. It is preferable to water because of the flavor it contributes. Stock does not add calories to a recipe, nor does it add cholesterol or fat, if you have defatted the stock.

• Evaporated skim milk adds creaminess to foods like mashed potatoes, so we've used it instead of nonfat milk in some recipes. Leftover evaporated milk can be kept for up to a week in a covered container in the refrigerator, or in the freezer. A word of warning: Evaporated skim milk has more than twice the protein content and calories of nonfat milk. So if you want larger portions of a dish that calls for it, try substituting nonfat milk in the recipe.

• Bread crumbs made from acceptable whole-grain bread are an ingredient in many recipes. To make them, use an electric blender or food processor.

Procedures

• Don't hesitate to individualize the recipes for your particular needs and preferences. For instance, you may wish to double or halve the recipe size or to modify the seasoning. Just make sure that whatever changes you make don't conflict with the nutritional guidelines (pages 191 to 199).

• With many recipes it is critically important that the dish be placed in a *preheated oven*. When an oven temperature is given, wait to put the dish in until the oven has reached the specified temperature.

• Although it is not mentioned in the recipes, some preliminary preparation of ingredients is essential. All vegetables and fruits should be washed thoroughly before they are used. If they have been waxed, peel before using whenever possible. When grated orange or lemon rind is called for, if the fruit has been waxed or colored with artificial coloring, peel the fruit and grate the inside of the rind to avoid the wax or coloring on the outside.

• Fresh or frozen fish and poultry should be rinsed in cold water, then patted dry with paper towels. Instructions for preparation of legumes and grains follow.

COOKING GRAINS, BEANS, AND VEGETABLES— SOME BASIC INFORMATION

You will need to be well acquainted with some methods for cooking grains, beans, and vegetables, which are the basis of the Pritikin diet. Unfortunately, the idea of preparing grains and beans from scratch is unappealing to many people. Yet nothing could be simpler once you know a few basic rules. So bear with us on this.

How to Cook Grains

To cook grains, you need merely add a specified quantity of the grain to a specified amount of boiling liquid, then just let them cook unsupervised. What could be simpler? Also, since cooked grains can be kept in the refrigerator for days and reheated, cooking large quantities is recommended. Cooked brown rice, in particular, is called for in many of the dinner menus, to be served plain or as an ingredient in another dish. So do prepare larger quantities of rice in order to have leftovers for such occasions. While long-grain brown rice is specified in some of the recipes, if you prefer, you can substitute the softer-textured short-grain variety.

When you have no cooked grains on hand and are really in a hurry, cook *bulgur*. Bulgur derives from wheat which has been parboiled, dried, and broken up. It cooks in only 15 minutes and is very similar to rice in taste and appearance. Or, just pour boiling water over dry bulgur, let it stand for 20–30 minutes until it is soft and fluffy, then drain off the excess water, as they do in the Middle East for such dishes as *tabbouli*. Because it is precooked, bulgur expands less after cooking than whole grains, such as brown rice. A cup of uncooked bulgur yields about 2½ cups cooked grain; a cup of brown rice expands to 3 or more cups.

If grains have not been cleaned (the package will tell you), you may need to rinse and drain them before adding them to boiling liquid. To cook any whole grain, bring water or stock to a boil, add grains slowly, reduce temperature to low, and cook tightly covered for the required amount of time or until all the water is absorbed. Don't stir during the cooking, and allow the grain to rest, covered, at the end of the cooking period for another 10 minutes or longer to permit the grains to fluff. (Some cooks follow a different procedure—lifting the lid of the longer-cooking grains, like rice, to let the grains separate about 5 to 10 minutes before the end of the cooking period.)

The table that follows gives cooking time and liquid required in cooking various grains, though you may wish to vary slightly the amount of liquid used or the cooking time in certain recipes.

For Each Cup of Grain:

Grain	Water or Stock	Required Cooking Time
Brown rice	2 cups	40–45 minutes
Barley	3 cups	60 minutes
Buckwheat (kasha)	2 cups	15 minutes
Bulgur	2 cups	15 minutes
Millet	3 cups	45 minutes
Whole berries		50–60 minutes (then pour
Whole rye	3 cups	off excess liquid)
Whole triticale		

Oven-toasting of grains before adding them to the liquid is optional. It does seem to improve the flavor and texture of the cooked product and is desirable in some instances for certain grains, such as buckwheat or brown rice. Here is a recipe for brown rice in which the grains are first oven-toasted, which uses slightly more liquid. (Another, *Spiced Toasted Rice*, appears on page 370.)

BROWN RICE

⅔ cup brown rice
2 cups water or stock

Spread the rice in a baking dish with sides, and place in a 350° oven for 20 minutes, or until lightly browned. Combine the toasted rice and liquid, and bring to a boil. Reduce heat, cover, and simmer for 40–45 minutes.

YIELD: ABOUT 4 CUPS

How to Cook Beans

It is very handy to keep cooked beans on hand in your refrigerator or freezer to be used in bean spreads and soups, or reheated for quick tacos or other recipes. So do prepare large quantities when you cook beans so that you'll have extras for future use.

Beans are also very easy to prepare from scratch. Rinse and sort through them; then measure them out and add water. With beans the amount of water added is less critical than with grains. Also, beans other than lentils, split peas, and black-eyed peas should be soaked before they are cooked.

To soak: Place beans in a pot, add plenty of water (about 2½ to 3 cups per cup of beans), and let the beans soak for 10 hours, or overnight, at room temperature. (In hot weather, place them in a cool spot to avoid their turning sour.) Long periods of soaking cause beans to swell and decreases the cooking time. For a quick alternative, add the water for soaking, bring to a boil, and let boil for 3–5 minutes; then turn off heat and let the beans soak for 1 hour, or up to 10 hours, if you wish.

Many cooks discard the water in which the beans soaked and replace it with fresh water for cooking. The advantage is a *small* reduction in the substances (oligosaccharides) that cause flatulence, or gas, in some people, but you will also lose some nutrients, flavor, and color.

To cook the soaked beans: Make sure the water level reaches at least an inch above the level of the beans. Simmer covered (watch to avoid boiling over) or with lid ajar until the beans are tender. Lentils and split peas cook fastest—in about 45 minutes; baby limas and black-eyed peas take about an hour; navy, white, and kidney beans take about an hour to an hour and a half; large limas, black beans, and red beans require about 1½ hours to cook; pintos take about 1½ to 2 hours, and garbanzos 2 hours or more.

A *pressure cooker* is useful for reducing the cooking time of beans, but should not be used for cooking lentils or split peas because they tend to foam and clog the safety valve, which could cause an explosion (and a splattered ceiling). Navy and lima beans will cook in a pressure cooker in about 20 minutes, kidney beans and pintos in about 30 minutes, and garbanzos in 35–45 minutes.

How to Cook Vegetables

In developing the Pritikin cuisine, we have evolved several cooking techniques for vegetables such as dry-sautéing or liquid-sautéing to replace the conventional method of sautéing in butter or oil. Either dry- or liquid-sautéing can be done using a nonstick or stainless-steel skillet or pan. In dry-sautéing, chopped onions, celery, mushrooms, or other watery vegetables are cooked directly in the skillet or pan over low heat, stir-fried until tender, and if desired, slightly browned. To liquid-sauté, use a little nonfat liquid, such as water, vegetable or chicken stock, or wine. For 1 cup chopped vegetables, bring about ¼ cup of liquid to a boil in a large pan or skillet. Turn down the heat to medium-low and add the vegetables. Stir-fry until sufficiently cooked, from 2 to 15 minutes, depending upon the vegetables used, size of cut, and degree of doneness desired. A little extra liquid may be added during liquid-sautéing if the vegetables seem too dry.

You will also be preparing a lot of steamed vegetables. Properly cooked, steamed vegetables are tender-crisp and retain most of their nutrients. A collapsible steamer basket that adapts to pots of different sizes is very convenient to steam vegetables. Make certain that the steamer basket is above the level of the water, and that the water is boiling rapidly before the vegetables are covered. The table below suggests steaming times for vegetables that will produce a crisp-tender result and retain more nutrients than longer cooking times. If you wish to prepare vegetables in advance, steam them, then plunge them under cold running water to stop the cooking and preserve color and texture, and reheat briefly to serve.

Be sure to save the leftover liquid in the bottom of the cooking pot for later use in recipes requiring vegetable stock, or to substitute for chicken stock, when desired. Let the liquid cool; then store in a jar or heavy-duty seal-top plastic bag. The broth left from steaming several days' worth of vegetables can be saved in the refrigerator, then frozen in 1-cup portions in plastic bags. When a recipe calls for 1 or 2 cups of vegetable stock, you'll be ready to go without further measurement.

Steaming whole potatoes takes more time than covering them with water and boiling them, but some nutrients otherwise lost are retained. In recipes in this book requiring whole cooked potatoes, we have not specified steaming, but it would be slightly preferable to boiling.

Baked potatoes are a Pritikin diet mainstay; in fact, the

THE PRITIKIN PROMISE
Fresh-Vegetable Steaming Times

Vegetable	Minutes	Vegetable	Minutes
Asparagus	5	Lettuce	1–2
Beans:		Mint	1–2
green	5	Mushrooms	2
lima	5	Mustard, fresh	1–2
string or snap	5	Okra	5
Bean sprouts	1–2	Onions:	
Beets, quartered	15	green tops	3
Broccoli	5	whole	5
Brussels sprouts	5	Parsley	1–2
Cabbage, quartered	5	Pea pods (snow peas)	3
Carrots, ½-inch slices	5	Peas	3–5
Cauliflower:		Peppers:	
florets	3	chile	2–3
whole	5	green and red bell	2
Celery root	3–4	Potatoes:	
Celery stalks	10	sweet: ½-inch slices	15
Chayote	3	white: ½-inch slices	10
Chicory	1–2	Pumpkin	5
Chives	2–3	Radishes	5
Collards	1–2	Romaine lettuce	1–2
Corn		Rutabagas	8
kernels	3	Shallots	2
on the cob	3	Spinach	1–2
Coriander (cilantro)	1–2	Squash:	
Cucumber	2–3	acorn	5
Dandelion greens	1–2	hubbard	5
Eggplant	5	spaghetti	5
Garlic	5	summer	3
Jerusalem artichokes	8	zucchini	3
Jicama	10	Tomatoes	3
Kale	1–2	Turnips, quartered	8
Kohlrabi, quartered	8–10	Watercress	1–2
Leeks	5		

Suitable herbs and spices for seasoning cooked vegetables are suggested in the following table.*

---

* Based on "Spices and Herbs, Vegetables in Family Meals," *Home and Garden Bulletin* No. 105, U.S. Department of Agriculture, 1965.

Cooked Vegetable	Suitable Herb or Spice for Seasoning
ASPARAGUS	Mustard seed, sesame seed, or tarragon
LIMA BEANS	Marjoram, oregano, sage, savory, tarragon, or thyme
SNAP BEANS	Basil, dill, marjoram, mint, mustard seed, oregano, savory, tarragon, or thyme
BEETS	Allspice, bay leaves, caraway seed, cloves, dill, ginger, mustard seed, savory, or thyme
BROCCOLI	Caraway seed, dill, mustard seed, or tarragon
BRUSSELS SPROUTS	Basil, caraway seed, dill, mustard seed, sage, or thyme
CABBAGE	Caraway seed, celery seed, dill, mint, mustard seed, nutmeg, savory, or tarragon
CARROTS	Allspice, bay leaves, caraway seed, dill, fennel, ginger, mace, marjoram, nutmeg, or thyme
CAULIFLOWER	Caraway seed, dill, mace, or tarragon
CUCUMBERS	Basil, dill, mint, or tarragon
EGGPLANT	Marjoram or oregano
ONIONS	Caraway seed, mustard seed, nutmeg, oregano, sage, or thyme
PEAS	Basil, dill, marjoram, mint, oregano, poppy seed, rosemary, sage, or savory
POTATOES	Basil, bay leaves, caraway seed, celery seed, dill, chives, mustard seed, oregano, or thyme
SPINACH	Basil, mace, marjoram, nutmeg, or oregano
SQUASH	Allspice, basil, cinnamon, cloves, fennel, ginger, mustard seed, nutmeg, or rosemary
SWEET POTATOES	Allspice, cardamom, cinnamon, cloves, or nutmeg
TOMATOES	Basil, bay leaves, celery seed, oregano, sage, sesame seed, tarragon, or thyme

NOTE: Parsley may be used with any of the above vegetables. Curry powder adds piquancy to vegetables.

midafternoon "mini-meal" served at the Pritikin Centers is a baked potato on most days. To bake potatoes, sweet potatoes, or yams, scrub the skins well and pierce them with the tines of a fork to allow steam to escape and prevent bursting. Don't wrap in foil, as this steams rather than bakes them (unless you prefer a softer skin). Yams and sweet potatoes have a tendency to splatter, so place them on a baking sheet or piece of foil to protect your oven. A medium white potato will bake in 40 to 45 minutes at 400 degrees, but you can bake your potatoes at temperatures ranging from 325 to 450 degrees, if you are baking other foods at the same time. Yams and sweet potatoes take about the same time to bake. When you can insert a fork easily into a potato, or when it yields to pressure from your fingers, they are done. Let them sit in a warm place, covered, until serving time. Baked potatoes are especially delicious accompanied with one of the following toppings: *Salsa* (page 407), *Mock Sour Cream* (page 408), *Mustard-Yogurt Topping* (page 407), or *Nonfat Yogurt* (page 409).

Now, the moment you've been waiting for. On to the dinner plans!

PART FOUR

THE
28-DAY
DIET

17
CHAPTER

Your
Most Important Meal:
28-Day Dinner Menus

For most of us, dinner is the most enjoyable and leisurely meal of the day. With this in mind, we have developed a 28-day dinner menu plan, around which you will build your own program for breakfasts, lunches, and snacks. You will find all the information you need for the 28-day program in this chapter—menu plans, recipes, and cooking methods. Dishes for which recipes or special instructions are given are shown in the menu plan in capital letters. Most of the time, the recipes immediately follow the menu-plan page. We have also included suggestions for menu simplifications or "Timesavers," as well as "Leftover Suggestions" and "Weight-Loss Suggestions," with each menu. Asterisks after certain dishes indicate that you should check for time-saving suggestions.

Breakfast and lunch menus need to be more flexible, so you will want to devise your own menus from day to day. The supplementary recipe chapters beginning on page provide recipes for breakfasts, lunches, snacks, salad dressings, and desserts. For a complete discussion of how to plan your breakfasts and lunches and utilize the dinner menus, see pages 191 to 217 in Chapter 16. Check the index in the back of the book for a complete listing of all the recipes by category (for example, soups or desserts).

In addition, you will find important points about the recipes and helpful information on cooking grains, beans, and vegetables on pages 219 to 226.

1 DINNER MENU

SPAGHETTI SAUCE I, II, or III* served over Whole-Wheat Spaghetti

> *ZUCCHINI, PARSNIPS, AND WATER CHESTNUTS ***
> *Tossed Green Salad with MARINATED BEETS ****

TIMESAVERS:
* Prepare the faster-cooking *Italian-Style Tomato Sauce*.
** Steam zucchini; sprinkle with dried parsley and garlic powder.
*** Omit the *Marinated Beets*.

LEFTOVER SUGGESTIONS:
Reheat leftover sauce and serve over a baked potato, rice, or freshly cooked pasta, or reheat the sauce and spaghetti from the original meal. Sauce may also be made up in large quantities for freezing.

WEIGHT-LOSS SUGGESTIONS:
Have a half-serving of the spaghetti, or serve the sauce over baked spaghetti squash or steamed bean sprouts. Have a double serving of the zucchini dish, topped with a little sauce, if desired.

I. BASIC SPAGHETTI SAUCE

Use this excellent sauce over other foods besides pasta, such as baked potatoes, steamed vegetables, or stewed lentils. Lots of parsley gives this long-cooking sauce its meatlike color and texture. Chopped mushrooms could also be added about an hour before the end of the cooking time, if you like.

> 2 bunches of parsley (leaves only), finely chopped
> 7 cloves garlic, finely chopped or crushed

4 onions, finely chopped
1 teaspoon rosemary
½ teaspoon thyme
¼ teaspoon each sage and cloves
⅛ teaspoon each oregano and basil
1 cup red wine (Burgundy, Chianti, or Zinfandel)
1 28-ounce can whole tomatoes
2 15-ounce cans tomato sauce
3 cups boiling water

Bring ½ cup water to a boil in a large pot. Add the parsley, garlic, and onions and stir and sauté until the vegetables are slightly browned. Add the seasonings and the wine and simmer until the liquid has cooked off. Stir in the tomatoes, breaking them up with a fork, and the tomato sauce and boiling water. Bring to a boil, reduce heat, and simmer, covered, for about 3 hours, stirring more frequently as the sauce thickens. If it becomes too thick, add small amounts of water from time to time as needed.

YIELD: ABOUT 7–8 CUPS   CALORIES: 47/½ CUP

II. ITALIAN-STYLE TOMATO SAUCE

1 cup chopped onions
½ cup chopped celery
2 large ripe tomatoes, peeled and chopped
1⅓ cups chopped mushrooms
2 15-ounce cans tomato sauce (or 1 28-ounce can)
1 6-ounce can tomato paste
2 tablespoons red or white wine
2–3 bay leaves
¼ teaspoon cayenne pepper

In a skillet, dry-sauté the onions and celery over medium heat for 3–4 minutes until the vegetables are soft, stirring frequently. Transfer to a large saucepan and stir in the remaining ingredients. Bring to a boil; then lower heat and

simmer, uncovered, for 30 minutes. Remove bay leaves before serving.

YIELD: ABOUT 6 CUPS   CALORIES: 52/½ CUP

III. BOLOGNESE SAUCE

Bolognese Sauce—*a culinary triumph from the Italian
city of Bologna—is made with beef, but very good results
can be obtained using ground turkey breast instead. Serve
the sauce hot over whole-wheat spaghetti or other pasta,
Polenta (page 333), Gnocchi (page 291), or even a baked
potato or brown rice.*

    ¾ pound ground raw turkey breast or very lean beef
    1 teaspoon chile powder
    1 teaspoon oregano
    1 teaspoon rosemary
    Dash cayenne pepper
    1 small onion, chopped
    3 cloves garlic, minced or crushed
    ¾ cup finely chopped celery
    ½ cup shredded carrots
    1 cup dry red wine
    1 28-ounce can Italian tomatoes, coarsely chopped in blender
    2 cups canned tomato sauce

Place a large skillet over moderate heat, add the ground
turkey or lean beef, and sprinkle the spices over the turkey.
Stir-fry the turkey and spices for about 10 minutes, mixing
well, and using the back of the mixing spoon to break up
clumps of turkey as they cook. Add the onions, garlic, celery, and carrots and stir-fry another 5 minutes until the vegetables are partially cooked. Stir in the wine, cover, and
cook over moderate heat for 10 minutes. Add the tomatoes
and tomato sauce, stir, bring to a boil, then lower heat and
simmer, covered, for about an hour.

YIELD: 6½ CUPS   CALORIES: 54/½ CUP
                          POULTRY: 1 OUNCE/½ CUP

THE PRITIKIN PROMISE
ZUCCHINI, PARSNIPS, AND WATER CHESTNUTS

The different textures and flavors in this unusual vegetable combination are very appealing.

   3 large parsnips, peeled and cut diagonally into ½-inch-thick
      slices
   3 medium zucchini, cut diagonally into ¾-inch-thick slices
   1 small onion, chopped
   ¼ cup dry sherry
   1 8-ounce can water chestnuts, drained
   1 tablespoon finely chopped parsley
   1 tablespoon garlic powder

Place the parsnips and zucchini in a steamer basket over boiling water in a saucepan and steam, covered, for 5 minutes. Add the onions, cover again, and continue steaming another 5 minutes. Remove the steamer basket and vegetables, discard the liquid (or save for use as vegetable stock in another recipe), and place the wine in the saucepan. Bring the wine to a boil, add the water chestnuts and steamed vegetables, sprinkle with the parsley and garlic powder, and heat through.

MAKES 4 SERVINGS   **CALORIES:150/SERVING**

MARINATED BEETS

   2 cups sliced, cooked, and peeled fresh beets
      or canned beets
   ½ cup tarragon vinegar (or use rice vinegar plus
      1 teaspoon tarragon)
   ⅓ cup frozen apple-juice concentrate
   ¼ cup water
   1 teaspoon cornstarch
   ½ teaspoon allspice
   ¼ teaspoon cloves

Place the beets in a bowl or glass jar. Combine the other ingredients in a saucepan, mixing well. Bring to a boil; then lower heat and cook, stirring constantly, for about 3 min-

utes. Pour the mixture over the beets and let cool. Cover
the container and refrigerate. The flavors will improve each
day as the beets continue to marinate. (The beets will keep
refrigerated for at least 2 weeks.)

YIELD: 2 CUPS   CALORIES: 74/½ CUP

2 DINNER MENU

VEGETABLE CURRY I or *II served over Hot Brown Rice*
             CUCUMBERS WITH YOGURT or *CHILLED*
             CUCUMBER SOUP*
             MINT CHUTNEY**
             CHAPATIS***

TIMESAVERS:
* Omit cucumber recipe and substitute a simple tossed green salad.
** Omit chutney and serve the curry with slices of fresh fruit such as mango, papaya, or pineapple.
*** Omit *Chapatis* and substitute oven-warmed pita-bread halves.

LEFTOVER SUGGESTIONS:
Reheat the curry and serve plain or over rice.
Chilled Cucumber Soup keeps well for several days (but *Cucumbers with Yogurt* is best when eaten shortly after preparation).

WEIGHT-LOSS SUGGESTIONS:
Omit the rice.
Omit *Chapatis* or pita bread.

VEGETABLE CURRY

Two versions are offered, based on different vegetable combinations and somewhat different spicing. Both are moderately hot, suitable for use as an entrée, plain or over rice. If you like a hotter curry, or plan to serve smaller portions as a side dish alongside fairly bland foods, increase the curry powder in each recipe by half.

I.

2 cups sliced onions
⅓ cup vegetable stock or defatted chicken stock
1½ tablespoons curry powder

½–1 tablespoon soy sauce
2 teaspoons ground cumin
Dash cayenne pepper
1 eggplant, peeled and cut into 1-inch cubes
3 carrots, thinly sliced
1 large green pepper, thinly sliced
3 cloves garlic, minced or crushed
3 cups chopped tomatoes
⅓ cup raisins
2 tablespoons canned tomato paste
½ cup frozen green peas, rinsed in hot water and drained

In a large skillet, dry-sauté the onions over moderate heat until softened; remove them from the skillet and set aside. Bring the stock to a boil in the skillet, reduce the heat, and stir in the curry powder, soy sauce, cumin, and pepper. Add the eggplant, carrots, green pepper, and garlic. Return to a boil; then lower the heat to moderate and cook, stirring frequently, for about 15 minutes, or until vegetables are tender. Stir in the tomatoes, raisins, and tomato paste; cover, and simmer for about 5 minutes, stirring occasionally. Mix in the onions and green peas, and heat thoroughly.

MAKES 5 SERVINGS   CALORIES: 159/SERVING

II.

In this version, potatoes, cauliflower, green beans, and carrots are used. If desired, you could substitute other vegetable combinations, including bell pepper and eggplant, but keep the total number of cups of vegetables constant.

1 tablespoon turmeric
1 tablespoon whole-wheat pastry flour
2½ cups peeled and diced potatoes
2½ cups cut green beans
1½ cups cauliflower florets
¾ cup carrot strips (about 2 inches long)
1½ cups vegetable stock or water, divided
3 onions, chopped
2 apples, peeled and sliced

1 tablespoon curry powder
2 cups canned tomatoes, chopped, with juice
1½ teaspoons ground coriander
1 cup home-cooked or canned garbanzo beans, drained

Mix the turmeric and flour together in a large bowl. Add the vegetables and toss to coat lightly with the mixture. Place ⅔ cup of the stock in a large skillet, bring to a boil, and add the vegetables. Return to a boil, then reduce heat and stir-fry the vegetables for 3–4 minutes. Remove the vegetables from the skillet and set them aside. Add another ⅓ cup stock to the skillet with the onion and apple and stir-fry 3–4 minutes. Add the curry powder and continue to stir-fry another 2–3 minutes. Stir in the tomatoes, remaining stock, coriander, vegetables, and garbanzos. Bring to a boil, lower the heat, and simmer, covered, about 25 minutes or until the vegetables are tender, stirring occasionally to prevent sticking. If the skillet gets too dry, add a little more stock or water.

MAKES 6 SERVINGS   CALORIES: 211/SERVING

CUCUMBERS WITH YOGURT

¾ cup nonfat yogurt
¼ cup finely cut green onions
2½ tablespoons chopped fresh mint or 1 tablespoon
   dried mint
2 tablespoons lemon juice
1 clove garlic, crushed to a paste
1 cucumber, peeled and thinly sliced or diced

Combine the yogurt with all the ingredients except the cucumber, stirring to mix well. Add the cucumber (drain the cucumber first if watery) and toss thoroughly. If not served immediately, keep chilled in refrigerator and stir a few times to restore smooth consistency, if necessary, just before serving.

MAKES 4 SERVINGS   CALORIES: 32/SERVING

CHILLED CUCUMBER SOUP

4 cucumbers, peeled, seeded (if there are coarse, large seeds),
  and chopped
1 small onion, chopped
2 cups defatted chicken stock, divided
1 teaspoon dillweed
1 teaspoon basil
Dash cayenne pepper
1 teaspoon grated lemon rind
2 cups nonfat yogurt

Place the chopped cucumbers and onions in a skillet with 1
cup of the stock. Bring to a boil, lower the heat, and simmer,
covered, for 10 minutes. Transfer the skillet contents to a
blender, add the rest of the stock and the dried spices, and
blend until pureed. Pour the mixture into a bowl and, when
cooled, stir in the lemon rind and yogurt.

YIELD: ABOUT 7 CUPS   CALORIES: 56/CUP

MINT CHUTNEY

2 tablespoons lemon juice
1½ cups chopped fresh mint (loosely packed)
2 green onions, coarsely chopped
1 fresh green chile, seeded and coarsely chopped
1 tablespoon grated fresh ginger

Place lemon juice in a blender and blend in mint, a little at a
time. Add the other ingredients and continue blending until
mixture is smooth.

YIELD: ABOUT ½ CUP   CALORIES: 16/TABLESPOON

CHAPATIS

1 cup whole-wheat pastry flour
Pinch salt
½ cup water

Combine the flour and salt in a bowl. Add the water gradually, stirring to form a firm dough. Transfer the dough to a floured bread board and knead for 5 minutes. Roll the dough into a ball and cover with a damp cloth. Set aside to rest for 30 minutes or more. (You can leave the dough in the refrigerator overnight, if desired.)

Divide the dough into 6 pieces, forming each piece into a ball. Cover again with a damp cloth. Shape and bake one piece at a time before starting the next, according to the following procedures. Place the ball of dough on a floured bread board or countertop, and using a rolling pin, flatten it into a circle. Roll from the center of the circle to the edges, applying equal pressure on all sides to form a circle about 8 inches in diameter. Place it on a nonstick baking pan and set under a broiler to bake and brown for 1–2 minutes. Keep the oven door ajar and watch closely to avoid overbrowning. Turn the chapati and brown the other side, again watching closely. Repeat procedure with the other dough balls until all are baked.

YIELD: 6 CHAPATIS   CALORIES: 75/CHAPATI

3 DINNER MENU

*OVEN-BAKED BREADED FILLET OF SOLE served with
SPICY FISH SAUCE**

> *MASHED POTATOES** and Steamed Green
> Cabbage Wedges, or COLCANNON***
> *BAKED WINTER SQUASH WITH RAISIN
> SAUCE****
> *Tossed Green Salad*

TIMESAVERS:

* Omit *Spicy Fish Sauce* or serve fish with bottled hot sauce.

** Omit *Mashed Potatoes* or *Colcannon,* but boil potatoes (as directed in either of those recipes) or steam them and serve whole or halved. (Steamed new potatoes in their jackets would be excellent.) Serve steamed green cabbage wedges alongside the potatoes.

*** Prebake squash, as directed, earlier in the day or when starting meal preparations; return it to the oven with the sauce to finish baking when the fish is in the oven. If desired, omit the sauce and finish baking with only a sprinkling of pumpkin-pie spice; or substitute baked yam or sweet potato for the squash.

LEFTOVER SUGGESTIONS:

Use leftover fish for sandwiches.

Make potato patties with leftover *Colcannon* (especially delicious with *Colcannon*) or *Mashed Potatoes*. For every 2 cups leftovers, mix in 1 fork-beaten egg white, ¼ cup matzo meal, some onion powder, and a little pepper. Form into patties 3–4 inches across (they should be rather flat) and dip the bottom surface into additional matzo meal to prevent them from sticking while baking. Arrange patties on a nonstick pan and bake in a 400° oven for about 25–30 minutes, or until browned. Serve with leftover *Spicy Fish Sauce,* bottled hot sauce, or prepared mustard.

Eat leftover squash hot or cold.

WEIGHT-LOSS SUGGESTIONS:
Omit potato dish and substitute an extra serving of cabbage.
Omit *Raisin Sauce* on the squash, using only the sprinkling
of pumpkin-pie spice.

OVEN-BAKED BREADED FILLET OF SOLE

*We wanted to devise a recipe that was as close as possible
to the fried fish fillets most people adore. This is the excellent result.*

BREADING:
⅓ cup whole-wheat pastry flour
¼ cup canned evaporated skim milk
2 egg whites, whisked
1 teaspoon lemon juice
1 teaspoon onion powder
¼ teaspoon garlic powder
1⅓ cups fine whole-wheat bread crumbs (from acceptable
    bread), sprinkled with 1 teaspoon onion powder

About 8 fillets of sole (total weight about 1 pound)

Combine all the breading ingredients except the bread
crumbs in a shallow bowl; stir well to mix. Place the seasoned bread crumbs in another shallow bowl. Coat the fillets
by dipping them, one by one, in the flour mixture and then
in the bread crumbs, covering both sides. Arrange the fillets
in a nonstick baking pan. Bake uncovered in a 350° oven for
about 30–35 minutes (the breading should be browned and
crisp-looking). Serve plain or with *Spicy Fish Sauce*
(below).

MAKES 4 SERVINGS   CALORIES: 172/SERVING
                          FISH: 4 OUNCES

SPICY FISH SAUCE

½ cup canned green chile salsa
2 tablespoons water
1 tablespoon prepared mustard

1½ teaspoons frozen apple-juice concentrate
1 teaspoon soy sauce
1 teaspoon chile powder
½ teaspoon cornstarch
Dash Tabasco

Combine all ingredients in a saucepan, mixing well. Bring to a boil, stirring constantly, reduce heat and continue cooking until the mixture thickens. Serve hot or cold with fish.

YIELD: ⅔ CUP   CALORIES: 6/TABLESPOON

MASHED POTATOES

4 large boiling potatoes
¾ cup canned evaporated skim milk (preferred) or nonfat milk, heated
2 teaspoons lemon juice
1 teaspoon soy sauce
1 tablespoon onion powder
1 teaspoon dillweed

Place the unpeeled potatoes in a large saucepan and cover them with water. Bring to a boil, lower the heat, and simmer, partially covered, until tender (about 35–45 minutes). Remove the potatoes from the pot, cool briefly, and peel. Mash them with a potato masher and whip in the milk and seasonings; beat until the potatoes are fluffy, using an electric or hand mixer. Mound the mashed potatoes into a casserole dish and serve hot.

MAKES 4 SERVINGS   CALORIES: 191/SERVING

COLCANNON
(Mashed Potatoes with Cabbage)

Even the Irish get tired of plain potatoes. Two of their staple foods—potatoes and cabbage—are combined with excellent results in this recipe.

3 large boiling potatoes
½ teaspoon soy sauce
1 cabbage, cored and shredded
½ cup nonfat milk, heated
1 tablespoon lemon juice
2 teaspoons onion powder
2 tablespoons dried parsley

Place the potatoes in a large saucepan and cover them with water. Bring to a boil; then lower the heat and simmer, cover ajar, until tender (about 35–45 minutes). Remove the potatoes from the pot and set aside to cool briefly. In a large skillet, bring ½ cup water to a boil and stir in the soy sauce. Add the cabbage, stirring constantly over moderate heat for about 10 minutes or until tender. Peel the potatoes and mash them together with the milk, lemon juice, onion powder, and 1 tablespoon of the parsley; whip until fluffy using an electric or hand mixer. Beat in the cabbage and mound the mixture into a casserole dish. To garnish, make a 1-inch depression in the center of the casserole with the back of a spoon; fill with the remaining parsley. Serve hot.

MAKES 6 SERVINGS   CALORIES: 119/SERVING

BAKED WINTER SQUASH WITH RAISIN SAUCE

About 1½ pounds winter squash (whole or piece), such as butternut squash, banana squash, or other varieties

RAISIN SAUCE:
¼ cup frozen apple-juice concentrate
1 tablespoon pectin
1 teaspoon arrowroot
½ cup raisins
Sprinkling of pumpkin-pie spice

If a whole squash is used, cut it in half lengthwise and seed it. Place the squash, cut side down, in a baking dish. Set in a 400° oven to bake uncovered for 45 minutes. Pour the pan juice into a saucepan (there should be ¼ cup juice or more). Add the apple juice, pectin, arrowroot, and raisins. Cook until thickened, stirring constantly, for about 3–4 minutes. Turn the squash cut side up and pour the sauce over the top; sprinkle with pumpkin-pie spice. Bake the squash an additional 20 minutes at 350° or until the sauce appears to be "set" in the squash. (If the pan bottom becomes too dry, add a few tablespoons of water.)

MAKES 4 SERVINGS   **CALORIES: 153/SERVING**

4 DINNER MENU

CARROT-LEEK SOUP* or ORANGE-CARROT SOUP*
   JADE EMPRESS CHICKEN and Hot Brown
   Rice or
      CHINESE SESAME-CHICKEN SALAD and
      SNOW PEA AND RICE SALAD**

TIMESAVERS:
* Omit the soup.
** Omit *Snow Pea and Rice Salad* and substitute plain rice,
bread, or rolls.

LEFTOVER SUGGESTIONS:
Any of the foods can be eaten as leftovers. The chicken
salad loses a little of its eye appeal after the first day, but
retains good taste and texture.

WEIGHT-LOSS SUGGESTIONS:
Omit rice or rice salad and substitute a large serving of a
steamed green vegetable or steamed vegetable combination.
Snow peas, bok choy, asparagus, green beans, and bean
sprouts would be good choices singly or in combinations.

CARROT-LEEK SOUP

*Serve it hot or serve it cold; either way it's delicious and
different.*

> 3 cups defatted chicken stock, divided
> 1 cup sliced leeks, white part only
> 1 teaspoon grated fresh ginger
> 6 carrots (about 1 pound), thinly sliced
> Dash cayenne pepper

> GARNISH: minced parsley

Heat 1 cup of the stock in a large saucepan. Add the leeks,
ginger, and carrots, and cook and stir over medium heat
until the leeks are soft. Cover, and simmer over low heat
until the carrots are tender (about 30–35 minutes). Transfer

the mixture to a blender and blend until pureed. Return the puree to the saucepan and stir in the remaining 2 cups stock and the pepper, mixing well. Bring to a boil; then lower heat and simmer, covered, for 3 minutes. Serve hot or chilled, garnishing individual serving bowls with a sprinkling of minced parsley.

YIELD: 5 CUPS   CALORIES: 62/CUP

VARIATION: ORANGE CARROT SOUP
Add ½ cup orange juice to the soup together with the remaining 2 cups of chicken stock. Proceed as directed above.

YIELD: 5½ CUPS   CALORIES: 67/CUP

JADE EMPRESS CHICKEN

½ cup dry sherry
½–1½ tablespoons soy sauce
1 teaspoon grated fresh ginger
3 cloves garlic, minced or crushed
2 small boneless chicken breast halves, skinned and cut in 1-inch cubes
½ cup defatted chicken stock
1½ cups sliced mushrooms
1½ cups sliced celery
1 cup coarsely chopped onions
1 large green pepper, cut in chunks
2 8-ounce cans unsweetened pineapple chunks, juice-packed
2 tablespoons arrowroot
¾ cup sliced green onions

Combine the sherry, soy sauce, ginger, and garlic in a bowl. Place the chicken cubes in the mixture and marinate in the refrigerator for several hours or overnight. In a large skillet, bring the stock to a boil. Add the mushrooms and stir-fry for 2 minutes. Add the celery, onions, and green pepper and stir-fry an additional 2 minutes. Stir in the chicken and marinade, and cook until the chicken is opaque, about 2 minutes. Drain the pineapple, reserving the juice, and cut the chunks into thirds, setting them aside. Combine ¾ cup of the juice with the arrowroot. Stir the mixture into the skillet and cook, stirring constantly, until thickened. Fold in the pineapple and ½ cup of the green onions. Garnish with the remaining green onions. Serve over hot brown rice.

MAKES 4 SERVINGS   CALORIES: 276/SERVING
                          POULTRY: 4 OUNCES/SERVING

CHINESE SESAME-CHICKEN SALAD

Chinese cooks like to cut the cooked chicken with the grain into thin shreds for recipes of this type. The lettuce and green onions too should be shredded to give this dish its proper character.

2 tablespoons sesame seeds
2 cups finely shredded cooked chicken breasts
2 tablespoons hot Chinese-type dry mustard
1½ teaspoons garlic powder
1 teaspoon onion powder
¼ cup orange juice
2 teaspoons soy sauce
2 cups finely chopped celery
2 cups finely shredded green onions cut into 1½-inch lengths
½ cup coarsely chopped fresh cilantro (Chinese or Mexican
     parsley)
5 cups shredded crisp iceberg lettuce

GARNISH: orange slices, tomato wedges, cilantro sprigs

Toast the sesame seeds until lightly browned by placing them in a small pan in a moderately hot oven for a few minutes; let them cool. Put the chicken in a bowl and sprinkle it with the mustard, garlic and onion powders, orange juice, soy sauce, and sesame seeds; toss well. Place the chicken in the refrigerator to marinate and chill. Meanwhile, prepare the celery, green onions, cilantro, and lettuce. Stir the celery, green onions, and cilantro into the marinated chicken. Arrange the lettuce on a flat platter and mound the chicken salad over it. Garnish the platter with orange slices, tomato wedges, and cilantro sprigs.

MAKES 4 SERVINGS   CALORIES: 241/SERVING
POULTRY: 4 OUNCES (RAW WEIGHT)

SNOW PEA AND RICE SALAD

Pectin in the dressing substitutes for oil, giving the salad a glossiness as well as a little extra tang. You'll find pectin in all supermarkets. (It's an ingredient used in making jams and jellies.) If you use frozen snow peas, the package will probably say "Chinese pea pods."

4 cups cooked long-grain brown rice, cold
¾ cup coarsely cut fresh snow peas (or 1 6-ounce package frozen snow peas, thawed and well drained)
⅔ cup chopped green onions
¼ cup minced parsley
¼ cup diced red bell pepper or 1 2-ounce jar chopped pimiento

DRESSING:
¼ cup orange juice
2 tablespoons rice vinegar
1 tablespoon pectin
2 teaspoons soy sauce

Combine the rice and vegetables, tossing to mix well. In a separate container, mix the dressing ingredients thoroughly. Pour the dressing over the rice and vegetables, tossing well. Serve chilled.

YIELD: ABOUT 6 CUPS   CALORIES: 134/CUP

5 DINNER MENU

MEXICAN RED BEANS* or MEXICAN BLACK BEANS* or
TURKEY CHILI*

CORN BREAD**
Baked Sweet Potato or Yam
SALAD SALSA or Tossed Green Salad

TIMESAVERS:
* Soak and cook the beans earlier in the day or in the preceding day, or use cooked beans that have been stored in
the freezer and thawed.
** Choose the faster-cooking of the two corn bread recipes,
Basic Corn Bread, or substitute warmed leftover brown rice
and oven-warmed corn tortillas.

LEFTOVER SUGGESTIONS:
Reheat either of the bean dishes or the chili, or freeze for
later meals. Consider doubling the recipe when making bean
dishes; it is little trouble to do so and well worth the effort.
Leftover beans are like money in the bank—so useful! Try
some of the ideas below for use with leftover beans. The
first requires leftover corn bread; the others use packaged
corn tortillas.

Corn Bread–Bean Casserole: Cut leftover corn bread in
half horizontally, arranging the pieces in a baking pan.
Cover with leftover beans, and top with canned tomato
sauce that has been seasoned with a little ground cumin
and garlic powder. (Leftover spaghetti sauce or *Eggplant-
Tomato Stew,* page 279, are also suitable sauces.) Bake uncovered for 15 minutes in a hot oven, removing the cover
near the end.

Taco: Heat a corn tortilla in a hot oven until it is hot and
still a little soft. Place a few tablespoons of hot beans in the
center, fold in half, then stuff in a topping of shredded lettuce and chopped tomatoes, onions or green onions, and, if
you have it, cilantro. Add a few drops of bottled hot sauce
or taco sauce and a dollop of nonfat yogurt over the vegetables for additional flavor. Eat out of hand, sandwich style.

Tostada: Heat a corn tortilla in a hot oven until it is lightly browned and rather crisp. Pile a few tablespoons of hot beans in the center, and top with raw vegetables and condiments as for the taco (above). Eat out of hand like an open-faced sandwich.

Burrito: Make "bean rolls" by placing hot beans in the center of an oven-warmed (but still soft) corn tortilla and rolling up, tucking in the ends to seal securely. Accompany with tossed green salad. If you wish, wrap each bean roll individually in aluminum foil for use later in home or take-out lunches. Bean rolls may be frozen, then reheated in an oven.

WEIGHT-LOSS SUGGESTIONS:
Beans, corn bread, and sweet potato or yam are all relatively high-calorie foods. Reduce the total calories of the meal by omitting the corn bread and sweet potato or yam, substituting steamed vegetables such as broccoli, green beans, or carrots. Or make low-calorie tacos or tostadas using a minimum of beans and lots of raw vegetables.

MEXICAN RED BEANS

2 cups dried red beans
1 large onion, chopped
1 7-ounce can green chile salsa
2 teaspoons ground coriander
1 teaspoon each: onion powder, garlic powder, and chile powder
Dash cayenne pepper

Put the beans in a large pot and cover them with water (about 6 cups). Bring to a boil, lower heat, and cook for 5 to 10 minutes. Turn off the heat, cover, and let the beans soak for about an hour. Add the other ingredients and bring to a boil; set cover ajar and simmer until the beans are tender (approximately an hour), stirring occasionally to prevent sticking. (If the beans seem too dry near the end of the cooking period, add a little more water.)

YIELD: ABOUT 6 CUPS (4–6 SERVINGS)   CALORIES: 237/CUP

THE PRITIKIN PROMISE
MEXICAN BLACK BEANS

2 cups dried black beans
1 large onion, chopped
1 green pepper, chopped
⅓ cup coarsely chopped fresh cilantro (Mexican or Chinese parsley)
3 large cloves garlic, minced or crushed
1 7-ounce can green chile salsa
1½ tablespoons ground cumin
2 teaspoons ground coriander
½ teaspoon oregano
½ cup canned tomato sauce

Place the beans in a large pot with 7 cups of water. Bring to a boil, lower the heat, and cook for 5 to 10 minutes. Turn off the heat, cover, and let the beans soak for about an hour. Add the other ingredients to the pot, except the tomato sauce. Heat to boiling; then reduce the heat to low and simmer beans, with cover ajar, until they are very tender (about an hour). Stir occasionally to prevent sticking, and add a little water to the pot toward the end of the cooking period if the beans seem too dry. Stir in the tomato sauce and simmer another 5 minutes.

YIELD: ABOUT 6 CUPS (4–6 SERVINGS)   CALORIES: 271/CUP

TURKEY CHILI

This is a simplified and improved version of a recipe that appeared in an earlier Pritikin book. Turkey Chili is a delicious dish, very suitable for freezing. It should be made with freshly ground turkey.

3½ cups defatted chicken or turkey stock, divided
1¼ cups ground raw turkey breast
1–2 tablespoons soy sauce
2 tablespoons chile con carne seasoning
2 tablespoons ground cumin
1 tablespoon onion powder
1 tablespoon garlic powder

1 teaspoon ground coriander
¼ teaspoon allspice
Dash cayenne pepper
1⅔ cups chopped onions
½ cup chopped green pepper
4 cloves garlic, minced or crushed
1 cup cooked pinto beans
1 cup cooked kidney beans
1 16-ounce can diced tomatoes in juice
1 15-ounce can tomato sauce
1½ teaspoons oregano

Heat ½ cup of the stock to a boil in a skillet. Add the ground turkey and the soy sauce; then sprinkle all the dried seasonings, except the oregano, over the turkey. Stir-fry over moderate heat for about 10 minutes, or until the turkey is cooked, using the back of the mixing spoon to break up clumps of turkey. Set the skillet aside. In a large pot, bring the rest of the stock to a boil. Add the onions, green pepper, and garlic; lower the heat, and cook the vegetables about 5–7 minutes over moderate heat until softened. Chop the pinto beans a bit and add them to the pot together with the kidney beans, tomato products, oregano, and cooked turkey and juices in the skillet. Simmer the chili uncovered over low heat for about 15 minutes, stirring frequently.

YIELD: 9 CUPS

CALORIES: 152/CUP
POULTRY: 1 OUNCE/CUP

CORN BREAD

A hearty corn bread makes a wonderful accompaniment to bean dishes and soups. Two versions are provided. The sweet and spicy Chili Corn Bread *has a definite Mexican flavor. Serve them hot from the oven.*

BASIC CORN BREAD

1½ cups sifted whole-grain yellow cornmeal
¾ cup whole-wheat pastry flour or finely ground corn flour
1 tablespoon baking powder

1 teaspoon baking soda
1 teaspoon onion powder
1 cup skimmed buttermilk
¼ cup frozen apple-juice concentrate
3 egg whites

Combine the dry ingredients, stirring to mix well. Stir in the other ingredients, except the egg whites. Beat the egg whites until soft peaks form; fold them into the batter. Transfer the batter to a nonstick 8-by-10-inch baking pan and bake uncovered for 20 minutes in a 400° oven. Remove from oven and cover pan with foil. Let cool; then cut into squares.

YIELD: 16 SQUARES　　　　　　**CALORIES: 78/SQUARE**

CHILI CORN BREAD

1½ cups sifted whole-grain yellow cornmeal
¾ cup whole-wheat pastry flour or finely ground corn flour
1 tablespoon baking powder
1 teaspoon baking soda
1 tablespoon chile powder
1 teaspoon ground cumin
1 teaspoon Schilling-brand Mexican seasoning, or increase
　chile powder and cumin by ½ teaspoon each
1 teaspoon ground coriander
½ cup seeded, chopped fresh green chiles
1 small onion, finely chopped
¾ cup frozen apple-juice concentrate
¾ cup skimmed buttermilk
¼ cup canned tomato sauce
3 egg whites

Combine the dry ingredients, mixing well. Add the other ingredients, except the egg whites, and mix again. Beat the egg whites until soft peaks form; fold them into the batter. Transfer the batter to a nonstick 8-by-10-inch baking pan, cover the pan with aluminum foil, and place in a 400° oven to bake. Remove the foil after 20 minutes and continue baking for an additional 15 or 20 minutes. Remove from oven and cover pan with foil. Let cool; then cut into squares.

YIELD: 16 SQUARES   CALORIES: 98/SQUARE

SALAD SALSA

This unusual recipe combines the flavors and textures of salsa and salad in one easily prepared dish. Serve it as a salad, as a raw-vegetable topping for bean tacos or other tortilla-based dishes, or by itself as a filling rolled in an oven-warmed corn tortilla, for a quick snack.

    1 head iceberg lettuce, finely shredded
    3 ripe tomatoes, diced
    1¼ cups chopped green onions
    ½ cup finely chopped fresh cilantro (Mexican or Chinese
        parsley)
    ½ jalapeño chile, seeded and finely minced
    3 cloves garlic, minced or crushed
    ½–1 tablespoon soy sauce
    1 teaspoon each garlic powder and onion powder
    ½ teaspoon ground cumin

Combine the lettuce, tomatoes, green onions, and cilantro. In a separate container, mix together the jalapeño chile, garlic, soy sauce, and spices. Add the seasoning mixture to the salad vegetables and stir gently but thoroughly. Serve chilled.

YIELD: ABOUT 8 CUPS   CALORIES: 32/CUP

6 DINNER MENU

*CHICKEN AND POTATOES IN MUSHROOM-TOMATO
SAUCE or BREADED CHICKEN WITH TOMATO-CHEESE
                SAUCE
                with Boiled, Baked, or MASHED POTATOES
                (page 243)
                ROMAINE SUCCOTASH**
                or *Tossed Green Salad*

TIMESAVERS:
* Substitute frozen lima beans and corn sprinkled with dried
dillweed.

LEFTOVER SUGGESTIONS:
Reheat cooked dishes. For suggestions for leftover baked
potatoes, see pages 206 and 209.

WEIGHT-LOSS SUGGESTIONS:
Omit potatoes and substitute steamed zucchini wedges.
Omit the lima beans from *Romaine Succotash*, substituting
another quart of the cut strips of romaine.

CHICKEN AND POTATOES IN MUSHROOM-TOMATO SAUCE

    5 potatoes (boiling variety)
    ½ cup whole-wheat pastry flour
    ½ teaspoon paprika
    5 small boneless chicken breast halves, skinned
    1¼ cups defatted chicken stock
    1 large onion, chopped
    ¾ cup chopped mushrooms
    ½ cup chopped green pepper
    ½ cup chopped celery
    3 large cloves garlic, minced or crushed
    ½–1 tablespoon soy sauce
    ⅛ teaspoon cayenne pepper
    ½ cup dry white wine
    1 16-ounce can diced tomatoes in juice

Place the potatoes in a pot of boiling water and cook for about 25 minutes over moderate heat until partially done. Remove the potatoes from the pot and cool briefly; peel and halve lengthwise. Combine the flour and paprika in a shallow bowl, mixing well. Coat the chicken breasts with the flour mixture, one at a time, by rolling them in the flour. Shake off excess flour and set the chicken aside.

Bring the chicken stock to a boil in a large skillet. Add the onion, mushrooms, green pepper, celery, and garlic. Cook the vegetables over moderate heat for 5 minutes, stirring occasionally; then add the soy sauce, pepper, and chicken breasts. Cover and simmer for 5–10 minutes, stirring if needed. Stir in the wine and tomatoes. Bring the sauce to a boil; then lower the heat. At this stage, if desired, the skillet contents may be transferred to a baking dish for oven-baking. In either case, arrange the potatoes around the chicken, cover, and simmer (or bake at 325°) for 25 minutes, or until the chicken and potatoes are tender. Stir occasionally, basting the chicken and potatoes with the sauce.

MAKES 5 SERVINGS

CALORIES: 338/SERVING
POULTRY: 4 OUNCES/SERVING

BREADED CHICKEN WITH TOMATO-CHEESE SAUCE

TOMATO-CHEESE SAUCE:
½ onion, coarsely chopped
2 cloves garlic, coarsely chopped
½ teaspoon dillweed
1 cup canned tomato sauce
1 cup canned crushed tomatoes in puree
3 tablespoons canned tomato paste
¼ cup dry white wine
2 tablespoons grated Sapsago cheese
1½ teaspoons basil
½ teaspoon oregano

5 small boneless chicken breast halves, skinned
⅓ cup nonfat milk or canned evaporated skim milk
1 cup fine whole-wheat bread crumbs (from acceptable bread)

THE PRITIKIN PROMISE

Place the onion, garlic, dill, and tomato sauce in a blender and blend at low speed for about a minute. Add the other tomato products and the wine. Lightly brown the cheese by placing it in a small aluminum-foil holder and setting it in a hot oven for a few minutes. Add the cheese to the blender. Blend the sauce mixture until smooth and transfer to a saucepan. Stir in the basil and oregano, and cook over medium heat for 5 minutes. Spread 1 cup of the sauce in a baking dish, reserving the rest of the sauce.

Dip the chicken breasts in the milk, then roll in the bread crumbs, covering well. Arrange breasts in the baking dish; pour the remaining sauce over them. Cover the dish and bake in a 350° oven for an hour.

MAKES 5 SERVINGS

CALORIES: 220/SERVING
POULTRY: 4 OUNCES/SERVING

ROMAINE SUCCOTASH

If you have never cooked romaine lettuce, you will be pleasantly surprised to find that it makes a wonderful cooked green. In this recipe, it is teamed with succotash (lima beans and corn), dill (preferably fresh), and other seasonings to make an unusual and good-tasting dish. Kale or bok choy could be substituted for romaine lettuce, if you prefer.

    1 onion, diced
    1 clove garlic, minced or crushed
    1 10-ounce package frozen baby lima beans
    4 cups (packed) cut strips of romaine lettuce leaves
    ½ cup chopped fresh dill (avoid coarse stems), or 2½
        teaspoons dried dillweed
    ⅔ cup frozen corn kernels
    Juice of ½ lemon

Bring ⅓ cup water to a boil in a medium skillet. Add the onion and garlic, reduce the heat, and stir-fry them until tender. Separate the frozen beans (put them in a colander and pour warm water over them, if necessary) and add them to the skillet. Continue to stir-fry for a minute or two. Add the romaine and dill, and stir-fry another couple of minutes. Add ⅓ cup water, cover, and simmer the vegetables for 10 minutes. Add the corn and lemon juice, and simmer 5 minutes longer, stirring occasionally as required.

MAKES 5 SERVINGS   CALORIES: 104/SERVING

7 DINNER MENU

EASY BAKED FISH IN SAUCE
        ORANGE-MINT RICE*
        Steamed Green Beans sprinkled with basil
        and lemon juice
        COLE SLAW,** or BANANAS WITH
        YOGURT** and Tossed Green Salad

TIMESAVERS:
* Serve plain brown rice or baked potatoes. Start baking potatoes 15 to 20 minutes or longer before putting fish in same oven. (Medium-size potatoes bake in about 45 minutes in a 400° oven.)
** Serve only the green salad (omit either of other two dishes).

LEFTOVER SUGGESTIONS:
Reheat fish, rice, or green beans.

WEIGHT-LOSS SUGGESTIONS:
Omit the rice. Substitute steamed carrots and celery.

EASY BAKED FISH IN SAUCE

In California, we use red snapper fillets for this recipe. You could substitute varieties of rockfish (striped bass) or Eastern cod with equally good results.

    About 1½ pounds fish fillets, cut into 6 serving pieces
    ¼ cup dry white wine
    3 tablespoons orange juice
    2 tablespoons lemon juice
    1 teaspoon soy sauce
    1 teaspoon arrowroot
    1 teaspoon dillweed
    1 teaspoon onion powder
    Dash cayenne pepper
    ¼ cup chopped green onion

Arrange the fillets in a baking dish. Mix together the other ingredients, except the green onion, and pour over the fillets; sprinkle with the green onion. Cover the dish and bake in a 400° oven for about 25 minutes. Transfer the fish and sauce to a serving dish. Garnish with lemon slices and parsley sprigs.

MAKES 6 SERVINGS

CALORIES: 174/SERVING
FISH: 4 OUNCES/SERVING

ORANGE-MINT RICE

Festive-looking and good to eat, yet it can be quickly prepared using cold cooked rice (leftover is fine) and a few other simple ingredients.

¾ cup finely chopped onion
⅔ cup finely chopped celery
2 cups cooked long-grain brown rice
¼ cup orange juice
2 teaspoons finely chopped fresh mint (or 1 teaspoon dried mint)
1½ teaspoons onion powder ·
Orange slices, cut in half

Place ⅓ cup water in a medium skillet and bring to a boil. Add the onion and celery, sautéing over medium heat until the vegetables are tender and the water has evaporated. Add the rice, and continue cooking and stirring for about 2 minutes, using the back of the mixing spoon to break up any clumps of rice. Add the orange juice; stir and cook for another 1 or 2 minutes. Stir in the mint and onion powder. Transfer the rice mixture to a baking dish, stand the half-orange slices around the inside edge of the dish, cover, and bake in a 350° oven for 15 minutes. Serve warm.

MAKES 4 SERVINGS

CALORIES: 119/SERVING

THE PRITIKIN PROMISE
COLE SLAW

DRESSING:

½ cup cottage cheese, 1 percent fat (by weight) maximum
½ cup nonfat yogurt, divided
¼ cup frozen apple-juice concentrate
2 tablespoons rice vinegar
1 tablespoon lemon juice
1 teaspoon grated fresh ginger

SLAW:

2 cups shredded cabbage (coarse-grated)
1 cup shredded carrots (medium-grated)
½ cup shredded parsnips (medium-grated)
½ cup raisins
¼ cup canned unsweetened crushed pineapple, juice-packed, drained

Place the cottage cheese and half the yogurt in a blender. Add the other dressing ingredients and blend until smooth. Combine the vegetables, raisins, and pineapple and stir in the blended mixture, tossing gently. Add the remaining nonfat yogurt and toss again. Chill before serving.

MAKES ABOUT 6 SERVINGS   **CALORIES: 108/SERVING**

BANANAS WITH YOGURT

This interestingly flavored side dish, known as a raita in Indian cuisine, adds novelty and zip to the right menu. It's excellent with baked fish as well as with Indian recipes. For variation, substitute 1½ cups diced mango or melon balls for the bananas.

1 cup nonfat yogurt
½ fresh green chile, seeded and finely chopped
1½ teaspoons frozen apple-juice concentrate
½ teaspoon soy sauce
Dash cayenne pepper
2 ripe, firm bananas, peeled and sliced

Combine the yogurt with all the ingredients except the bananas, mixing thoroughly. Gently stir in the sliced bananas. Serve immediately or cover and refrigerate briefly until serving time.

MAKES ABOUT	CALORIES: 87/SERVING
4 SERVINGS	DAIRY: ½ *DAIRY SERVING*/SERVING

8 DINNER MENU

Two different menus are offered, each based on a grain entrée. The first entrée, "Fried" Rice, makes a good choice for a quick meal, served vegetarian style or, if desired, with the optional ingredient of chopped chicken.

I.
"FRIED" RICE
Baked Yam or Sweet Potato, or Baked Potato
Tossed Green Salad

II.
BULGUR WHEAT WITH CHICK-PEAS AND VEGETABLES*
BAKED EGGPLANT WITH YOGURT** and Steamed Frozen
Green Peas, or CAULIFLOWER AND PEAS**
Baked Yam or Sweet Potato, or Baked Potato
Tossed Green Salad
CHAPATIS*** (page 239)

TIMESAVERS (FOR MENU II):
* Use canned products for mushrooms, tomatoes, and chick-peas.
** Omit recipe choice and serve only steamed frozen green peas.
*** Substitute oven-warmed pita halves.

LEFTOVER SUGGESTIONS:
Reheat any of the recipes. The bulgur wheat entrée is also good eaten cold as a salad, served with a wedge of lemon.

WEIGHT-LOSS SUGGESTIONS:
If using menu I, have half serving of *"Fried"* Rice and steam a large cabbage wedge to eat alongside rice dish. If using menu II, omit *Chapatis* or pita bread. Substitute steamed greens such as kale, mustard or turnip greens, or bok choy for the potatoes on both menus.

"FRIED" RICE

Many different combinations of vegetables may be used in this recipe; just be sure to cut the pieces small enough so they cook quickly. Other choices besides those used in the recipe would be green pepper, celery, green onion, and bean sprouts. Bean sprouts should be kept whole, however, and both they and green onion should be added near the end of the vegetable cooking period.

1 teaspoon grated fresh ginger or ½ teaspoon ground ginger
½ teaspoon dry mustard
1 cup carrots, chopped in small strips
1 cup onions, coarsely chopped
1 cup broccoli, chopped in small strips
½–1 tablespoon soy sauce
2 cups cooked long-grain brown rice
½ cup chopped cooked chicken (optional)
⅓ cup raisins (optional)
⅓ cup sliced canned water chestnuts (optional)

Mix the ginger and mustard with ½ cup water, and heat the mixture to boiling in a large skillet. Add the vegetables, and stir-fry over moderate heat until tender, about 10–15 minutes. Add the soy sauce and rice, mix well, and heat thoroughly, stirring as needed. Stir in the chicken, raisins, and water chestnuts, if used, while the rice is heating.

MAKES 2 SERVINGS (AS MAIN DISH) OR 4 SERVINGS (AS SIDE DISH)   **CALORIES: 260/½ RECIPE (WITHOUT OPTIONAL INGREDIENTS)**

BULGUR WHEAT WITH CHICK-PEAS AND VEGETABLES

1½ cups vegetable stock or defatted chicken stock, divided
1 onion, chopped
3 cloves garlic, minced or crushed
2 cups coarsely chopped mushrooms (about ½ pound)
2 tomatoes, peeled and finely chopped, or 1 cup canned tomatoes
1 cup cooked, drained chick-peas (garbanzo beans), home-cooked or canned

½ cup minced fresh cilantro (Chinese or Mexican parsley)
⅓ cup seeded chopped green chiles, fresh or canned
1 teaspoon soy sauce
Dash cayenne pepper
1 cup medium- or coarse-grained bulgur wheat

In a large skillet, heat ½ cup of the stock to a boil. Add the onion, garlic, and mushrooms, and stir-fry for about 5 minutes or until the vegetables are tender. Add all the rest of the ingredients except the bulgur wheat and the remaining stock, and cook over low heat another 10 minutes, stirring frequently. Add the bulgur wheat and the remaining 1 cup stock, bring to a boil, cover, reduce heat to low, and cook for 35 minutes. (If a drier texture is preferred, place in a baking dish at the end of the cooking period and bake uncovered in a 375° oven for 10–15 minutes.)

MAKES 6 SERVINGS   CALORIES: 160/SERVING

BAKED EGGPLANT WITH YOGURT

1 large eggplant
¼ teaspoon black mustard seeds
¼ teaspoon each ground cumin and ground coriander
Dash cayenne pepper
2 cloves garlic, crushed
¼ cup nonfat yogurt

Pierce the eggplant with a fork, place it in a baking pan, and set the pan in a 400° oven. Bake for 40–50 minutes, or until the eggplant is dark and well wrinkled on the outside, and the inside is soft and thoroughly cooked. Cool briefly, then remove stem and skin. Mash the pulp in a bowl with a potato masher until smooth. Toast the mustard seeds by setting them in a hot oven (use a tiny aluminum-foil holder) or in a heated skillet until they begin to pop. Set them aside. In a skillet, bring 3 tablespoons of water to a boil; add the mustard seeds and other spices, garlic, and mashed eggplant. Cook and stir over medium heat for 5 minutes. Turn down heat to low and stir in the yogurt, mixing well. Cook, covered, for another 2–3 minutes.

YIELD: ABOUT 2½ CUPS   CALORIES: 44/½ CUP
(4–6 SERVINGS AS A SIDE DISH)

CAULIFLOWER AND PEAS

    1 head cauliflower
    ¼ teaspoon black mustard seeds
    ¼ teaspoon each: turmeric, ground coriander, and cumin
      seeds
    Dash cayenne pepper
    1 teaspoon arrowroot
    1 cup frozen green peas
    1 tablespoon lemon juice

Core the cauliflower and cut it into individual florets, cutting the larger florets in half lengthwise. Wash and drain them and set them aside. Lightly toast the black mustard seeds in a hot oven (use a tiny aluminum-foil holder) or in a hot skillet until they begin to pop. Set them aside. Heat a cup of water in a skillet and stir in the mustard seeds, turmeric, coriander, cumin seeds, and cayenne pepper. When the water is boiling, add the cauliflower, and cook, covered, over medium heat for 5–7 minutes or until the cauliflower is almost tender. Make a smooth paste of the arrowroot with 2 tablespoons of water and stir it into the skillet. Cook and stir the cauliflower for a few minutes to coat it well with the thickening liquid; continue cooking until almost all the liquid is gone. Add the peas, and cook and stir for another 4 minutes. Pour the lemon juice over all and toss lightly to mix well.

MAKES 4 SERVINGS   CALORIES: 90/SERVING

9 DINNER MENU

TURKEY BALLS IN TOMATO SAUCE or TURKEY LOAF WITH TOMATO SAUCE
Served with Whole-Wheat Noodles
CAPONATA *
Steamed Broccoli Spears
Tossed Green Salad

TIMESAVERS:
* Omit the *Caponata*.

LEFTOVER SUGGESTIONS:
Reheat the turkey dish and serve with *Mashed Potatoes* (page 243), with rice, or with the whole-wheat noodles. Or make a sandwich with the balls or loaf, adding lettuce, tomato, and cucumber, and spreading a little of the sauce on the bread. The leftover balls or loaf can also be frozen.

WEIGHT-LOSS SUGGESTIONS:
Omit the noodles. Serve with steamed, sliced crookneck squash or over steamed bean sprouts.

TURKEY BALLS IN TOMATO SAUCE

1 pound raw deboned turkey breast or turkey breast slices, ground
1½ cups whole-wheat bread crumbs (from acceptable bread)
1 cup finely chopped onions
¾ cup finely chopped green pepper
½ cup grated carrots
1 cup canned tomato sauce
¼ cup frozen apple-juice concentrate
1 teaspoon cider vinegar
1 teaspoon ground sage

TOMATO SAUCE:
3 cups canned tomato sauce
4 tablespoons canned tomato paste

1 large apple, peeled and coarsely chopped
⅓ cup sherry
Dash cayenne pepper

Combine all ingredients for the turkey balls in a bowl, mixing well. Shape into balls about 1½ inches in diameter and place them on a nonstick cookie sheet; bake in a 400° oven for about 30 minutes. To remove the turkey balls from the sheet, pour about ¼ cup water around balls onto sheet and wait 2–3 minutes; then loosen them with a spatula and transfer them to a baking dish, arranging them in a single layer.

Sauce: Place the tomato products in a saucepan. Combine the apple with ½ cup water in a blender and blend until smooth. Add the blended apple, wine, and pepper to the saucepan, stir, bring to a boil, then reduce heat and simmer over medium-low heat for 10 minutes, stirring as necessary. Pour the sauce over the turkey balls and bake uncovered in a 375° oven for 20 minutes. Serve over whole-wheat pasta, *Mashed Potatoes* (page 243), or brown rice.

YIELD: ABOUT
36 TURKEY BALLS
WITH SAUCE

CALORIES: 165/4 TURKEY BALLS AND
¼ CUP SAUCE
POULTRY: 2 OUNCES/4 TURKEY BALLS
AND ¼ CUP SAUCE

TURKEY LOAF WITH TOMATO SAUCE

1 pound raw deboned turkey breast or turkey breast slices,
   ground
2 cups whole-wheat bread crumbs (from acceptable bread)
2 egg whites, lightly beaten
1 cup chopped onions
1 cup chopped celery
1 cup chopped green pepper
¾ cup finely chopped carrots
½ cup canned evaporated skim milk
½ cup canned tomato juice
2 teaspoons ground thyme
1 teaspoon ground sage
Dash cayenne pepper

TOMATO SAUCE:

1 cup canned tomato sauce

¾ cup canned tomato paste

2 tablespoons Picante hot sauce (optional)

Place all the loaf ingredients in a large bowl and mix thoroughly. Shape into a loaf (or 2 smaller loaves) on a 10-by-14-inch nonstick pan. Cover the pan with aluminum foil shaped into a dome and set in a 400° oven for 30 minutes. Prepare the sauce by mixing the tomato sauce and tomato paste until smooth. Remove the pan from the oven and spread about half the sauce over the top of the loaf or loaves. Continue to bake, uncovered, for another 30 minutes. Transfer to a serving platter and garnish with parsley sprigs and lemon slices. Offer the rest of the sauce on the side, having spiced it up a bit, if you like, by stirring in the Picante sauce.

MAKES 10 TO   CALORIES: ABOUT 150/SERVING
12 SERVINGS   POULTRY: ABOUT 1½ OUNCES/SERVING

CAPONATA

This sweet-sour eggplant dish of Sicilian origin is good served any number of ways, besides its traditional use as part of an antipasto course (preceding pasta dishes). Serve it hot, as a side dish; or chilled as a relish or appetizer on crackers or lettuce leaves.

½ cup vegetable stock or water

⅓ cup dry white wine

2 eggplants, cubed (unpeeled)

2 onions, chopped

2 stalks celery, chopped

1 28-ounce can Italian plum tomatoes, drained, or 6 large ripe tomatoes, peeled, seeded, and quartered

2 tablespoons canned tomato paste

1 tablespoon capers

½ cup frozen apple-juice concentrate

⅓ cup red wine vinegar

Few drops Tabasco

Combine the stock and wine; place about ⅓ cup of the mixture in a large skillet and bring to a boil. Add the eggplant and sauté over moderate heat for 10–15 minutes or until tender, stirring constantly. Remove the eggplant from the skillet and set it aside. Add the remaining wine mixture and sauté the onions until soft. Stir in the celery, tomatoes, tomato paste, and capers and cook another 5 minutes, stirring as required. Add the cooked eggplant, apple juice, vinegar, and Tabasco. Continue to cook, stirring frequently, for 10–15 minutes.

MAKES 8 SERVINGS　　　　　**CALORIES: 100/SERVING**

10 DINNER MENU

TOFU-and-SNOW PEA SOUP *
> *LOBSTER SZECHUAN STYLE (or*
> *SCALLOPS or TUNA SZECHUAN STYLE)*
> *RICE WITH CHINESE VEGETABLES* **
> *Hot Corn-on-the-Cob*

TIMESAVERS:
* Omit the soup and substitute a simple tossed green salad.
** Serve plain hot brown rice.

LEFTOVER SUGGESTIONS:
Reheat any of the cooked dishes.

WEIGHT-LOSS SUGGESTIONS:
Have half serving of rice dish and omit the corn. Substitute
steamed broccoli spears.

TOFU-AND-SNOW PEA SOUP

4 cups defatted chicken stock
1 4-ounce cake tofu, cubed
¼ cup thinly sliced mushrooms
¼ cup minced green onions
¼ cup finely chopped carrot
1 large clove garlic, minced or crushed
1 teaspoon grated fresh ginger
Pinch anise
1 teaspoon soy sauce
1 cup fresh snow peas (Chinese pea pods)

Place all the ingredients except the snow peas in a saucepan.
Bring to a boil, lower the heat, and simmer, covered, for 20
minutes or until the vegetables are tender. Add the snow
peas and cook briefly until just tender. Garnish, if desired,
with additional chopped green onions.

YIELD: 4 CUPS   **CALORIES: 40/CUP**

LOBSTER SZECHUAN STYLE
(or Scallops or Tuna Szechuan Style)

While lobster may be your preferred choice for making this dish, you can also get good results by substituting 1 cup cooked scallops, coarsely shredded, or 1 cup canned tuna, coarsely flaked.

½ cup chopped dried mushrooms, soaked in water for 10–15 minutes, then drained, or ½ cup chopped fresh mushrooms
⅓ cup chopped green onions (white part only)
2 cloves garlic, minced or crushed
1 teaspoon grated fresh ginger
1 cup cooked lobster chunks, coarsely shredded
¼ teaspoon hot dried crushed red pepper (or, for a less hot sauce, use a seeded dried red pepper, removing it at end of cooking period)
1⅓ cups defatted chicken stock
¼ cup dry sherry
1 teaspoon soy sauce
1 tablespoon cornstarch

Place a medium skillet over moderate heat and add the mushrooms, onions, garlic, and ginger; stir constantly for about 1 minute. Add the lobster and pepper. Stir in the stock, bring to a boil, lower the heat, and simmer for 2 minutes. Mix the sherry and soy sauce into the cornstarch to make a smooth paste. Add the cornstarch mixture to the skillet, stirring constantly until sauce is thickened.

YIELD: 2 CUPS   CALORIES: 142/CUP
(2–3 SERVINGS)   SHELLFISH (OR FISH): 3.4 OUNCES/CUP

RICE WITH CHINESE VEGETABLES

2 cloves garlic, minced or crushed
4 stalks celery, thinly sliced
2 bunches green onions, chopped
1 8-ounce can water chestnuts, drained and sliced
1 teaspoon oregano
½ teaspoon basil
2 tablespoons grated fresh ginger

THE PRITIKIN PROMISE

¼ cup frozen apple-juice concentrate
2 tablespoons lemon juice
½–1 tablespoon soy sauce
2 cups bean sprouts
4 cups cooked long-grain brown rice

In a large skillet or wok bring ¼ cup water to a boil. Add the garlic and celery and cook over medium heat, stirring constantly, for about 2 minutes. Add the green onions and continue cooking and stirring another 2 minutes. Turn the heat low and stir in the water chestnuts, oregano, and basil Combine the ginger, apple juice, lemon juice, and soy sauce, and stir into the mixture. Add the bean sprouts and rice and mix well, continuing to cook for about 5 minutes, stirring as required, until the mixture is heated through.

MAKES 6 SERVINGS   CALORIES: 180/SERVING

11 DINNER MENU

*MOROCCAN CHICKEN AND VEGETABLE STEW
(COUSCOUS)* * or *VEGETABLE STEW and CORN BREAD
(page 253)* **
Tossed Green Salad

TIMESAVERS:
* Start the Moroccan stew earlier in the day or the preceding
day, but do not add the zucchini, green peas, raisins, and
chick-peas until ready to finish cooking. Choose fast-cooking couscous for the grain.
** Omit corn bread and serve with purchased bread of
choice.

LEFTOVER SUGGESTIONS:
Reheat either entrée.

WEIGHT-LOSS SUGGESTIONS:
Omit the cooked grain if serving the Moroccan stew; omit
the corn bread or other bread choice if serving the vegetable
stew. Substitute a steamed cabbage wedge.

MOROCCAN CHICKEN AND VEGETABLE STEW
(Couscous)

*Couscous—a wonderfully festive party dish easy enough
for the most casual meal—is also the name of the coarsely
ground form of hard wheat used to accompany the stew.
But if you wish, you could substitute other grains for couscous. Millet, also widely eaten in Africa, resembles couscous in appearance and taste (though not in texture), and
would be slightly preferable nutritionally to couscous, which
is partially refined. Look for whole hulled millet or packaged
parboiled couscous in health- or natural-food stores or spe-
cialty-food sections of supermarkets. Or you could use a
staple like bulgur wheat, brown rice, or even whole-wheat
noodles.*

    2 cups cubed raw chicken breast
    2 large onions, chopped

1 green pepper, chopped
3 carrots, cut in ½-inch rounds
2 large potatoes, peeled and cut in 1-inch chunks
4 cups chopped tomatoes or 1 16-ounce can diced tomatoes in juice
½ cup raisins
1 teaspoon soy sauce
1 teaspoon ground ginger
¼ teaspoon turmeric
⅛ teaspoon cayenne pepper
1/16 teaspoon saffron (optional)
2 cups cooked chick-peas (garbanzo beans), drained, home-cooked or canned
4 cups thickly sliced zucchini
½ cup frozen green peas
2 cups (about 1 pound) parboiled dry couscous or 1 cup uncooked hulled millet

In a large pot, place the chicken, onions, green pepper, carrots, potatoes, tomatoes, raisins, and seasonings. Add just enough water to barely cover: 2 cups if using fresh tomatoes, 3 cups if using canned tomatoes; bring to a boil, reduce heat, and simmer, covered, for 40 minutes. Add the chick-peas and zucchini and cook another 20 minutes. Just before the end of the cooking period, stir in the green peas, then turn off heat.

Cook couscous or millet, as desired, in a saucepan as follows: *Couscous:* Bring 2 cups water to a boil, turn off heat, add couscous, cover, and let stand 5 minutes. Uncover and fluff with a fork. *Millet:* Bring 3 cups water to a boil; add the millet, cover, reduce heat, and simmer for 30 minutes. Fluff with a fork before serving.

Arrange the cooked grain on a large platter, making a well in the center. Using a slotted spoon, remove vegetables and chicken and place them in and around the well, forming a mound of stew surrounded by a ring of grain. Moisten the grain ring with a little of the broth from the pot and serve the extra broth in a bowl on the side. If desired, the dish may be eaten in individual soup bowls, with lots of broth added to the servings of grain and stew. Bottled hot pepper sauce is good with the dish.

MAKES 6–8 SERVINGS

Stew
CALORIES: 300/⅛ RECIPE
POULTRY: 2 OUNCES/⅛ RECIPE

Couscous
CALORIES: 205/1 CUP COOKED

Millet
CALORIES: 150/1 CUP COOKED

VEGETABLE STEW

2½ cups defatted chicken stock or vegetable stock
4 red- or white-skinned variety boiling potatoes, peeled and
   cubed
4 carrots, coarsely chopped
3 turnips, peeled and cubed
3 tomatoes, chopped
5 stalks celery, sliced
3 onions, quartered, or 12 whole baby onions
4 cloves garlic, minced or crushed
1 7-ounce can diced green chiles, drained
1–2 tablespoons soy sauce
2 tablespoons minced parsley
1 tablespoon basil
¼ cup cornstarch
2 cups fresh or frozen green peas

Bring the stock to a boil in a large pot. Add all the other
ingredients, except the cornstarch and green peas, and simmer, covered, until tender (about 25 minutes). Stir ¼ cup
cold water into the cornstarch and mix until smooth. Add
the cornstarch paste slowly to the stew, stirring constantly
as the stew thickens. Add the green peas and simmer for a
few more minutes.

MAKES 8–10 SERVINGS   CALORIES: 132/1/10 RECIPE

12 DINNER MENU

SPICY MEXICAN LENTILS or *EGGPLANT-TOMATO STEW*
or *HEARTY LENTIL SOUP*
> *SPANISH RICE**
> *GREEN BEAN GUACAMOLE***
> Corn Tortillas, oven-warmed, for tacos,
> tostadas, or chips
> Tossed Green Salad
> or Taco Topping Raw Vegetable Assortment
> and Garnishes (shredded lettuce, diced
> tomatoes, chopped green onion, and
> shredded carrot; and nonfat yogurt and
> grated Sapsago cheese)

TIMESAVERS:
* Substitute plain brown rice or baked potato.
** Substitute steamed green beans seasoned with a little
oregano.

LEFTOVER SUGGESTIONS:
Reheat or freeze lentils, stew, soup, or rice. (The guacamole
does not freeze well.) The lentils, stew, or guacamole all
make excellent fillings for tacos for a quick meal of leftovers.

WEIGHT-LOSS SUGGESTIONS:
Omit the rice. Substitute steamed cauliflower and red or
green bell peppers.

SPICY MEXICAN LENTILS

*This dish is tremendously versatile. Serve it over rice,
baked potatoes, or even yams or sweet potatoes. Or use it
to make Mexican tacos or tostadas. For tacos, warm corn
tortillas in the oven until hot but still pliable, then spoon
some of the lentil mixture into the center of each tortilla.
Garnish with assorted chopped salad ingredients, fold in
half, and top with a dollop of nonfat yogurt and a few drops
of bottled salsa or taco sauce. For tostadas, warm tortillas*

in the oven until lightly browned and crisp, spread some of the lentil mixture on top, followed by the salad ingredients, and end with the yogurt and salsa or taco sauce. (Eat tacos as you would a regular sandwich; tostadas are eaten as open-faced sandwiches.)

> 1½ cups lentils
> 1 onion, chopped
> 5 cloves garlic, minced or crushed
> ½ cup chopped fresh cilantro (Mexican or Chinese parsley)
> ½ fresh green chile, seeded and minced; or 1 teaspoon chile powder
> 1½ teaspoons ground cumin
> 1 teaspoon ground coriander
> 1 7-ounce can green chile salsa
> 2 cups canned tomato sauce
> 2 cups water

Place all the ingredients in a pot. Bring to a boil; then reduce heat to moderate, cover, and cook until the lentils are tender (about 30–40 minutes), stirring frequently

MAKES 6–8 SERVINGS (6 CUPS)   CALORIES: 103/CUP

EGGPLANT-TOMATO STEW

A satisfying combination of vegetables that can be used in so many ways: tucked inside an oven-warmed tortilla for an instant vegetable taco; to top a baked potato, brown rice, beans, or noodles; cold over a tossed green salad; and more. Keep a supply of this basic dish in your refrigerator, if it pleases your palate.

> 1 large eggplant, peeled and diced
> 1 large green pepper, chopped
> 1 large onion, chopped
> 4 cloves garlic, minced or crushed
> 1 cup vegetable stock or water
> 1 16-ounce can diced tomatoes in juice
> ¼ cup canned tomato paste
> 1½ teaspoons soy sauce

1½ teaspoons chile powder
1 teaspoon each: garlic powder, onion powder, curry powder, and ground cumin

Place the eggplant, green pepper, onion, garlic, and ¼ cup of the stock in a large skillet. Bring the stock to a boil, lower the heat to moderate, and sauté the vegetables for approximately 10 minutes, stirring constantly. (The stock should evaporate, but the vegetables must not be permitted to scorch.) Add the remaining stock and all the other ingredients, stir well, and return to a boil. Reduce the heat to low and cook, covered, for 25 minutes.

YIELD: ABOUT 6 CUPS   CALORIES: 100/CUP

HEARTY LENTIL SOUP

5 cups vegetable stock or water
1 cup lentils
1 onion, finely chopped
1 stalk celery, finely chopped
1 carrot, finely chopped
1 clove garlic, minced or crushed
1 small green pepper, finely chopped
1 small potato, peeled and diced
2 cups canned tomato sauce
½ teaspoon curry powder
½ teaspoon basil

Combine the stock, lentils, onion, celery, carrot, and garlic in a large pot and bring to a boil. Lower the heat and simmer, covered, until the vegetables are tender, about 30 minutes. Add the green pepper, potato, tomato sauce, and spices, stir, cover again, and continue to simmer until the potatoes are cooked, about 15 minutes longer.

YIELD: ABOUT 8 CUPS   CALORIES: 125/CUP

SPANISH RICE

1 cup long-grain brown rice
1 cup chopped onions
¾ cup chopped red or green bell pepper
3 cloves garlic, minced or crushed
⅔ cup canned diced green chiles
1 cup canned tomato sauce
1 scant tablespoon ground cumin
1 teaspoon mild chile powder, or more, to taste

GARNISH: fresh cilantro or parsley sprigs

Place the rice in a large dry skillet over medium heat. Toast the rice for 3–4 minutes, stirring frequently. Add 2⅓ cups water, bring to a boil, cover, reduce heat to low, and cook for 45–50 minutes until all the water is absorbed. Turn off the heat, but leave the skillet on the burner, covered, to steam the rice for approximately 10 minutes. Do not stir.

While the rice is cooking, prepare the sauce. Bring ½ cup water to a boil in a small skillet and add the onions, bell pepper, and garlic. Sauté the vegetables, stirring frequently, for about 4–5 minutes, or until tender. Add the remaining ingredients and heat to a simmer. Let cook for about 10 minutes, stirring often. When the rice has finished steaming, add the sauce, and mix well. Serve immediately or transfer to a casserole and keep warm in a slow oven, or refrigerate, then reheat. Garnish with cilantro or parsley, if desired.

YIELD: ABOUT 5 CUPS   CALORIES: 185/CUP

GREEN BEAN GUACAMOLE

The combination of blended green beans and hard-boiled egg whites works very well in replicating the color and texture of the oil-rich avocado, which is not Pritikin-OK. The addition of Mexican spicing makes a surprisingly good "guacamole." Serve this dip with corn chips (page 398, Chip 'n' Dip), crackers, or raw vegetables, or try it as a topping for a salad. For a special snack, spread the guacamole on an oven-warmed corn tortilla, garnish as you would a taco, then roll or fold, and enjoy.

1 20-ounce package frozen green beans
3 hard-boiled eggs, yolks discarded
½ cup nonfat yogurt
¼ cup canned green chile salsa
¼ cup chopped green onions
2 tablespoons chopped celery
1 tablespoon onion powder
½ tablespoon finely chopped seeded jalapeño chile
1 teaspoon dry mustard
1 teaspoon garlic powder

Place the green beans in a steamer basket and set over boiling water in a saucepan. Cover and cook until the beans are tender. Place the beans in a colander and, using a potato masher or the back of a large spoon, press out some of the liquid so that the beans are quite dry. Place the beans in a blender with the other ingredients and blend at moderate speed until the mixture is smooth. Chill before serving.

YIELD: 2 CUPS   CALORIES: 10/TABLESPOON

13 DINNER MENU

TOMATO BOUILLON* or TOMATO ASPIC*
   TUNA-VEGETABLE CASSEROLE
   served over Whole-Wheat Noodles
   or TUNA-LINGUINE SALAD
   Hot or Chilled Steamed Asparagus Spears
   with lemon wedge
   Tossed Green Salad

TIMESAVERS:
* Omit, or serve chilled tomato juice.

LEFTOVER SUGGESTIONS:
Reheat or freeze leftover soup. *Tomato Aspic* will last for days refrigerated. Serve *Tuna-Vegetable Casserole* over toasted whole-wheat English muffins. Pack leftover *Tuna-Linguine Salad* for a takeout lunch.

WEIGHT-LOSS SUGGESTIONS:
If serving hot tuna casserole, omit noodles and substitute steamed rutabaga slices. If serving tuna salad, have small serving of salad, and supplement with steamed rutabaga.

TOMATO BOUILLON

   5½ cups canned tomato juice
   2 large tomatoes, quartered
   1 clove garlic, coarsely chopped
   1 small or medium green chile, seeded
   2 tablespoons finely chopped parsley
   ½ bay leaf
   ¼ teaspoon oregano
   ¼ teaspoon dill seed
   ¼ teaspoon curry powder

Place 4 cups of the tomato juice in a saucepan. Put the other 1½ cups in a blender with the tomatoes and garlic. Cut the chili in half and coarsely chop one half and add to the blender; finely chop the other half chili and add to the saucepan. Process the vegetables and juice in the blender at moderate speed until pureed. Transfer the blender contents to the saucepan. Add the parsley and bay leaf, bring to a boil, reduce heat, and simmer for 30 minutes. Add the seasonings and continue to simmer another 5 minutes.

YIELD: ABOUT 6½ CUPS   CALORIES: 60/CUP

TOMATO ASPIC

2 tablespoons lemon juice
2 tablespoons frozen apple-juice concentrate
2 envelopes unflavored gelatin
1 cup boiling water
1 cup canned tomato sauce
2 tablespoons cider vinegar
1½ teaspoons grated onion
⅛ teaspoon cloves
2 cups diced celery

Place the lemon juice and apple juice in a bowl. Sprinkle the gelatin over the juices; let soak a few minutes. Add the boiling water and stir to completely dissolve the gelatin. Mix in the tomato sauce, vinegar, onion, and cloves. Chill until partially set, then fold in the celery. Transfer to a 1-quart ring mold or other suitable container and chill until firm. Unmold and garnish with lettuce leaves and watercress or parsley sprigs; or cut into slices and serve on individual salad plates garnished as above.

MAKES 6–8 SERVINGS   CALORIES: 40/⅙ RECIPE

TUNA-VEGETABLE CASSEROLE

This recipe is ideal for a quick brunch, lunch, or late light supper, and is especially good over toasted whole-wheat English muffins.

3½ cups defatted chicken stock
1 large onion, chopped
½ cup chopped celery

1 green pepper, chopped
¾ cup nonfat dry milk
1½ teaspoons each: onion powder, garlic powder, tarragon, and cumin
½ teaspoon curry powder
1 2-ounce jar sliced pimiento, chopped
2 6½-ounce cans water-packed tuna, drained and flaked
3 tablespoons cornstarch
¼ cup vermouth or other dry white wine
2 cups frozen peas and carrots (10-ounce package)
3 tablespoons fine whole-wheat bread crumbs (from acceptable bread)
2½ tablespoons grated Sapsago cheese
Paprika

Bring ½ cup of the stock to a boil in a large skillet. Add the onions and celery and sauté until just tender. Add the green pepper and continue to sauté until partially cooked. Combine the dry milk and the remaining stock, stirring well to dissolve the dry milk, and add to the skillet. Stir in the spices, pimiento, and flaked tuna. Cook over medium heat, stirring occasionally, until it begins to simmer; lower the heat. Mix the cornstarch and vermouth into a smooth paste and stir into the skillet mixture. Continue to cook over low heat, stirring constantly, until thickened. Mix in the peas and carrots.

Transfer the skillet contents to a 9-by-13-inch baking dish and sprinkle with the bread crumbs, cheese, and a little paprika. Cover loosely with aluminum foil and bake in a 375° oven for 15–20 minutes, removing the foil after 10 minutes. Serve over toasted whole-wheat English muffins, whole-wheat noodles, mashed potatoes, or brown rice.

MAKES ABOUT 6 SERVINGS   CALORIES: 185/⅙ RECIPE
                                FISH: 1.7 OUNCES/⅙ RECIPE

TUNA-LINGUINE SALAD

DRESSING:
½ cup rice vinegar
⅓ cup water

1 tablespoon pectin
½–1 tablespoon soy sauce
1 teaspoon garlic powder
1 teaspoon onion powder
1 teaspoon basil
½ teaspoon curry powder
½ teaspoon arrowroot

½ cup frozen green peas
½ cup canned (water-packed) tuna, drained and flaked
4 canned (water-packed) artichoke hearts, halved
1 small red bell pepper, seeded and thinly sliced into 2-inch
    lengths, or 1 2-ounce jar sliced pimiento, drained
1 small tomato, chopped
½ cup finely chopped green onion
2 cups cooked and drained whole-wheat linguine (flat pasta
    without egg yolks), cooled

GARNISH: lettuce leaves, grated Sapsago cheese to taste
    (optional)

Put the dressing ingredients in a small bowl; beat vigorously
with a fork. Soak the frozen green peas briefly in hot water
and drain them in a strainer. Combine the tuna, peas, and
other vegetables in a large bowl. Add the dressing, tossing
gently to coat ingredients well. Mix in the noodles carefully
to avoid breakage. Chill. To serve, line an attractive dish
with lettuce and arrange the pasta salad in the center. Top
with a sprinkling of Sapsago cheese.

YIELD: ABOUT 4 CUPS   CALORIES: 130/CUP
                                       FISH: 1 OUNCE/CUP

VARIATION: LINGUINE SALAD
Follow above directions omitting tuna and Sapsago cheese.

14 DINNER MENU

TURKEY-"FRIED" STEAK or OVEN-BAKED BREADED CHICKEN

> *MASHED POTATOES (page 243)* *
> *ONION GRAVY***
> *Steamed Frozen Baby Limas*
> *Tossed Green Salad*

TIMESAVERS:
* Serve plain boiled or steamed potatoes, whole or halved; or bake potatoes in a 425° oven until partially done; then turn down heat, put in turkey or chicken, and finish baking together.
** Omit the *Onion Gravy*.

LEFTOVER SUGGESTIONS:
Reheat any of the recipes for later meals. The leftover refrigerated chicken could be used to make sandwiches.

WEIGHT-LOSS SUGGESTIONS:
Omit the potatoes and substitute cooked frozen collards, turnip greens, or kale. Omit the limas and substitute a medley of steamed zucchini, crookneck squash, and red bell pepper.

TURKEY-"FRIED" STEAK

1 cup fine whole-wheat bread crumbs (from acceptable bread)
1 tablespoon onion powder
1 teaspoon garlic powder
½ teaspoon paprika
⅛ teaspoon cayenne pepper
6 raw turkey breast slices (about 2½ to 3 ounces per slice)
½ cup canned evaporated skim milk or nonfat milk (or water)
¾ cup water
½ cup dry white wine
2 teaspoons soy sauce
1 cup defatted chicken or turkey stock or vegetable stock (or water)

Combine the bread crumbs with the dry spices and mix well. Pound the turkey slices with a mallet to tenderize them. Dip each slice in the milk, then in the bread crumbs, covering well. Reserve the leftover bread crumbs. Combine the water, wine, and soy sauce in a large skillet and bring to a boil. Lay the breaded turkey slices in the skillet and cook, covered, over medium heat for 8–10 minutes. Transfer the turkey slices to a flat casserole and sprinkle them with the leftover bread crumbs. Place the stock in the skillet, bring to a boil, stir, and pour the skillet contents over the turkey slices. Cover and bake in a 400° oven for 20 minutes. Serve hot with *Mashed Potatoes* (page 243), whole-wheat noodles, or brown rice.

MAKES 6 SERVINGS   CALORIES: 185/⅙ RECIPE
                            POULTRY: 3 OUNCES/⅙ RECIPE

OVEN-BAKED BREADED CHICKEN

You may use chicken breasts that have the bones in, or boneless breasts, for this recipe.

BREADING:

⅓ cup whole-wheat pastry flour
¼ cup canned evaporated skim milk
2 egg whites, beaten lightly
½–1 tablespoon soy sauce
1½ teaspoons lemon juice
1½ teaspoons onion powder
½ teaspoon garlic powder
Dash cayenne pepper
1⅓ cups fine whole-wheat bread crumbs (from acceptable bread), sprinkled with 1½ teaspoons onion powder

4 small chicken breast halves, skinned

Combine all the breading ingredients except the bread crumbs in a bowl; stir well to mix. Place the seasoned bread crumbs in a separate bowl. Coat each breast by dipping in the flour mixture, then in the bread crumbs, covering both sides. Arrange the chicken on a nonstick baking pan. Cover the pan with aluminum foil and bake in a 375° oven for 35 minutes. Remove foil, turn heat up to 425°, and continue baking another 15–20 minutes to crisp the coating.

MAKES 4 SERVINGS   CALORIES: 305/SERVING
                                    POULTRY: 4 OUNCES/SERVING

VARIATION: TARRAGON OVEN-BAKED BREADED CHICKEN

Sprinkle 1 teaspoon tarragon over the unbaked breaded chicken before covering pan with foil.

ONION GRAVY

Toasted dried minced onions give this gravy color, flavor, and texture.

- 1 teaspoon dried minced onions or ready-toasted dried minced onions
- 1 cup defatted chicken stock or vegetable stock, or water
- ½–1 tablespoon soy sauce
- 1 tablespoon cornstarch
- 1 tablespoon whole-wheat pastry flour
- ¼ cup nonfat dry milk

To toast dried minced onions: place them in an aluminum-foil holder in a hot oven for a few minutes, stirring as needed, until lightly browned. Put the toasted onions in a saucepan with ½ cup of the stock and the soy sauce. In a small bowl, combine the cornstarch, flour, and dry milk, and blend in the other half-cup stock, stirring until smooth. Bring the contents in the saucepan to a boil; then stir in the cornstarch mixture. Reduce heat to low and cook, stirring constantly, until the gravy is thickened. If a thinner gravy is desired, stir in another ¼ cup stock or water and simmer another minute.

YIELD: ABOUT 1 CUP   CALORIES: 30/¼ CUP

15 DINNER MENU

GARBANZO MINESTRONE*
>   *POTATO GNOCCHI IN TOMATO SAUCE***
>   or *PRITIKIN PIZZA*** or *QUICK PITA-BREAD*
>   *PIZZA***
>   Tossed Green Salad

TIMESAVERS:
* Omit the soup. If desired, substitute a side dish of cooked whole-wheat pasta topped with some of the sauce prepared for the gnocchi or pizza. (Make extra sauce for this purpose when preparing the gnocchi or pizza.)
** Make the *Quick Pita-Bread Pizza* for the fastest meal.

LEFTOVER SUGGESTIONS:
Freeze leftover sauce, pizza crust, or completed dishes. Leftover pizza is a great takeout lunch item.

WEIGHT-LOSS SUGGESTIONS:
Modify the recipe for the minestrone soup by omitting beans and noodles and increasing vegetable quantities. Have half-portions of the gnocchi or pizza, and supplement with a larger serving of the calorie-reduced soup or with steamed broccoli spears or zucchini.

GARBANZO MINESTRONE

The base of pureed garbanzo beans gives this minestrone a flavorful, smooth body that blends beautifully with the other ingredients.

> 2 cups dried garbanzo beans, or 4 cups drained canned
>   garbanzo beans (reserve liquid)
> 2 cups defatted chicken stock or vegetable stock
> 1 cup diced carrots
> 1 cup chopped celery
> 1 cup chopped onions
> 1 cup chopped green pepper
> 1½ cups diagonally sliced green beans, or frozen French-cut
>   green beans

1 16-ounce can diced tomatoes in juice
1 8-ounce can tomato sauce
1 tablespoon soy sauce
1 tablespoon garlic powder
1½ teaspoons Italian seasoning
1⅓ cups uncooked whole-wheat or corn noodles

If using dried garbanzos, place the beans in a saucepan and cover them with water (about 8 cups). Bring to a boil and cook about 10 minutes, then turn off the heat and allow beans to soak for 1 hour or more. Discard the water and replace with 8 cups fresh water. Bring to a boil, lower the heat, and simmer the beans with cover ajar until tender, about 1½ hours or longer. Drain the beans, reserving the cooking liquid, and set aside.

Place the stock and 5 cups water in a large pot. Add the carrots, celery, onions, green pepper, and green beans. (If frozen green beans are used, add them later with the tomato products.) Bring to a boil, then cook over medium heat, uncovered, until vegetables are almost tender (about 20 minutes). Stir in the tomato products, seasonings, and 2 cups of the garbanzos. Place the remaining garbanzos in a blender with 1 cup of the reserved garbanzo liquid and blend until smooth. Stir the blended mixture into the soup. Return the soup to a boil, reduce heat, and simmer until the vegetables are tender, stirring as necessary. Add the noodles about 5 minutes before the end of the cooking time

YIELD: ABOUT 14 CUPS   CALORIES: 145/CUP

POTATO GNOCCHI IN TOMATO SAUCE

These tender little dumplings take some time to prepare but are fun to make. Served with an Italian-style tomato sauce, they are a nice alternative to pasta.

1½ pounds red- or white-skinned variety boiling
    potatoes
½ cup whole-wheat pastry flour
½ cup unbleached all-purpose flour

SAUCE:

1 28-ounce can crushed tomatoes in puree
1 15-ounce can tomato sauce
1 tablespoon chopped fresh or dried basil
1 teaspoon oregano
1 teaspoon garlic powder

Place the potatoes, unpeeled, in a pot with water to cover. Bring to a boil and cook, cover ajar, over moderate heat for about 45 minutes, or until potatoes are tender but still firm. While the potatoes are cooking, prepare the sauce: simmer sauce ingredients in a saucepan for 10–15 minutes. Ladle a little of the sauce into a large baking dish, and set the baking dish and the rest of the sauce aside.

Drain the cooked potatoes and peel when cool enough to handle. While still warm, put them through a food mill or potato ricer, or use a potato masher to mash thoroughly. Mix the flours together in a small bowl; then work the flour a little at a time into the potatoes to form a smooth, firm dough. Transfer the dough to a floured bread board and knead it gently for about 4–5 minutes, adding a little more whole-wheat flour from time to time if necessary. Sprinkle a little additional flour over the dough and cut it into 4 equal pieces. Using your hands, roll out each piece into a rope about ¾ inch in diameter; then press the top surface of each rope all along its length to flatten slightly. Cut each flattened rope into 1-inch sections; then press down lightly around the cut edges of each piece with the tines of a fork.

Cook the gnocchi in approximately 3 batches in a large pot of boiling water. Lower them carefully into the boiling water, a few at a time, using a long wooden spoon to loosen any that stick to the bottom. When the gnocchi float to the surface, let them cook for another 10 seconds; then remove them with a slotted spoon, shaking off excess water. Arrange the gnocchi in the baking dish and pour over them another 1½ to 1¾ cups sauce (or more, if desired). Bake in a 350° oven, uncovered, for 15–20 minutes.

MAKES 6 SERVINGS   CALORIES: 230/SERVING

VARIATION: SPINACH-POTATO GNOCCHI IN TOMATO SAUCE

Follow the recipe for *Potato Gnocchi*, but blend into the mashed potatoes a spinach-and-onion mixture: in a dry skillet over medium heat stir-fry 4 cups chopped fresh spinach or 1 10-ounce package frozen chopped spinach (thawed) and 3 tablespoons finely minced onion. Cook until the spinach seems dry; then sprinkle with ½ teaspoon nutmeg. Transfer the cooked vegetables to a strainer and use the back of a spoon to press out any residual liquid. Stir the vegetables into the potatoes, mixing well. Proceed as for *Potato Gnocchi*.

PRITIKIN PIZZA

This first cousin to a real pizza boasts a lot of veggies and a delicious crust. Since making the crust is a bit of an operation, it's a good idea to make more than one ahead of time and freeze what you don't use. This recipe makes enough dough for 4 12–14-inch pizzas, or you can use part of the dough to make a delicious Onion Mini-Loaf, *according to the directions at the end of the pizza recipe.*

CRUST:

4 cups whole-wheat pastry flour, plus a little additional flour, if needed

1 tablespoon dried minced onions

⅛ teaspoon soy sauce

2 tablespoons (2 packages) active dry yeast

1¾ cups lukewarm water

Mix 3 cups of the flour with the onions and soy sauce in a large bowl. In a small bowl, dissolve the yeast in the water, stirring well. Stir the dissolved yeast gradually into the flour mixture; blend thoroughly. Cover the bowl with a wet tea towel and set in a warm oven. (Preheat the oven to 200°; then turn off just before putting in the bowl.) Let the dough rise for about 2 hours. Turn the dough out onto a lightly floured bread board or counter top and knead the reserved cup of flour into the dough. Continue to knead for a few minutes, adding a little additional flour, if needed to make dough workable. Divide the dough into 4 equal parts and shape into balls. (At this point you can put whatever you're not using into the freezer, or set aside half the dough to make the *Onion Mini-Loaf*.) Roll out two of the balls to fit 2 12- to 14-inch nonstick round pizza pans. Crimp the edges of the crusts and prick bottoms in several places; then place pans in a 350° oven for 5 minutes to prebake the crusts. Set the crusts aside.

PIZZA SAUCE:

½ onion, quartered
3 cloves garlic, coarsely chopped
½ teaspoon anise seed
1 15-ounce can tomato sauce
1 cup canned tomato paste
1 tablespoon onion powder
1 teaspoon each: garlic powder, Italian seasoning, and ground coriander
1 tablespoon cornstarch

Place the onion, garlic, anise seed, and tomato sauce in a blender; blend until smooth. Transfer the mixture to a saucepan and add the tomato paste and seasonings. Mix the cornstarch with 2 tablespoons cold water, stirring to make a smooth paste, and add it to the saucepan. Stir the sauce and bring it to a boil; then reduce the heat and simmer for about 10 minutes, stirring as required. Spread a generous amount of sauce on each pizza crust. Top with Vegetable-Cheese topping.

VEGETABLE-CHEESE TOPPING:

1 cup chopped onion
1 cup chopped green pepper
1 cup thinly sliced mushrooms
1 4-ounce jar sliced pimiento, chopped
1 cup dry cottage cheese, 1 percent fat (by weight) maximum, crumbled if in brick form
4 tablespoons grated Sapsago cheese

Sprinkle the vegetables, then the cottage cheese, over the pizza crusts. Top with the Sapsago cheese. Bake uncovered at 400° for about 30 minutes. Slice each pizza into 6–8 pie-shaped wedges and serve hot.

YIELD: 2 MEDIUM PIZZAS   CALORIES: 96/SLICE (⅛ PIZZA)
(6–8 SLICES PER PIZZA)

ONION MINI-LOAF:
Roll out the leftover dough and spread with about ½ cup chopped onion and 1 teaspoon garlic powder. Brush with 1 teaspoon of soy sauce, if desired. Roll over, jelly-roll fashion, and bake for 20 minutes uncovered at 400°. Wrap tightly in aluminum foil while still hot to keep soft.

QUICK PITA-BREAD PIZZA

2 large whole-wheat pita breads

SAUCE AND TOPPING:
½ teaspoon Italian seasoning
1½ cups canned tomato sauce
1 small onion, thinly sliced
1 zucchini, shredded
½ cup diced or sliced bell pepper
½ cup sliced mushrooms
½ cup sliced canned artichoke hearts, water-packed
1 cup dry cottage cheese, 1 percent fat (by weight) maximum,
   crumbled if in brick form
2 tablespoons grated Sapsago cheese

Separate each pita bread at edges to make two rounds. Place the four rounds smooth side down on a nonstick baking sheet.

Stir the Italian seasoning into the tomato sauce; spread the pita crusts with the sauce. Spread the vegetables over the crusts, then the cottage cheese and a sprinkling of Sapsago cheese. Bake the pizzas at 425°, uncovered, until bubbling hot (approximately 15 minutes).

YIELD: 4 PITA PIZZAS   CALORIES: 175/PIZZA
(2 SERVINGS AS MAIN DISH;
4 SERVINGS AS SNACK)

16 DINNER MENU

SRI LANKA CHICKEN CURRY with FRUIT CHUTNEY or
CHICKEN-FRUIT CURRY or POTATOES PUNJAB STYLE*
>   Hot Brown Rice
>   DAL (with potato entrée only) or Steamed
>   Frozen Green Peas
>   TOMATO-CUCUMBER INDIAN RELISH**

TIMESAVERS:
* Omit the *Fruit Chutney*.
** Substitute for the Indian relish sliced tomatoes and cucumbers with a dressing of lemon juice mixed with a little ground cumin and dash of cayenne pepper.

LEFTOVER SUGGESTIONS:
Reheat either of the curries, the potatoes, or the *dal,* and serve with rice.

WEIGHT-LOSS SUGGESTIONS:
Omit the rice, and green peas or *dal*. Substitute baked eggplant slices: cut unpeeled eggplant into slices about ½ inch to ¾ inch thick or into wedge-shaped pieces like thick French-fries. Mix onion powder and coriander leaves and sprinkle over the eggplant. Bake the eggplant on a nonstick baking sheet in a 400° oven for about 40–45 minutes or until cooked through and lightly browned.

SRI LANKA CHICKEN CURRY

>   2½ cups defatted chicken stock or vegetable stock
>   3 small boneless chicken breast halves, skinned and cut in 1-inch cubes
>   2 onions, chopped
>   2 potatoes, peeled and diced
>   1 green pepper, chopped
>   2 tablespoons canned tomato paste
>   2 teaspoons soy sauce
>   1 teaspoon grated fresh ginger

1 teaspoon each chile powder and curry powder
½ teaspoon each cardamom and turmeric
¼ teaspoon cloves
1 stick cinnamon (or 1 teaspoon ground cinnamon)
3 drops Tabasco (optional)
⅓ cup raisins

CONDIMENTS (optional): Nonfat yogurt, fresh or canned
unsweetened pineapple chunks, *Fruit Chutney* (page 298)

In a large skillet, bring ½ cup of the stock to a boil. Add the chicken, onions, potatoes, and green pepper, and cook over medium heat until the chicken is opaque (about 3–5 minutes). Stir in the remaining stock and the other ingredients and bring to a boil. Lower heat and simmer, uncovered, until the vegetables are tender and the mixture has desired consistency. Remove cinnamon stick. Serve with hot brown rice and condiments.

MAKES 6 SERVINGS   CALORIES: 240/SERVING
                                    POULTRY: 4 OUNCES/SERVING

CHICKEN-FRUIT CURRY

If you enjoy Indian-style food but don't like to fuss, this one-pot curry is just for you. The yogurt will break down, but the sauce looks fine by the end of the cooking period.

1½ cups defatted chicken stock or water
¾ cup finely chopped onions
3 cloves garlic, minced or crushed
3 tablespoons curry powder
2 bay leaves
4 small boneless chicken breast halves, skinned
1 cup drained canned whole tomatoes
3 apples, peeled, cored, and cut into chunks
2 slightly green bananas, peeled and cut into chunks
1 cup nonfat yogurt
1 teaspoon soy sauce (optional)
Dash cayenne pepper

Heat the chicken stock to a boil in a medium skillet. Add the onions, garlic, curry powder, and bay leaves; reduce heat to medium, and sauté the vegetables for 7–10 minutes. Add the chicken and continue to cook another 5 minutes, stirring as needed and turning the chicken once or twice. Add the remaining ingredients and simmer about 45 minutes, stirring occasionally. (The sauce will become smooth by the end of the cooking period.) Serve with hot brown rice.

MAKES 4 SERVINGS

CALORIES: 325/SERVING
POULTRY: 4 OUNCES/SERVING

FRUIT CHUTNEY

8–10 large ripe mangoes or 3 pounds apples, apricots, or other fruit
2 large dried chiles, seeded and coarsely chopped
1 cup rice vinegar
2 cloves garlic, coarsely chopped
1 teaspoon chopped fresh ginger
1 teaspoon *garam masala* (Indian spice available at specialty food stores)
1 cup unsweetened apple juice (not concentrate)
1 cup raisins, chopped
Grated lemon or orange rind (optional)

Peel the mangoes or other fruit and slice thickly, discarding the seeds. Soak the chiles in a little of the vinegar for 10 minutes. Put the chiles, undrained, in a blender with the garlic, ginger, and *garam masala* and blend. Transfer the mixture to a saucepan, add the remaining vinegar and apple juice, and bring to a boil. Lower heat and simmer, uncovered, for 15 minutes. Add the mangoes and other fruit, raisins, and lemon or orange rind, if used, and simmer until thick and syrupy. Chill.

YIELD: ABOUT 5 CUPS

CALORIES: 90/¼ CUP

POTATOES PUNJAB STYLE
(Aloo Punjabi)

This flavorful potato dish in an Indian-spiced tomato-based sauce is unique and delicious. You can cut the potatoes rather small, as for a potato salad, into large chunks, or just quartered as preferred.

    6 potatoes, red- or white-skinned boiling variety
    2 cups defatted chicken stock or vegetable stock
    ½ onion, chopped
    1 teaspoon minced or crushed garlic
    1 teaspoon grated fresh ginger
    1 16-ounce can tomatoes, pureed in electric blender
    1 8-ounce can tomato sauce
    ½ cup medium-fine-chopped fresh cilantro (Chinese or
        Mexican parsley)
    ½ teaspoon turmeric
    ½ teaspoon ground coriander
    ¼ teaspoon cayenne pepper
    1/16 teaspoon saffron (optional)
    ½ cup nonfat yogurt
    ¼ teaspoon *garam masala*, an Indian spice (or substitute
        equal parts ground cloves, cinnamon, and cardamom to
        make up ¼ teaspoon)
    ⅛ teaspoon dried mint, crushed

Peel the potatoes, cut them to the desired size, and place them with the chicken stock in a saucepan. Bring to a boil, reduce heat, and cook over moderate heat, cover ajar, until potatoes are just done. Transfer about 3 tablespoons of the stock from the saucepan to a large skillet; add the onion, garlic, and ginger, and stir-fry until soft. Add the blended tomatoes, tomato sauce, cilantro, and dried spices, except the *garam masala* and mint. Cook over low heat for a few minutes, stirring occasionally. Add the potatoes and the remaining stock from the saucepan and stir to coat the potatoes well. Stir in the yogurt, *garam masala*, and mint. Heat without boiling for a few minutes to blend flavors, stirring as needed.

MAKES 4–6 SERVINGS   CALORIES: 135/⅙ RECIPE

THE PRITIKIN PROMISE

DAL
(with yellow split peas)

Throughout India, dals—varieties of dried beans and peas cooked in an infinite number of ways—are eaten in one or another form almost every day. This version uses yellow split peas and is quite thick, although often dals are rather soupy. Use it as a side dish or accompaniment with rice.

3 cups defatted chicken stock or water, or a combination
1 cup yellow split peas
1 clove garlic, minced or crushed
¼ teaspoon black mustard seeds
¼ teaspoon each: ground cumin, ground coriander, cayenne
  pepper, and turmeric
1 tablespoon lemon juice

Heat the stock or water to a boil in a saucepan. Add the split peas and garlic and bring to a boil again. Cover, and cook over low heat until the split peas are very soft, about 30 minutes. Lightly toast the black mustard seeds by setting them in a hot oven (use a tiny aluminum-foil holder) until they begin to pop. Add them to the saucepan together with the other spices and the lemon juice, stirring to combine well. Cook uncovered for 5 minutes, stirring from time to time. (If the *dal* thickens too much upon standing, thin it with a little hot water.) Serve hot.

YIELD: ABOUT 2½ CUPS   CALORIES: 145/½ CUP
(5 SERVINGS)

TOMATO-CUCUMBER INDIAN RELISH

1 tomato
1 cucumber, peeled
2 tablespoons minced fresh cilantro (Chinese or Mexican
  parsley)
1½ tablespoons lemon juice
1 teaspoon ground cumin
Cayenne pepper to taste

Dice tomato and cucumber fine. Combine all ingredients in a bowl and mix well. Cover and refrigerate to chill thoroughly.

MAKES 4 SERVINGS　　　　　　　　　　　**CALORIES: 19/SERVING**

17 DINNER MENU

BAKED FISH WITH PLUM TOMATOES or *VERACRUZ RED SNAPPER*

> CONFETTI RICE*
> BOK CHOY (I or II) or *Steamed Cabbage*
> *Wedges*
> *Tossed Green Salad*

TIMESAVERS:
* Serve plain brown rice; or bake potatoes, starting them in a 425° oven early enough to finish baking at a lower temperature with the fish.

LEFTOVER SUGGESTIONS:
Reheat any of the recipes, or serve cold.

WEIGHT-LOSS SUGGESTIONS:
Omit the rice and substitute steamed carrot and zucchini rounds.

BAKED FISH WITH PLUM TOMATOES

SAUCE:
1 tablespoon dry white wine
¼ large onion, chopped
1 clove garlic, minced or crushed
¼ cup finely chopped parsley
1 28-ounce can Italian plum tomatoes
1 cup sliced mushrooms
1 teaspoon basil
1 bay leaf
1 teaspoon frozen orange-juice concentrate
1 tablespoon capers

1 to 1¼ pounds fillets of halibut, bass, or cod (not rock cod)
about 1 inch thick
2 teaspoons Dijon mustard
¼ cup whole-wheat pastry flour
1 tablespoon paprika
1 teaspoon dillweed

Place the wine in a heated skillet; add the onion, garlic, and parsley, and sauté the vegetables over moderate heat for a few minutes, stirring frequently. Drain the tomatoes, keeping them intact, and reserve ½ cup of the juice. Add the tomatoes, half-cup juice, mushrooms, basil, bay leaf, and orange juice to the skillet and simmer, stirring occasionally, for 5 minutes. Remove half of the tomatoes from the skillet and arrange them around the edges of a baking dish. Place the other tomatoes in a blender to puree; then return the pureed tomatoes to the skillet. Stir in the capers. Pour the sauce over the bottom of the baking dish.

Cut the fish fillets into 4–5 serving pieces. Spread the mustard over one side of the fillets. In a shallow bowl, combine the flour, paprika, and dill; dip each fillet in the mixture, coating both sides. Place the fillets (mustard side up) over the sauce in the baking dish, but do not cover with sauce. Cover the baking dish with an aluminum-foil dome and bake in a 350° oven for 35–40 minutes.

MAKES 4–5 SERVINGS

CALORIES: 220/SERVING
FISH: 4 OUNCES/SERVING

VERACRUZ RED SNAPPER

4–5 red snapper fillets (or rockfish or Eastern cod variety), about 1¼ pounds total
2 tablespoons dry white wine
2 tablespoons lime juice
½ cup stock (defatted fish or chicken, or vegetable), or water
1 large onion, coarsely chopped
1 green pepper, coarsely chopped
⅔ cup chopped celery
3 cloves garlic, minced or crushed
⅓ cup canned tomato paste
1 16-ounce can diced tomatoes in juice
1 7-ounce can green chile salsa
1 tablespoon capers
1 teaspoon oregano
¼–½ teaspoon chile powder, or to taste

GARNISH: lime slices and parsley sprigs

Marinate the fish fillets in a mixture of the wine and lime juice for an hour or more. Bring the stock to a boil in a skillet, and add the onion, celery, green pepper, and garlic. Reduce the heat to moderate and stir-fry the vegetables for about 10 minutes; then stir in the tomato products, capers, and spices. Cook over medium-high heat until the sauce has reduced slightly, about 10 minutes. Place the fish and marinade in a baking dish, pour the sauce over the fish, and bake uncovered in a 350° oven for about 35 minutes. Garnish with lime slices and parsley.

MAKES 5 SERVINGS

CALORIES: 195/SERVING
FISH: 4 OUNCES/SERVING

CONFETTI RICE

Colorful, flavorful, and quickly made using already-cooked rice!

1 onion, chopped
1 green pepper, chopped
2 cups frozen corn kernels
1 4-ounce jar sliced pimiento, chopped
1 teaspoon oregano
½ teaspoon paprika
½–1 tablespoon soy sauce
1 cup frozen green peas
4 cups cooked long-grain brown rice

In a large skillet, dry-sauté the onion and green pepper over medium heat, stirring constantly, until the vegetables are tender-crisp (about 5 minutes). Add the corn, pimiento, and seasonings, and continue cooking for 2–3 minutes, stirring as needed. Stir in the green peas and rice, and heat thoroughly for about 5 minutes, stirring occasionally as required.

MAKES 6 SERVINGS

CALORIES: 205/SERVING

Bok choy, commonly used in Chinese dishes, is also a wonderful cooked green by itself (version I) or combined with other vegetables (as in version II). It has a delicate flavor, somewhat like that of Swiss chard, and is highly nutritious. Use the white stem with the green leaves when cutting it for cooking.

I.

1 large head bok choy
1½ cups vegetable stock or water
1 teaspoon soy sauce
1 tablespoon lemon juice
½ teaspoon garlic powder
½ teaspoon onion powder

Cut the bok choy into coarse diagonal slices. Heat the stock and soy sauce to a boil in a large pot, add the bok choy, cover, and cook over moderate-low heat for 5 minutes. Add the lemon juice and seasonings, cover again, and continue cooking for 5–10 minutes.

MAKES 4–5 SERVINGS   CALORIES: 20/SERVING

II.

1 large head bok choy
1 large head Savoy cabbage, quartered
2 cups vegetable stock or water
½–1 tablespoon soy sauce
1 teaspoon onion powder

Cut the bok choy and cabbage in coarse diagonal slices. Combine the remaining ingredients in a large pot, bring to a boil, and add the vegetables. Cover, lower the heat, and simmer for about 20 minutes.

MAKES 8 SERVINGS   CALORIES: 25/SERVING

18 DINNER MENU

BOSTON BAKED BEANS*
    SWEET POTATO BREAD** or PUMPKIN
    BREAD**
    Hot Corn-on-the-Cob
    CARAWAY SLAW or Tossed Green Salad

TIMESAVERS:
* Soak and cook the beans earlier in the day or on the preceding day, or use cooked beans that have been stored in
the freezer and thawed.
** Omit home-baked bread and substitute a good-quality
purchased bread and/or baked yams or sweet potatoes
placed in the oven about the time the beans are put in to
bake.

LEFTOVER SUGGESTIONS:
Reheat or freeze leftover beans. Use *Sweet Potato Bread* or
Pumpkin Bread for snacks or sandwiches.

WEIGHT-LOSS SUGGESTIONS:
Omit bread and corn. Substitute a steamed artichoke,
cooked in water with a little red wine vinegar and served
with wedge of lemon or with *Vinaigrette* or other low-calorie
dressing of choice.

BOSTON BAKED BEANS

*These beans are so delicious you may want to double the
recipe when you prepare them in order to have enough for
other meals or for freezing. You may have a cup or more of
beans left over after measuring out the cooked beans for the
recipe, depending upon soaking time and other factors. If
so, why not add them to a soup?*

  2 cups dried navy beans
  1 onion, chopped
  ⅔ cup canned tomato paste
  ½ cup canned tomato sauce

¼ cup frozen apple-juice concentrate
¼ cup white wine
¼ cup water
2 tablespoons cider vinegar
1 teaspoon grated fresh ginger
1 teaspoon dry mustard
¼ teaspoon garlic powder
¼ teaspoon ground cloves
⅛ teaspoon cardamom
Dash cayenne pepper

Place the beans in a pot and add water to cover (about 5 cups). Bring the water to a boil, reduce the heat, and cook the beans for 5–10 minutes. Turn off the heat, cover, and let the beans soak for an hour. Return to a boil and cook over moderate heat, cover ajar, until the beans are tender, about an hour. Stir occasionally to prevent sticking. If necessary, add a little water toward the end of the cooking period if the beans seem too dry. Measure off 4 cups beans and mix them with all the other ingredients. Pour the bean mixture into a casserole, cover, and bake in a 350° oven for about an hour.

YIELD: ABOUT 5 CUPS   CALORIES: 130/½ CUP

SWEET POTATO BREAD

1 cup mashed sweet potato or yam, cooled
¾ cup canned evaporated skim milk or nonfat milk
⅓ cup frozen apple-juice concentrate
1 teaspoon soy sauce
1 tablespoon cinnamon
¼ teaspoon nutmeg
1 envelope active dry yeast, dissolved in ½ cup lukewarm
    water
4 cups whole-wheat pastry flour
1 tablespoon nonfat milk

Blend the potato, evaporated milk, apple juice, soy sauce, and spices in a food processor or blender. Transfer the mixture to a large bowl and stir in the dissolved yeast. Slowly add 3¼ cups of the flour, stirring to combine well. Knead for 3 to 5 minutes, gradually adding the rest of the flour. Shape into a loaf (the dough will be sticky), place in a nonstick loaf pan, and set the pan in a warm place. (Preheat the oven to 150°, then turn off heat just before setting pan in oven.) Let the dough rise for 1 hour. Bake in a 425° oven for 10 minutes; then prick the surface with a fork in several places and brush with the tablespoon of nonfat milk. Lower the heat to 375° and continue baking for 35 to 40 minutes. Cool before slicing. Cover bread with foil or plastic wrap to keep moist.

YIELD: 1 LOAF (ABOUT 16 SLICES)   CALORIES: 125/SLICE

PUMPKIN BREAD

1¾ cups whole-wheat pastry flour
⅓ cup nonfat dry milk
½ teaspoon baking soda
½ teaspoon baking powder
½ teaspoon each: allspice, cinnamon, ground cloves, and
    nutmeg
⅓ cup frozen apple-juice concentrate
⅓ cup water
½ teaspoon vanilla
1 cup canned or fresh-cooked and mashed pumpkin
2 egg whites

Combine the dry ingredients in a mixing bowl. Combine the apple juice, water, and vanilla and mix with the dry ingredients, stirring just to blend. Stir in the pumpkin briefly so the batter is streaked. Beat the egg whites until stiff peaks form and fold into the batter. Pour the mixture into an 8-inch square or 9-inch round nonstick baking pan. Bake for 1 hour in a 350° oven. Cool before slicing. Cover bread with foil or plastic wrap to keep moist.

YIELD: 1 LOAF (ABOUT 12 SLICES)   CALORIES: 75/SLICE

CARAWAY SLAW

2 cups finely shredded green cabbage
½ cup cottage cheese, 1 percent fat (by weight) maximum
¼ cup skimmed buttermilk, or more if necessary
1 8-ounce can unsweetened crushed pineapple, juice-packed, drained
1 tablespoon white vinegar
1 teaspoon caraway seeds

Place the cabbage in a bowl of ice water to crisp. Blend the cheese and buttermilk in a blender until very smooth, adding a little additional buttermilk if necessary. Transfer the blended mixture to a bowl and stir in the pineapple and seasonings. Chill well. Drain the cabbage thoroughly in a colander and stir into the chilled dressing.

MAKES 3–4 SERVINGS   CALORIES: 67/¼ RECIPE

19 DINNER MENU

WHITE BEAN-AND-TURKEY SOUP or VEGETABLE-
BARLEY SOUP** or SWEET POTATO-VEGETABLE SOUP
          CHEF'S SALAD WITH TUNA OR BEANS
          (page 381)*

TIMESAVERS:
* If cooking the bean soup, start soaking the beans early in
the day.
** If making the barley soup, cook the barley ahead of time
and refrigerate, if necessary.

LEFTOVER SUGGESTIONS:
Freeze or reheat leftover soup.

WEIGHT-LOSS SUGGESTIONS:
Since the soups are thick, add up to 2 cups additional stock
or water to reduce calories per serving; or omit or reduce
the amount of beans or barley.

WHITE BEAN-AND-TURKEY SOUP

     2 cups dried small white beans
     2 bay leaves
     1 cup diced raw turkey breast (or raw chicken breast)
     1 tablespoon soy sauce
     1 tablespoon garlic powder
     2 cups defatted chicken or turkey stock
     1 cup chopped onions
     1 cup chopped leeks
     ¾ cup chopped celery
     ½ cup sliced mushrooms
     2 cloves garlic, crushed
     ½ fresh green chile, seeded and chopped
     ½ teaspoon dry mustard
     2 cups frozen French-cut green beans, coarsely chopped

Place the white beans and bay leaves in a soup pot. Add
water to cover and bring to a boil; let boil for 5 minutes.

Turn off heat, cover, and let beans soak for an hour. Discard the water and replace with 8 cups fresh water. Return to a boil and cook over moderate heat, cover ajar, until beans are tender, about an hour. Remove the cooked beans from the pot, draining off and reserving the liquid, and discard the bay leaves.

In a small skillet, stir-fry the turkey with the soy sauce over moderate heat for a few minutes; sprinkle with the garlic powder and continue to stir-fry until the turkey is cooked. Place the turkey and pan juices into the pot the beans were cooked in and add 2 cups of the beans. Cover with 4 cups of water and the stock. Stir in the raw vegetables and mustard; then bring to a boil, reduce heat, cover, and cook over moderate heat, stirring occasionally, until the vegetables are partially tender, about 15–20 minutes. Place the rest of the beans and 1 cup of the bean-cooking liquid in a blender and blend until smooth. Add the pureed beans to the soup along with any remaining liquid from cooking the beans and continue cooking for 10 minutes, stirring occasionally to prevent sticking. Add the green beans a few minutes before turning off the heat.

YIELD: ABOUT 12 CUPS   CALORIES: 150/CUP

POULTRY: ½ OUNCE/CUP

VEGETABLE-BARLEY SOUP

Turnips and turnip greens give this vegetable soup an especially appealing fresh vegetable flavor, even without added spices, herbs, or other seasonings. But if you wish, you can test the soup near the end of the cooking period and heighten its flavor by adding small amounts of seasonings such as marjoram or thyme, or soy sauce, or a tablespoon or two of chopped parsley.

½ cup whole barley
2 cups diced turnips
1 cup chopped turnip greens (tops)
1 large onion, chopped
2 cups diced carrots
¾ cup chopped celery

1 cup fresh or frozen cut green beans
1 16-ounce can diced tomatoes in juice

Bring 3¼ cups water to a boil in a soup pot and stir in the barley. Reduce the heat, cover, and cook for 45 minutes. Add 6 cups water and all the other ingredients except frozen green beans, if used, and the tomatoes. (If the green beans are fresh, add them now with the other vegetables.) Stir and bring the soup to a boil; then lower the heat and cook, covered, until the vegetables are tender, about 45 minutes. Add frozen green beans, if used, and the tomatoes about 20 minutes before the end of the cooking period.

YIELD: ABOUT 10 CUPS   CALORIES: 80/CUP

SWEET POTATO-VEGETABLE SOUP

For a change in vegetable soups, try this mildly sweet, very smooth-textured version. It looks rather like split-pea-vegetable soup, but the sweet potatoes and cloves give it a very individual character.

4 cups sweet potatoes, peeled and cut into 1-inch chunks
2 cups chopped celery
1½ cups sliced leeks
1½ cups sliced onions
1 cup frozen cut green beans
½ teaspoon thyme
¼ teaspoon cloves
Dash cayenne pepper
½ cup nonfat milk or canned evaporated skim milk

Place the vegetables, except the green beans, in a large pot with 6 cups water. Bring to a boil; then reduce the heat, cover, and simmer until the vegetables are tender. Using a ladle, transfer about half the contents of the pot, including half the vegetables, to a blender; blend until smooth. Return the pureed mixture to the pot and stir in the green beans and spices. Bring the soup to a boil again, lower the heat, cover, and cook until the beans are tender, stirring occasionally. Stir in the milk.

YIELD: 9 CUPS   CALORIES: 130/CUP

20 DINNER MENU

SWEET-SOUR CABBAGE ROLLS*
>   *(with choice of filling: Rice-Meat or Potato-*
>   *Grain)*
>   *Baked Potatoes, Steamed Potato Halves, or*
>   *MASHED POTATOES (page 243) ***
>   *Steamed Frozen Green Peas and Carrots*
>   *Tossed Green Salad*

TIMESAVERS:
* Use leftover cooked rice to make the cabbage rolls with
the rice-meat filling. (The grains used in the potato-grain
filling need to be cooked.)
** Make baked potatoes, placing them in the oven a little
while before cabbage rolls are put in to bake.

LEFTOVER SUGGESTIONS:
Leftover cabbage rolls may be frozen or reheated. See page
205 for suggestions for leftover baked potatoes. Reheat leftover mashed potatoes or steamed potato halves together
with leftover cabbage rolls and peas and carrots.

WEIGHT-LOSS SUGGESTIONS:
Have only one cabbage roll. Substitute for the potatoes a
steamed medley of crookneck squash and zucchini or other
summer squash combination. Substitute cauliflower, or cauliflower and snow peas, for the peas and carrots.

SWEET-SOUR CABBAGE ROLLS

*Fill the rolls with either a rice-meat mixture (filling I) or a
potato-grain mixture (filling II) and top with the tangy sauce
before baking.*

   1 large head cabbage, cored

   SAUCE:
   2 onions, chopped
   1 28-ounce can tomatoes
   1 8-ounce can tomato sauce

⅓ cup lemon juice
¼ cup frozen apple-juice concentrate
1 tablespoon soy sauce
¼ teaspoon cayenne pepper
⅓ cup raisins

FILLING I: Rice-Meat
2¾ cups cooked long-grain brown rice
¾ pound lean ground beef
¼ cup grated onion
1 egg white, fork-beaten
2 teaspoons chopped fresh or dried mint
1 teaspoon each basil and thyme

FILLING II: Potato-Grain
½ cup long-grain brown rice
½ cup whole buckwheat groats
1 tablespoon soy sauce
1 tablespoon ground coriander
1 teaspoon dillweed
¼ teaspoon fennel seed, ground in blender
2 cups peeled potatoes, diced medium-fine
1½ cups chopped onions
1½ cups chopped celery
½ cup chopped green pepper
2 egg whites, fork-beaten

GARNISH: lemon slices

Set the cabbage core side down in a steamer over boiling water, covered, for about 10 minutes, or until cabbage leaves are soft. Let cool and separate leaves. Prepare the sauce by sautéing the onions in ½ cup boiling water in a large skillet. Cook, stirring frequently, until the water has evaporated and the onions are slightly browned. Stir in the other ingredients, bring to a boil, reduce heat, and simmer, covered, for about 10 minutes.

Filling I. Mix together all of the ingredients. Place about ⅓ cup of the rice-meat mixture on each cabbage leaf, using 2 leaves when one is too small. Tuck in the sides and roll up carefully. Arrange the rolls seam side down in a nonstick baking pan and pour the sauce over and around the rolls. Bake covered in a 350° oven for an hour and a quarter. Serve the cabbage rolls garnished with lemon slices.

Filling II. Spread the buckwheat and rice in a baking pan and place in a 400° oven for about 10 minutes to toast, stirring occasionally so the grains brown evenly. Bring 2½ cups water to a boil in a saucepan. Stir in the soy sauce, spices, and toasted grains. Return to a boil; then turn heat low, cover tightly, and cook for 40–45 minutes. Keep covered for an additional 10 minutes to permit grains to fluff from steam. Combine the cooked grains, potatoes, vegetables, and egg whites, mixing well. Fill the rolls and bake as directed for filling I.

YIELD: 12
CABBAGE ROLLS

CALORIES: 183/MEAT-FILLED ROLL
MEAT: 1 OUNCE/MEAT-FILLED ROLL
CALORIES: 165/POTATO-GRAIN–
FILLED ROLL

21 DINNER MENU

*Turkey breast is utilized in these menus in three very dif-
ferent recipes. Two of them start with raw turkey breast
slices, available prepackaged at most markets. The menu
featuring a whole breast of turkey "complete with all the
trimmings" is designed for use at Thanksgiving or other
festive occasions.*

I.
*TURKEY BREAST SLICES WITH POTATOES IN WINE-
CAPER SAUCE or BREADED TURKEY SLICES ITALIANA
WITH POTATOES*
> *GLAZED CARROTS* *
> Tossed Green Salad

II.
*ROAST BREAST OF TURKEY
HERBED WILD RICE WITH BROWN RICE* * ONION GRAVY
(page 289)* ***
> *CRANBERRY-APPLE COMPOTE or
> MOLD* ***
> *SWEET POTATO-ORANGE MERINGUE
> PUDDING* *****
> French-Cut Green Beans with Sliced Water
> Chestnuts or Steamed Brussels Sprouts
> Tossed Green Salad*

TIMESAVERS:
Menu I: * Omit carrot recipe; substitute a frozen vegetable
of choice.
Menu II: * Omit wild-rice dish; substitute plain brown rice.
** Omit gravy. Defat pan juices from turkey, adding a little
defatted chicken stock, if needed, and serve turkey "au
jus."
*** Omit cranberry-apple dish and substitute *Baked Apples*
(page 412), put in oven to bake while turkey is roasting.
**** Omit sweet-potato dish; substitute baked sweet potatoes or yams, put in oven while turkey is roasting.

LEFTOVER SUGGESTIONS:
Menu I: Reheat or freeze leftover turkey dish and carrots.
Menu II: Use leftover carved turkey for sandwiches or for making dinner menu entrée 26, *Chicken or Turkey Tacos*. It could also be substituted for the chicken in *Chicken-Salad-Stuffed Tomatoes* (page 380). Enjoy any of the other leftovers reheated or served chilled, as appropriate.

WEIGHT-LOSS SUGGESTIONS:
Menu I: Choose the lower-calorie turkey recipe, *Turkey Breast Slices in Wine-Caper Sauce*, and omit the potato variation. Supplement the meal with steamed green beans, broccoli, or cabbage.
Menu II: Omit either the rice or the sweet-potato dish, and have only a half-serving of the other. Supplement the meal with steamed bean sprouts and Chinese snow peas.

To follow the menu plan, use the variation that includes potatoes (following) when making either *Turkey Breast Slices with Potatoes in Wine-Caper Sauce* or *Breaded Turkey Slices Italiana with Potatoes*.

TURKEY BREAST SLICES IN WINE-CAPER SAUCE

6 raw turkey breast slices (about 2½ to 3 ounces per slice)
¾ cup vermouth or other dry white wine
¾ cup bottled white grape juice
¾ cup water
3 tablespoons lemon juice
2 tablespoons Dijon mustard
1 tablespoon arrowroot
1 tablespoon coarsely chopped capers
½ teaspoon onion powder
¼ teaspoon garlic powder

Pound the turkey slices with a mallet to tenderize them. Place them with ¼ cup water in a large skillet. Bring to a boil; then turn down the heat and simmer, covered, for 5 minutes. Turn the turkey slices over and add the wine, grape juice, and water (¾ cup). In a small bowl, combine the lemon juice and mustard, stirring well, and add 1 tablespoon water to dilute slightly. Blend in the arrowroot until smooth. Add this mixture to the skillet together with the remaining seasonings, stir, and return to a boil. Reduce the heat to low, cover, and cook for 35 minutes. During the cooking period, turn the slices over again once or twice, and stir gently to keep them covered with the sauce and to prevent sticking. Serve garnished with lemon slices and parsley sprigs.

MAKES 5–6 SERVINGS   CALORIES: 185/⅙ RECIPE
                                  POULTRY: 3 OUNCES/⅙ RECIPE

VARIATION: TURKEY BREAST SLICES WITH POTATOES IN WINE-CAPER SAUCE

Place 3 long white boiling potatoes in a pot with water to cover. Bring to a boil, reduce heat, and cook, cover ajar, until just tender. Remove potatoes from the pot, cool, peel, and cut into halves or thirds, as desired. Follow the above recipe for the preparation of the turkey breast slices. Near the end of the cooking period, place the potatoes in the skillet with the turkey slices, spooning the sauce over all. Cover and finish cooking as directed above.

BREADED TURKEY SLICES ITALIANA

SAUCE:
½ onion, cut into chunks
2 cloves garlic, coarsely chopped
1 cup canned tomato sauce
⅓ cup canned tomato paste
2 cups canned crushed tomatoes in puree
2 teaspoons each basil and ground sage
Dash cayenne pepper
¼ cup red Burgundy

6 raw turkey breast slices (about 2½ to 3 ounces per slice)
1½ cups fine whole-wheat bread crumbs (from acceptable bread)
1 teaspoon each: onion powder, garlic powder, and paprika
½ cup nonfat milk or canned evaporated skim milk
2 tablespoons grated Sapsago cheese

Place the onion and garlic in a blender with the tomato sauce and tomato paste; blend until pureed and transfer to a saucepan. Stir in the crushed tomatoes, basil, sage, pepper, and wine. Bring to a boil, reduce heat, and simmer the sauce for about 10 minutes. Spread half the sauce in a 10-by-14-inch baking dish and reserve the other half.

Pound the turkey slices with a mallet to tenderize them. Combine the bread crumbs with the onion and garlic powders and paprika in one container; place the milk in another container. Dip the slices, one by one, first in the milk, then in the breading mixture, covering both sides. Arrange the breaded slices over the sauce in the baking dish and cover them with the reserved sauce. Cover the baking dish with an aluminum-foil dome and place in a 350° oven for an hour. About 15 minutes before the end of the baking time, sprinkle the turkey slices with the Sapsago cheese. Cover again with the foil and finish baking.

MAKES 6 SERVINGS

CALORIES: 270/SERVING
POULTRY: 3 OUNCES/SERVING

VARIATION: BREADED TURKEY SLICES ITALIANA WITH POTATOES

Place 4–6 red boiling potatoes in a pot with water to cover. Bring to a boil, reduce heat, and cook, cover ajar, until almost tender. Remove potatoes from the pot, cool, peel, and cut into halves, if desired. Follow the above recipe for the preparation of the breaded turkey breast slices. Arrange the cooked potatoes around the turkey slices near the end of the baking time (when adding the Sapsago cheese), ladling some of the sauce over the potatoes. Cover and continue baking as directed.

GLAZED CARROTS

8 large carrots, sliced in thin rounds
¼ cup frozen apple-juice concentrate
1 tablespoon grated orange rind
2½ teaspoons cornstarch
1 teaspoon ground ginger

Place the carrots in a steamer basket over 1½ cups boiling water in a saucepan; cover and cook over medium heat until tender. Reserve ⅔ cup of the cooking water from the carrots. Combine the apple juice, orange rind, cornstarch, and ginger in another saucepan; mix until smooth; then stir in the carrot water. Cook, stirring constantly, until the mixture has thickened and cleared. Add the carrots, stirring well to coat with the sauce.

MAKES 6 SERVINGS   **CALORIES: 65/SERVING**

ROAST BREAST OF TURKEY

    2 stalks celery with leaves
    1 onion
    1 5- to 6½-pound turkey breast
    Garlic powder
    Ground sage
    Poultry seasoning

Chop the vegetables and place them in a large baking pan to make a "bed" for the turkey. Remove the skin and any visible fat from the turkey and rub the breast meat with the seasonings. Place the turkey, breast side up, over the vegetables and add 1 cup water to the pan. Cover the pan with an aluminum-foil dome and place in a 375° oven for 1¾ to 2¾ hours. Baste the turkey with the pan juices every half-hour and if necessary add a little more water. Test for doneness by inserting a fork into the meat. When done, the meat will be tender and the juices will be clear, not pink. Do not overcook. Remove the cooked turkey breast from the oven and let stand for about 10 minutes before slicing.

MAKES 12 OR MORE SERVINGS   **CALORIES: 175/3½ OUNCES POULTRY**

HERBED WILD RICE WITH BROWN RICE

    3 cups defatted chicken stock
    ½ cup wild rice
    ½ cup long-grain brown rice

2 tablespoons minced green onions
2 cloves garlic, minced or crushed
1 teaspoon soy sauce
1 teaspoon each: thyme, marjoram, and basil
3 bay leaves
Dash cayenne pepper

In a medium saucepan, bring ¼ cup of the stock to a boil. Add the rice, green onions, garlic, and soy sauce and stir-fry for 2–3 minutes until the vegetables are soft. Add the remaining stock and seasonings, bring to a boil, reduce heat to low, cover, and cook for 1 hour until the rice is tender. Discard the bay leaves and continue to cook uncovered until any remaining liquid has evaporated. Fluff lightly with a fork and serve.

MAKES 4 TO 6 SERVINGS　　　　**CALORIES: 110/⅙ RECIPE**

CRANBERRY-APPLE COMPOTE

You'll find this delicious cooked fruit combination excellent as an accompaniment with roast turkey or chicken, as a sweet spread on bread, or as a dessert topping over yogurt or frozen desserts. Or gelatinize it to make a mold, as instructed in the recipe variation (page 322). You can use fresh or frozen cranberries with equally good results.

2 cups fresh or frozen unsweetened raw cranberries
½ cup water
½ cup frozen apple-juice concentrate
5 apples, peeled and sliced thin
3 tablespoons pectin
1 tablespoon cornstarch
1 tablespoon vanilla extract
¼ teaspoon lemon extract

Combine the cranberries, water, and apple juice in a saucepan. Bring to a boil, add the apples and pectin, reduce heat to moderate, and continue cooking, uncovered, for 8–10 minutes, stirring as required. Mix the cornstarch with 2 tablespoons water until smooth. Stir the flavor extracts and

321

cornstarch paste into the simmering fruit and cook for another 2 minutes, stirring constantly as the mixture thickens. Serve hot or cold.

YIELD: 4 CUPS   CALORIES: 190/CUP

VARIATION: CRANBERRY-APPLE MOLD
Follow instructions for *Cranberry-Apple Compote* with these changes:
1. Omit the cornstarch mixture.
2. Increase water from ½ cup to 1¼ cups.
3. Increase frozen apple-juice concentrate from ½ cup to ¾ cup.
4. Sprinkle 2 envelopes plus 1 teaspoon unflavored gelatin over ½ cup cold water. Add the softened gelatin to the saucepan at the end of the 8–10-minute cooking period; stir well to dissolve; then pour the cooked fruit mixture into a 1-quart mold. Chill until firm. Unmold onto a lettuce-lined plate and garnish with orange wedges and grapes and/or other fruits.

SWEET POTATO-ORANGE MERINGUE PUDDING

The natural affinity of sweet potatoes for oranges is exemplified in this delicious recipe. Make sure the oranges are sweet, and avoid using the white membrane, which could be bitter.

2 teaspoons vanilla extract
1 teaspoon grated orange rind
½ teaspoon nutmeg
1½ cups mashed cooked sweet potatoes or yams, or a combination
1⅓ cups seeded orange pulp (from 2–3 large oranges), cut into chunks, white membranes removed
2 tablespoons cornstarch
2 egg whites, beaten until stiff peaks form

Combine the vanilla, orange rind, and nutmeg with the mashed sweet potatoes, mixing thoroughly. Spread the mixture over the bottom of a pie pan or other shallow baking dish. Place the orange pulp and cornstarch in a saucepan, stir well, and bring to a boil. Lower the heat and cook, stirring constantly, for about 3 minutes, until thickened. Layer the orange mixture over the sweet potatoes; then top with a layer of beaten egg whites swirled decoratively. Finish with a light sprinkling of additional nutmeg. Bake in a 400° oven for a few minutes, until the egg white is lightly browned. Serve warm or at room temperature.

MAKES 8 SERVINGS   CALORIES: 65/SERVING

22 DINNER MENU

STEAMED SALMON STEAKS (served hot or chilled)

> With Hot Fish
> MUSTARD-YOGURT TOPPING (page 407) or
> SPICY FISH SAUCE (page 242)
> Steamed Asparagus   Boiled Potatoes
> BAKED TOMATOES*
> Tossed Green Salad

> With Chilled Fish
> CHILLED MARINATED VEGETABLES*
> POTATO SALAD VINAIGRETTE
> Sliced Tomatoes
> MOLDED FRESH CUCUMBER-MINT
> SALAD**

TIMESAVERS:
Hot-fish menu: * Omit baked tomatoes; add fresh tomatoes to tossed green salad. Chilled-fish menu: * Omit marinated vegetables. ** Omit molded salad. Substitute a tossed green salad.

LEFTOVER SUGGESTIONS:
Most of the prepared foods make fine leftovers, but you can do some simple but special things with leftover fish or potatoes.

Leftover fish: Bone and flake leftover salmon and serve on a bed of finely shredded lettuce topped with *French Dressing* (page 403) on individual salad plates or in sea scallop shells, if you happen to have them. Or place the flaked salmon on a bed of rice in a shallow baking dish or in the sea scallop shells, cover with *Mustard-Yogurt Topping,* and set under a hot broiler for 7–8 minutes (or omit the topping, cover, bake until heated through, and serve with *Spicy Fish Sauce*).

Leftover potatoes: Make a quick potato salad (page 208) or mock "French Fries" (page 372).

WEIGHT-LOSS SUGGESTIONS:
Hot-fish menu: Substitute steamed turnip and rutabaga slices for the potatoes. Chilled-fish menu: Substitute *Cucumbers with Yogurt* (page 238) for the potato salad.

STEAMED SALMON STEAKS

3 8-ounce salmon steaks
Juice of ½ lemon
1 lemon, sliced
1 green onion, chopped

Sprinkle the salmon steaks with the lemon juice, cover, and refrigerate until ready to cook. Place a steamer basket in a large pot, making sure that the steaks will fit in the basket without overlapping. (If more than 3 steaks are to be cooked, cook them in batches, 3 at a time.) Add a few inches of water to the pot to reach just below the steamer basket. Arrange the salmon steaks in the basket, sprinkle them with the green onion, and lay the lemon slices over and around the fish. Bring the water to a boil, cover tightly, and cook for 6–7 minutes, or until the salmon is opaque throughout. To test, pull one of the salmon steaks slightly apart in the center, using the tines of a fork. If the flesh is still bright pink and translucent, steam 1 or 2 minutes longer. (But do not overcook, or salmon will be dry.) Remove the salmon from the steamer, cut each steak in half lengthwise, and place on individual plates or a serving platter. Garnish with parsley sprigs and lemon wedges. Serve hot or chilled with *Mustard-Yogurt Topping* (page 407) or *Spicy Fish Sauce* (page 242).

MAKES 6 SERVINGS   CALORIES: 140/⅙ RECIPE
FISH: 4 OUNCES/⅙ RECIPE

NOTE: An alternative method for steaming salmon or other fish is to lay the fish in a heatproof pie pan, then set the pan over a rack to steam in a pot filled with a few inches of boiling water and covered.

THE PRITIKIN PROMISE
BAKED TOMATOES

3 large tomatoes, halved
2 tablespoons dried parsley
2 tablespoons dried minced onion
1 tablespoon basil
2 tablespoons grated Sapsago cheese

Place the halved tomatoes cut side up in a shallow nonstick baking pan. Sprinkle the parsley, onion, basil, and cheese over the tomatoes. Bake in a 325° oven until tender, about 20 minutes, or longer if a softer consistency is preferred.

MAKES 6 SERVINGS   **CALORIES: 30/SERVING**

CHILLED MARINATED VEGETABLES

4–6 cups fresh or frozen vegetables of choice, such as
  asparagus spears, whole green beans, Brussels sprouts,
  whole mushrooms, carrot sticks or baby carrots, cherry
  tomatoes, or others

MARINADE:
1⅓ cups apple-cider vinegar
⅔ cup water
2 cloves garlic, minced or crushed
2 teaspoons thyme
1 teaspoon dried parsley
1 small red onion, thinly sliced

Place the vegetables in a steamer basket set over boiling water in a pot; cover and cook briefly until tender but still firm. If several vegetables are used, add them to the pot according to their required cooking times (see page 224); or cook them in batches, if preferred. Cool the vegetables and lay them in a broad, shallow container. Combine the marinade ingredients and pour the marinade over the vegetables. Refrigerate for several hours or overnight. To serve, arrange the vegetables attractively on a serving platter and drizzle with the marinade. (Leftover marinade may be used as a dressing with a green salad.)

MAKES 6–8 SERVINGS   CALORIES: 55/⅙ RECIPE

POTATO SALAD VINAIGRETTE

6 long white potatoes
¾ cup *Vinaigrette Dressing* (page 403)
1 2-ounce jar sliced pimiento, chopped
¼ cup finely chopped onion
2 tablespoons minced parsley

Place the potatoes in a vegetable steamer set in a pan of boiling water. Cook, covered, until potatoes are just tender when pierced with a fork. Peel the potatoes while still warm, then slice them lengthwise in thirds or fourths, and crosswise into chunks. Put the potatoes in a bowl and toss them with the *Vinaigrette Dressing*. Mix in the pimiento, onion, and parsley. Serve warm or chilled.

MAKES 6–8 SERVINGS   CALORIES: 195/⅙ RECIPE
                                      145/⅛ RECIPE

MOLDED FRESH CUCUMBER-MINT SALAD

3 envelopes unflavored gelatin
3 medium cucumbers, peeled
2½ cups nonfat yogurt
1 teaspoon finely chopped seeded jalapeño chile
3 tablespoons grated onion
1 tablespoon finely chopped fresh mint
½ teaspoon ground coriander
Dash cayenne pepper

Sprinkle the gelatin over ½ cup cold water in a small bowl; let soak for a few minutes. Set the bowl inside a saucepan filled with a few inches of boiling water and stir until the gelatin dissolves. Cut the cucumbers in half lengthwise, removing any large, coarse seeds; then slice the cucumbers into medium-sized chunks (there should be about 6 cups).

Place the cucumbers in a blender with 1 cup of the yogurt and the chile, and blend until pureed. Stir in the rest of the yogurt, onion, mint, and spices, mixing well. Using a rubber spatula, add the dissolved gelatin, again mixing well. Transfer to a 1½-quart ring mold and chill until firm. Unmold and garnish with mint sprigs.

MAKES ABOUT 12 SERVINGS   **CALORIES: 40/SERVING**

23 DINNER MENU

Two unusual breaded-chicken recipes are featured in these menus that are perfect for picnic or patio party (They'll meet with approval indoors, too!)

I.
COLD CURRIED ZUCCHINI SOUP*
MUSTARD-BREADED CHICKEN
          FRUITED RICE SALAD (page 382)
          Tossed Green Salad

II.
BREADED CINNAMON CHICKEN
RICE WITH SWEET POTATOES
          ZUCCHINI BOURGUIGNON*
          Tossed Green Salad

TIMESAVERS:
Menu I: * Omit soup: substitute zucchini, carrot. and celery sticks, if desired.
Menu II: * Omit *Zucchini Bourguignon;* substitute plain steamed zucchini.

LEFTOVER SUGGESTIONS:
Either kind of leftover chicken may be reheated or served cold. The zucchini soup keeps well for days in the refrigerator. Reheat *Zucchini Bourguignon.* Reheat *Rice with Sweet Potatoes* or eat cold.

WEIGHT-LOSS SUGGESTIONS:
Have large servings of green salad and small servings of chicken and rice dishes. Supplement with a steamed artichoke or raw vegetable relishes.

COLD CURRIED ZUCCHINI SOUP

    4–5 zucchini, chopped
    1 cup chopped green onions
    1 tablespoon curry powder

1 tablespoon ground cumin
2 cups defatted chicken stock
3 cups skimmed buttermilk

Place the zucchini and green onions in a steamer basket set over boiling water in a saucepan. Cover and steam until the zucchini is tender. Transfer the cooked vegetables to a blender, add the spices and the stock, and blend until pureed. Place the puree in a saucepan and cook over low heat for 3–4 minutes. Transfer to a large bowl and let cool; then stir in the buttermilk. Chill the soup for several hours or overnight. Serve garnished with a sprinkling of minced green onion.

YIELD: ABOUT 9 CUPS   CALORIES: 55/CUP

MUSTARD-BREADED CHICKEN

The flavorful thick breading suggests Southern Fried Chicken! It would be preferable to use a Dijon-style mustard without added salt (this is available), since the recipe requires a large quantity of mustard.

½ cup Dijon mustard
¼ cup nonfat dry milk
2 tablespoons water
1 cup fine whole-wheat bread crumbs (from acceptable bread)
6 small boneless chicken breast halves, skinned
¼ cup finely chopped parsley

Combine the mustard, dry milk, and water in a bowl, mixing well. Stir in the bread crumbs. Using a rubber spatula, spread the mixture over the chicken breasts, leaving one side unbreaded. Place the chicken, breaded side up, in a nonstick baking pan. Sprinkle with the parsley. Bake uncovered in a 350° oven for an hour. If coating starts to brown too much, tent the pan loosely with foil. Serve warm or cold.

MAKES 6 SERVINGS   CALORIES: 220/SERVING
                                 POULTRY: 4 OUNCES/SERVING

BREADED CINNAMON CHICKEN

2–3 cloves garlic, crushed
1½ tablespoons frozen apple-juice concentrate
½–1 tablespoon soy sauce
6 small boneless chicken breast halves, skinned
1½ cups fine whole-wheat bread crumbs (from acceptable
    bread)
1 tablespoon cinnamon
½ cup white wine

Combine the garlic, apple juice, and soy sauce in a small bowl and rub the chicken in the mixture, moistening all surfaces. Mix the bread crumbs and cinnamon together in another bowl and roll the chicken in the seasoned crumbs. Place the breaded chicken in a nonstick baking pan, sprinkle lightly with some additional cinnamon, cover with foil, and set in a 400° oven. After half an hour, remove the foil and baste with the wine. Reduce heat to 350° and continue baking, uncovered, another half-hour. Transfer to a serving platter and garnish with chopped parsley, parsley sprigs and orange wedges. Serve warm or cold.

MAKES 6 SERVINGS CALORIES: 210/SERVING
                  POULTRY: 4 OUNCES/SERVING

RICE WITH SWEET POTATOES

Just by cooking brown rice with sweet potatoes, you can add another flavor and texture dimension. Enjoy this simple dish as a snack or lunch item, too.

1½ cups long-grain brown rice
1 tablespoon cinnamon
1 teaspoon soy sauce
3¼ cups water
2 cups peeled sweet potatoes, in 1-inch chunks

Spread the rice in a baking pan and place in a moderately hot oven to brown lightly. Combine the cinnamon, soy sauce, and water in a large skillet and bring to a boil. Transfer the rice to the skillet and stir in the sweet potatoes. Return to a boil, cover, reduce heat to low, and cook for 40–45 minutes, or until the water is absorbed. Serve hot or chilled.

MAKES 6 TO 7 SERVINGS   **CALORIES: 235/⅙ RECIPE**

ZUCCHINI BOURGUIGNON

The lowly zucchini achieves surprising heights in this dish.

> 4 zucchini, trimmed
> ½ cup defatted chicken stock or vegetable stock, or water
> 1 1-pound package fresh mushrooms, sliced
> 1 red onion, sliced thin
> 2 large cloves garlic, sliced thin
> 1 tablespoon arrowroot
> ¼ cup water
> 1 tablespoon red Burgundy
> ½ tablespoon soy sauce
> 1 2-ounce jar sliced pimiento, chopped

Place the zucchini in a steamer basket set over boiling water in a saucepan and steam, covered, for a few minutes. Remove the zucchini (it should still be quite firm) and slice in ½-inch slightly diagonal rounds. In a skillet, bring the stock to a boil and add the mushrooms, onion, and garlic; sauté over medium-low heat for about 8–10 minutes. Mix the arrowroot with the ¼ cup water, wine, and soy sauce, making a smooth paste. Add the arrowroot paste to the simmering vegetables, stirring constantly until thickened. Add the pimiento and zucchini and heat for several minutes, stirring occasionally.

MAKES 4 SERVINGS   **CALORIES: 85/SERVING**

24 DINNER MENU

POLENTA WITH ITALIAN SAUCE AND VEGETABLES * or
"ONE OLIVE" TAMALE PIE * or *QUICK TAMALE PIE* *
Steamed Broccoli
Tossed Green Salad

TIMESAVERS:
* Make the *Quick Tamale Pie*.

LEFTOVER SUGGESTIONS:
Reheat either of the tamale pies or the polenta. You can also
make different toppings for the polenta, each with its own
special character (pages 333–35). *Quick Tamale Pie,* made
into muffins or patties, makes a good lunch-box selection.

WEIGHT-LOSS SUGGESTIONS:
Have small servings of polenta or tamale pie. The other
foods on the menu, including the vegetables and sauce
served with the polenta, are low-calorie and unrestricted. If
desired, supplement the menu with steamed cauliflower.

A CORNMEAL BASE is featured in both Italian polenta and
Mexican tamale pie—two dishes otherwise very distinctive
in flavor and ethnic origin. Both recipes are quite simple and
fun to make. Polenta is a perfect partner to Italian sauces
and can be a welcome change from pasta. You can prepare
polenta in advance, refrigerate it for days, then reheat it with
any of the excellent sauces and toppings suggested in the
recipe. Tamale pie combines cornmeal with corn kernels,
other vegetables, and Mexican seasonings to make a hearty
and memorable dish.

POLENTA

2 cups unsifted coarsely ground whole yellow cornmeal
Water, as required

Set up a double-boiler assembly in a large pot. If necessary,
use a stainless-steel bowl for the top. Add water to the bot-

tom pot, up to the base of the top, and heat to a boil In a separate pot, bring 5 cups water to a boil. Place the corn-meal in a saucepan with 1½ cups cold water, mixing well. and stir in the 5 cups boiling water. Cook over moderate heat, stirring constantly, until the cornmeal reaches a full boil. Transfer it to the double boiler, cover, and cook over moderate heat for 35 minutes

Pour the hot cornmeal onto a large cookie sheet and, using a spatula, flatten it out evenly to cover the entire surface Cool, cover loosely with plastic wrap, and refrigerate for several hours or overnight to thicken the polenta. When ready to use, cut the polenta into rectangles of the desired size for use as a base with any of the following topping recipes.

MAKES 12 OR MORE SERVINGS   CALORIES: 75/¹⁄₁₂ RECIPE

POLENTA WITH ITALIAN SAUCE AND VEGETABLES

12 3-by-3-inch squares cold *Polenta* (see above)

ITALIAN SAUCE WITH VEGETABLES:

2 cups canned tomato sauce
1½ teaspoons frozen apple-juice concentrate
1½ teaspoons basil
1 teaspoon ground cumin
½ teaspoon oregano
⅛ teaspoon ground fennel seed
1 cup chopped onions
1 cup chopped celery
1 cup chopped zucchini or other summer squash
½ cup chopped green pepper
½ cup chopped mushrooms

Place the polenta squares in a baking dish. Combine the sauce ingredients in a medium saucepan, mixing well, and bring to a boil. Lower the heat and simmer for about 10 minutes. until vegetables are tender-crisp. Ladle the sauce over the polenta. Bake uncovered for 25–30 minutes in a 400° oven.

MAKES 4 SERVINGS   CALORIES: 300/SERVING

POLENTA WITH TOMATO SAUCE AND BEANS

9 3-by-3-inch squares cold *Polenta* (page 333)
1½ cups cooked beans (kidney, pinto, etc.)

SAUCE:

1 15-ounce can tomato sauce
2 teaspoons onion powder
1½ teaspoons garlic powder
1 teaspoon oregano

Arrange the polenta squares closely in a nonstick baking pan. Layer the beans over the polenta. Combine the sauce ingredients, mixing well, and pour over the polenta and beans, using all or part of the sauce, as desired. Bake uncovered for 30 minutes in a 450° oven.

MAKES 3–4 SERVINGS   CALORIES: 285/¼ RECIPE

VARIATION: POLENTA CAKES WITH TOMATO SAUCE AND CHEESE

Arrange the polenta squares on a large nonstick cookie sheet or baking pan leaving spaces between the squares. Prepare the sauce as in the recipe above and top each square with 2 tablespoons sauce; then sprinkle 1 teaspoon grated Sapsago cheese over each square. Bake uncovered for about 30 minutes in a 450° oven.

POLENTA WITH BOLOGNESE SAUCE

8 3-by-3-inch squares cold *Polenta* (page 333)
1½ cups *Bolognese Sauce* (page 233)

Arrange the polenta squares closely in a baking dish. Ladle the sauce over the squares. Bake uncovered for 25–30 minutes in a 400° oven. (If sauce was cold before baking, increase baking time a few minutes, as necessary.)

MAKES 4 SERVINGS   CALORIES: 180/SERVING

THE PRITIKIN PROMISE

"ONE OLIVE" TAMALE PIE

*In his nutritional lectures, when asked about the accept-
ability of olives (which are high in fat), Nathan Pritikin
quips, "You can have one olive a day." Our experimental
kitchen took up the challenge and invented this delicious
"One Olive" Tamale Pie, with just one olive per serving.
You could, of course, omit the olives from the recipe,
though they do add both decorative and flavor appeal, even
in such small quantities.*

1 large onion, chopped
1 large green pepper, chopped
3 cloves garlic, minced or crushed
2 cups frozen corn kernels
2 16-ounce cans diced tomatoes in juice
1 teaspoon each: basil, chile powder, and ground cumin
¼ teaspoon oregano
8 pitted ripe green or black olives, sliced (reserve half of the
   sliced olives for garnish)
1¾ cups sifted whole-grain yellow cornmeal, divided
3 cups skimmed buttermilk
2 tablespoons frozen apple-juice concentrate
1 tablespoon baking powder
½ teaspoon baking soda
1 teaspoon onion powder
2 egg whites, beaten until stiff peaks form

In a large skillet, sauté the onion and green pepper in ¼ cup
water until softened. Add the garlic, corn, tomatoes, dried
spices (except the onion powder), and half the olives. Cook,
covered, over medium heat for 45 minutes, stirring occasionally, as required. Stir in ¾ cup of the cornmeal, mix
well, and continue to cook, stirring as necessary to avoid
sticking, for another 10–15 minutes. (Add a little water if
the mixture becomes too thick.)

In another skillet, mix together the buttermilk, apple
juice, and remaining cornmeal. Heat, stirring constantly,
until the mixture thickens (about 2–3 minutes). Combine the
baking powder, soda, and onion powder, and stir them into
the thickened cornmeal. Fold in the beaten egg whites
Transfer the batter to a 10-by-14-inch nonstick baking pan

and bake uncovered in a 375° oven for 20 minutes. Spread the vegetable topping over the corn bread, cover the pan with aluminum foil, turn up the heat to 400°, and continue baking. After 15 minutes, remove the foil and decorate the top with the reserved olive slices; bake uncovered for 15 minutes longer. Cool the tamale pie briefly; then cut into squares. It may also be served cold.

YIELD: 16 SQUARES   CALORIES: 225/2 SQUARES
OR 8 SERVINGS   OR ⅛ RECIPE

QUICK TAMALE PIE

In this simplified version, the cornmeal base and vegetable topping become one—but the taste doesn't suffer as a consequence. The recipe may also be used to make muffins or patties—handy for lunches and snacks.

1⅓ cups unsifted coarsely ground whole yellow cornmeal
1 28-ounce can crushed tomatoes
1 large onion, chopped fine
3 cups frozen corn kernels, thawed
½ cup chopped green or red bell pepper
1 tablespoon chile powder
1 teaspoon garlic powder
Dash cayenne pepper

Combine all ingredients, mixing well. Bake in a 9-by-13-inch baking pan for 30 minutes in a 375° oven, or make muffins by filling nonstick muffin tins ¾ full and baking at 375° for 20 minutes. (Let the muffins rest in the tins about 10 minutes before removing them.)

MAKES 6 SERVINGS OR
36 SMALL MUFFINS   CALORIES: 240/SERVING 40/MUFFIN

VARIATION: TAMALE PATTIES

Mix 3 whisked egg whites into the batter, form patties, and bake in a nonstick baking pan in a 425° oven, or in a nonstick skillet on the stove.

25 DINNER MENU

CREAMY FISH CHOWDER * or *CIOPPINO*
　　　　　Baked Potato with SALSA (page 407) **
　　　　　Hot Corn-on-the-Cob
　　　　　Steamed Artichoke with MUSTARD-
　　　　　YOGURT TOPPING (page 407)
　　　　　Tossed Green Salad

TIMESAVERS:
* If you don't have chicken or fish stock on hand, make the *Cioppino*.
** Omit the *Salsa* and moisten the potato with the *Mustard-Yogurt Topping* or some of the liquid from the fish entrée, or use a canned or bottled salsa.

LEFTOVER SUGGESTIONS:
Freeze or reheat either fish entrée. Reheat corn and artichoke or serve cold from refrigerator. See pages 205 and 208 for suggestions for leftover baked potatoes.

WEIGHT-LOSS SUGGESTIONS:
Omit the baked potato or the corn-on-the-cob.

CREAMY FISH CHOWDER

This delectable chowder rivals any of the conventional "Boston" or cream-style chowders in taste, texture, and overall appeal. You can get good results with many kinds of lean fresh fish (cod is excellent), or use a combination, such as half English sole and half red snapper.

　　　4 cups defatted chicken stock or fish stock
　　　1 bay leaf, crumbled
　　　⅛ teaspoon thyme
　　　⅛ teaspoon rosemary
　　　1 pound white fish fillets, cut in 1-inch cubes
　　　1 large onion, chopped
　　　1 cup chopped celery (include tender leaves)
　　　4 cups peeled potatoes, diced in ½-inch cubes
　　　1 10-ounce can clams, drained and chopped

1 13-ounce can evaporated skim milk
¼ cup cornstarch
1 teaspoon gumbo filé, optional
2 drops Tabasco, optional

GARNISH: ¼ cup chopped green onions

Place the stock, first 3 seasonings, and fish in a large pot; bring to a boil. Add the vegetables and clams. When mixture returns to a boil, reduce heat and simmer, covered, for 30 minutes. Transfer 2 cups of the chowder to a blender and puree; then return pureed contents to the pot. Stir the milk into the cornstarch until smooth and add the mixture to the simmering chowder, stirring constantly until thickened. Add optional seasonings, if desired. Serve hot, garnished with green onions.

MAKES 8 SERVINGS

CALORIES: 205/SERVING
FISH: 3⅓ OUNCES/SERVING

CIOPPINO

2 large onions, chopped
2 potatoes, peeled and diced
1 green pepper, chopped
2 cloves garlic, minced or crushed
2 cups canned tomato juice
1 28-ounce can tomatoes
½ cup red Burgundy
1 teaspoon oregano
1 teaspoon dried parsley
½ teaspoon basil
Dash cayenne pepper
1 pound halibut, bass, or other lean, firm white fish, cut in chunks

Put the onions, potatoes, green pepper, garlic, and tomato juice into a large saucepan. Heat to simmering and cook over medium heat for 10 minutes, until vegetables are tender-crisp. Add the tomatoes, wine, and seasonings, and cook, covered, for 10 minutes, until vegetables are fork-tender. Add the fish and simmer, covered, for 10 minutes, or until the fish flakes easily with a fork.

MAKES 6 SERVINGS

CALORIES: 245/SERVING
FISH: 2½ OUNCES/SERVING

26 DINNER MENU

CHICKEN OR TURKEY TACOS with Raw-Vegetable Garnishes

> *GAZPACHO* or GAZPACHO MOLD**
> *Baked Yam or Sweet Potato*

TIMESAVERS:
* Omit the *Gazpacho* or *Gazpacho Mold*.

LEFTOVER SUGGESTIONS:
Serve any of the recipes as leftovers. If desired, serve leftover taco filling chilled in a lettuce-lined bowl surrounded by corn chips (page 398, *Chip 'n' Dip*).

WEIGHT-LOSS SUGGESTIONS:
Omit the baked yam or sweet potato; substitute steamed broccoli spears. Fill tacos with ¼ cup instead of ⅓ cup of the filling and supplement with lots of extra raw-vegetable garnishes, eaten in the tacos or as a separate salad.

CHICKEN OR TURKEY TACOS

This is a convenient recipe to make if you have leftover chicken or turkey and some rice in the refrigerator. The chicken or turkey flavor comes through very well, even though the quantity of rice used is almost equal.

¼ cup defatted chicken or turkey stock or vegetable stock
1 cup finely chopped onions
¾ cup finely chopped green or red bell pepper
¼ cup chopped fresh cilantro (Mexican or Chinese parsley)
1 4-ounce can diced green chiles
1 tablespoon finely chopped seeded jalapeño chile
2 cups diced cooked chicken or turkey
1½ cups cooked brown rice
2 teaspoons soy sauce
1½ teaspoons basil
1 teaspoon garlic powder
Dash cayenne pepper
12 corn tortillas

341

RAW VEGETABLE GARNISHES: shredded lettuce, diced
tomatoes, and chopped green onions

In a skillet, bring the stock to a boil and add the onions and
bell pepper. Sauté the vegetables over medium heat until
softened (about 5–7 minutes). Add the cilantro, chiles,
chicken or turkey, rice, and seasonings; stir well, cover, and
cook over low heat for 4–5 minutes, or until thoroughly
heated. Heat the tortillas in the oven until hot but still pliable. Spoon about ⅓ cup of the filling into each warmed
tortilla, add raw-vegetable garnishes, fold tortilla in half, and
eat sandwich style. A dollop of nonfat yogurt, a few drops
of bottled hot sauce or Picante sauce, and a little chopped
fresh cilantro may be used as additional garnishes for extra
flavor.

YIELD: 12 TACOS   CALORIES: 125/TACO
(ABOUT 4–6 SERVINGS)   POULTRY: ABOUT 1 OUNCE/TACO

VARIATION: CHICKEN OR TURKEY ENCHILADA BAKE
Make filling as for the taco recipe above. Prepare a simple
sauce as for *Millet-Applesauce Enchiladas* (page 367); then
fill and roll oven-warmed corn tortillas, top with sauce, and
bake as directed in that recipe. Garnish with nonfat yogurt
or *Mock Sour Cream* (page 408) and a little chopped fresh
cilantro.

GAZPACHO

*This cold soup of Spanish origin offers a different and
delicious way to eat your dinner salad. You can also mold
the soup as in the next recipe for a festive variation.*

    4 large ripe tomatoes, peeled and seeded
    1 large cucumber, peeled and seeded (or ½ Burpless Hybrid
      cucumber or other long thin-skinned variety, no peeling or
      seeding required)
    1 green or red bell pepper
    ½ small red or white onion
    2 shallots
    1 large clove garlic

342

1 cup canned tomato juice
1 cup defatted chicken stock
⅓ cup red wine vinegar
1 tablespoon fresh dill, or 1 teaspoon dried dill
1 teaspoon oregano
1 teaspoon paprika
6 drops Tabasco

GARNISH: diced fresh vegetables and homemade garlic
croutons (see below); *Mock Sour Cream* (page 408) or
nonfat yogurt

Chop the vegetables coarsely and puree them in the blender.
Transfer the pureed vegetables to a bowl and add the tomato
juice, stock, vinegar, and seasonings. Mix thoroughly; chill.
Serve with a garnish of diced vegetables (such as bell pepper, cucumber, green onion, and tomato) and garlic croutons (made from cubed acceptable bread seasoned with
crushed garlic and herbs, then baked in a slow oven until
crisp). *Gazpacho* may also be served with a dollop of *Mock
Sour Cream* or nonfat yogurt.

YIELD: ABOUT 8 CUPS   CALORIES: 40/CUP
(WITHOUT GARNISHES)

GAZPACHO MOLD

2 cups canned tomato juice or V-8
2 envelopes plus 1 teaspoon unflavored gelatin
1 tablespoon red wine vinegar
⅛ teaspoon Tabasco
1⅓ cups peeled and diced tomatoes
1 cup peeled, partially seeded (remove large seeds) and
chopped cucumber
¾ cup diced carrots
½ cup chopped green pepper
¼ cup finely chopped red onions
¼ cup finely chopped green onions or chives
3 tablespoons canned green chile salsa

Place ¾ cup of the tomato juice in a saucepan and sprinkle in the gelatin. Let soak briefly, then set the saucepan over low heat and stir constantly until the gelatin is dissolved. Remove from heat and stir in the remaining tomato juice, vinegar, and Tabasco. Chill to the consistency of unbeaten egg white. Fold in the chopped vegetables and salsa, combining well. Pour the mixture into a 1½-quart mold and chill until firm. Unmold and garnish with watercress or parsley sprigs.

MAKES 8–10 SERVINGS   **CALORIES: 42/⅛ RECIPE**

27 DINNER MENU

PASTA E FAGIOLI (Pasta and Beans) *
Steamed Asparagus
Tossed Green Salad

TIMESAVERS:
* Soak the beans and cook them beforehand, or use cooked beans that have been stored in the freezer.

LEFTOVER SUGGESTIONS:
Reheat or freeze *Pasta e Fagioli.*

WEIGHT-LOSS SUGGESTIONS:
Have half serving of *Pasta e Fagioli* and large servings of asparagus and tossed green salad. Serve another vegetable, such as steamed yellow squash or cabbage, to supplement, if desired.

PASTA E FAGIOLI

    2 cups dried kidney beans
    ½ cup defatted chicken stock or vegetable stock or water
    2 large onions, finely chopped
    2 carrots, finely chopped
    3 cloves garlic, minced or crushed
    1 cup chopped parsley, divided
    2 tablespoons basil
    1 teaspoon oregano
    3 large tomatoes, peeled and chopped
    3 cups cooked whole-wheat pasta (cooked *al dente*; use elbow
        macaroni or corkscrew pasta, or a combination of the two)
    ¼ cup grated Sapsago cheese

Place the beans in a soup pot. Add 8 cups water and bring to a boil; lower heat and cook for 5–10 minutes. Turn off heat, cover, and let beans soak for an hour. Return the water to a boil and cook over low heat, cover ajar, for 45–50 minutes, or until the beans are tender but not too soft. Drain the beans and set them aside.

Heat the stock to a boil in a large pot and add the onions, carrots, garlic, ¾ cup of the parsley, basil, and oregano. Stir-fry the mixture over medium heat for about 6–8 minutes. Stir in the tomatoes; then cover and simmer over low heat for 8–10 minutes. Add the beans, mix well, and simmer another 20 minutes, stirring occasionally. Gently mix in the cooked pasta and heat thoroughly. Sprinkle the remaining parsley and the cheese over the top. If a spicy flavor is desired, serve a bottled hot sauce on the side.

MAKES 8 SERVINGS   **CALORIES: 255/SERVING**

28 DINNER MENU

I.

FRUITED FISH FILLETS
RICE WITH LEAFY GREENS AND TOMATOES
Tossed Green Salad

II.

FISH-BROCCOLI ROLLS IN WINE SAUCE
Baked Potatoes or *MASHED POTATOES* (page 243)*
MUSTARD-YOGURT TOPPING (page 407)**
Broiled Tomato Halves
Tossed Green Salad

TIMESAVERS (FOR MENU II):
* Serve baked potatoes instead of *Mashed Potatoes*.
** Omit Mustard-Yogurt Topping (and moisten baked potatoes and fish with the wine sauce).

LEFTOVER SUGGESTIONS:
Reheat either fish dish. Reheat rice dish or *Mashed Potatoes*. See pages 205 and 208 for suggestions for leftover baked potatoes.

WEIGHT-LOSS SUGGESTIONS:
Omit rice or potato and topping. Serve steamed leafy greens and broiled tomatoes with either fish dish.

FRUITED FISH FILLETS

4 fish fillets, 3–4 ounces each, or 1 pound fish fillets cut into 4
 serving pieces (use sole, red snapper, bass, or other lean
 white fish)
½ cup bottled white grape juice, divided
¼ cup orange juice
1 tablespoon lemon juice
2 tablespoons white wine
1 teaspoon soy sauce
½ teaspoon grated fresh ginger
1½ teaspoons arrowroot

1 teaspoon onion powder
½ teaspoon curry powder
Dash cayenne pepper
½ orange (cut lengthwise), cut into thin wedges
½ lemon (cut lengthwise), cut into thin wedges

Arrange the fish in a baking dish (a spoke pattern in a shallow round dish will be attractive). Mix half the grape juice with the other fruit juices, wine, soy sauce, and ginger, and pour the mixture over the fish. Cover the baking dish and bake in a 375° oven for 15 minutes. Remove cover, baste fish with the juices, and continue baking uncovered about 10–15 minutes longer, or until fish flakes easily with the tines of a fork. Remove from oven and pour the juices into a saucepan, taking care to avoid disturbing the fish. Combine the remaining grape juice with the arrowroot and spices, mixing well. Heat the contents of the saucepan to a boil and add the arrowroot mixture, stirring constantly until thickened and smooth. Spoon the sauce over the fish fillets, and lay the fruit wedges in a pleasing pattern between the fillets. Return fish to the oven briefly (2–3 minutes) to heat the fruit and combine flavors, if desired.

MAKES 4 SERVINGS

CALORIES: 110/SERVING
FISH: 3 OUNCES/SERVING

FISH-BROCCOLI ROLLS IN WINE SAUCE

WINE SAUCE:
⅔ cup water
½ cup dry white wine
½ cup bottled white grape juice
3 tablespoons lemon juice
1 tablespoon plus 1 teaspoon Dijon mustard
1 tablespoon arrowroot
2 teaspoons coarsely chopped capers
½ teaspoon onion powder
¼ teaspoon garlic powder
1 bay leaf
⅓ cup chopped green onions

5 fillets of sole, 3–4 ounces each
5 broccoli spears (with stems cut to about 3 inches in length)

GARNISH: 5 slices canned pimiento, 5–10 steamed broccoli
    spears, lemon slices

Combine all the sauce ingredients except the green onion in
a skillet; mix well. Cook over medium heat, stirring frequently, until thickened. Stir in the green onions. Roll each
sole fillet around the stem of a broccoli spear; lay the rolls
in the sauce, seam side down, and baste with spoonfuls of
sauce. Cook, covered, over medium heat for 12 minutes.
Transfer the fish rolls to a serving dish and pour the sauce
over them. Decorate each fish roll with a pimiento slice,
arrange the additional broccoli spears around the fish, and
finish garnishing with lemon slices.

MAKES 5 SERVINGS   CALORIES: 140/SERVING
FISH: 3 OUNCES/SERVING   WITHOUT GARNISH

RICE WITH LEAFY GREENS AND TOMATOES

*Pretty as a picture, this recipe can be made ahead, then
popped into the oven for baking while you proceed with
other meal preparations. It provides both grain and vegetable courses in one dish. For the leafy greens, you could use
any of several vegetables: the green parts of bok choy or
romaine lettuce leaves, or more common greens like mustard, turnip, or kale.*

    1 onion, chopped
    2 cups chopped leafy greens
    ½ to 1 tablespoon soy sauce
    1 teaspoon ground cumin
    ½ teaspoon ground coriander
    3 cups cooked long-grain brown rice
    2 ripe tomatoes, sliced

In a large skillet, bring ¼ cup water to a boil. Add the onion
and stir-fry over medium heat until softened. Add the
greens, cover, and steam over low heat until the greens are

barely tender (5–10 minutes). Add the soy sauce, cumin, coriander, and rice; mix well, and remove from heat. Press the mixture into a 9-inch square baking dish. Layer the sliced tomatoes over the top. Bake 25–30 minutes in a 350° oven.

MAKES 6 SERVINGS   **CALORIES: 110/SERVING**

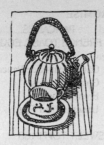

18
CHAPTER

Breakfast Fare

You will want a filling breakfast with good staying power to start each day. Although we will give you a variety of options, the best breakfast for most days on the Pritikin diet is simple: hot cereal topped with sliced bananas or other fresh fruit, a sprinkling of cinnamon, and, if you wish, a little nonfat milk. Those restricting calories should have a small portion of cereal and only half a banana. If you can skip the milk, you will be able to have more of your daily dairy-food allotment for lunch or dinner. An orange or a half grapefruit are good choices for a fruit course, and those not restricting calories might also want to add whole-grain toast, with or without a fruit spread, to round out the meal.

Breakfast is the meal at which most people can cut back on high-protein foods (dairy foods, legumes, and animal foods), permitting them a little more latitude for the rest of the day. For this reason, we have included in this section only breakfast foods that contain little or no dairy foods per serving. However, you will still find a good variety of recipes even for special occasions during the 28-day program. You'll find additional ideas for breakfasts in the discussion in Chapter 16, on pages 203 to 204.

HOT COOKED WHOLE-GRAIN CEREAL is your best breakfast
on the Pritikin diet. Favorites are cooked rolled oats or
cracked wheat, but you could also use different forms of
oatmeal or wheat, such as Scotch oats or bulgur wheat;
other cooked grains like brown rice, millet, barley, buckwheat, or cornmeal (see cooking chart, page 221); or any
acceptable whole-grain cereals found packaged as breakfast
hot cereals at supermarkets or health stores. Dieters can
make their cereal a little less thick (and less caloric per
serving) by reducing slightly the amount of oats or cracked
wheat added to the boiling water or by having smaller portions.

COOKED ROLLED OATS

⅔ cup regular rolled oats
1½ cups boiling water

Stir the oats into briskly boiling water. Reduce heat to moderate and cook 5 minutes or longer, uncovered, until oatmeal has desired consistency, stirring near end as necessary.
Cover, remove from heat, and let stand a few minutes. If
you wish, add a chopped, sliced, or grated apple or other
fresh fruit, or a few raisins, to the cereal a few minutes
before the end of the cooking period; cover and cook a little

longer over low heat until fruit and cereal reach desired consistency. Serve plain or with toppings of hot or cold skim milk, sliced fresh fruit, and a sprinkling of cinnamon, as desired.

MAKES 1 SERVING   208 CALORIES/SERVING

COOKED CRACKED WHEAT

½ cup cracked wheat
1½ cups boiling water

Stir the cracked wheat into briskly boiling water, reduce heat to low, cover, and cook for 7–10 minutes, stirring as necessary near the end of the cooking period; or cook in a double boiler over boiling water for 15–20 minutes. Serve with sliced fresh fruit or a few raisins, a sprinkling of cinnamon, and some hot or cold skim milk, if desired.

MAKES 1 SERVING   211 CALORIES/SERVING

GRANOLA

⅓ cup raisins or currants
¾ cup water
4 cups regular rolled oats
¼ cup frozen apple-juice concentrate
1 tablespoon vanilla extract
2 tablespoons whole-wheat pastry flour
2 tablespoons nonfat dry milk
1½ teaspoons cinnamon
⅛ teaspoon nutmeg

Soak the raisins or currants in the water for 20 minutes. Drain the raisins, reserving the water. Place the oats in a colander and pour the reserved water over them. Put the moistened oats in a mixing bowl and add the remaining ingredients, except the raisins or currants; mix well. Spread the granola in a thin layer on nonstick baking sheets. Bake in a 350° oven for 25 minutes. Add the raisins or currants to the granola for the last few minutes of baking.

YIELD: 5 CUPS   78 CALORIES/¼ CUP

APPLE-OAT CRUNCH

You can combine uncooked rolled oats with fruits to make an unusual fast-and-easy breakfast. (In Europe, particularly in Holland and Denmark, rolled oats are eaten uncooked as a ready-to-eat breakfast food.)

    1 cup regular rolled oats
    1 apple, sliced
    ½ cup unsweetened canned applesauce
    2 tablespoons raisins
    Dash cinnamon

Combine the uncooked oats and fruits, mixing well. Add the cinnamon.

YIELD: ABOUT 2½ CUPS
(1–2 SERVINGS)   246 CALORIES/½ RECIPE

FRUITED MILLET

Eat it hot as a cereal, or let it harden and cut it into bars to be eaten for snacks or packed in a lunch box.

    1 cup millet
    3 cups water
    ½ cup raisins
    1 apple, peeled and diced, or ½ cup drained canned crushed
      pineapple
    2 tablespoons grated orange peel
    3 tablespoons frozen pineapple-juice concentrate or apple-
      juice concentrate
    1 teaspoon vanilla extract
    2 teaspoons cinnamon
    ½ teaspoon nutmeg

354

Place the millet and water in the top of a double boiler. Add the raisins, apple or pineapple, and orange peel. Set over boiling water and cook, covered, over medium heat for 40 minutes or until all the water has been absorbed. Remove from heat and add the juice concentrate, vanilla, cinnamon, and nutmeg. Serve hot in cereal bowls; or spread cooked mixture out in a shallow pie plate to harden in refrigerator. Cut into bars or slices to be eaten cold or reheated in a moderate oven.

MAKES 6–8 SERVINGS   141 CALORIES/⅛ RECIPE

CINNAMON-RAISIN BREAD

¾ cup raisins, chopped
½ cup frozen apple-juice concentrate
1 tablespoon vanilla extract
1 tablespoon rum or brandy (optional)
3 cups whole-wheat pastry flour
2 tablespoons cinnamon
1 tablespoon ground coriander
½ teaspoon allspice
1 package or 1 tablespoon active dry yeast
¼ cup skimmed buttermilk

TOPPING:
¼ cup bran
1 tablespoon frozen apple-juice concentrate
1½ teaspoons ground coriander

Place the chopped raisins in a small bowl with the apple juice, vanilla, and rum or brandy, if used, and soak for at least 10 minutes. Combine the flour, cinnamon, coriander, and allspice in a large bowl and mix well. In a separate small bowl, stir the yeast into 1½ cups warm water until dissolved. Add the yeast solution to the flour mixture slowly, stirring continuously. Stir in the soaked raisins and liquids; then add the buttermilk, mixing well.

Cover the bowl with a damp towel and place it in a warm place (preheat oven to 150°, then turn off before putting bowl in). Let rise for 45 minutes. Transfer the dough to a

9-by-5-inch nonstick loaf pan (oiled very lightly unless the nonstick surface is very good). Stir together the topping ingredients; sprinkle topping over dough, patting it in gently with the back of spoon to adhere well. Cover the baking pan loosely with aluminum foil and bake at 400° for 30 minutes. Remove foil and bake uncovered for an additional 10 minutes. Take the baking pan out of the oven and cover tightly with foil while it cools for 20 minutes. Remove bread from pan and wrap tightly in foil to store.

YIELD: 1 LOAF (ABOUT 16 SLICES)   110 CALORIES/SLICE

OATMEAL BREAD

Version I of this recipe uses buttermilk but no sweetener; version II is milk-free but uses sweetener in the form of raisins, apple juice, and cinnamon. You'll like both versions.

I.

2 cups regular rolled oats
1½ cups skimmed buttermilk
1⅓ cup whole-wheat flour
1 teaspoon baking soda

Combine the oats and buttermilk. Cover and allow to soak for 1–2 hours. Combine the flour and soda and add to the oat mixture; knead to a smooth, stiff dough. Shape into a round ½ inch thick and place in a 9-inch round cake pan. Using a knife, slash the top of the dough twice to mark off four equal wedges. Bake in a 400° oven for 30 minutes; then reduce heat to 350° and continue baking for 10 minutes. Remove from oven, wrap in foil, and set on a wire rack to cool. Cut bread into quarters at slash marks; then cut each quarter in thin slices.

YIELD: 1 9-INCH ROUND LOAF
(MAKES ABOUT 24 THIN SLICES)   50 CALORIES/SLICE

II.

2 cups regular rolled oats
½ cup frozen apple-juice concentrate plus 1 cup water
½ cup raisins, coarsely chopped
1⅓ cups whole-wheat flour
1 teaspoon baking soda
1 tablespoon cinnamon.

Combine the oats, diluted apple-juice, and raisins. Cover and allow to soak for 1–2 hours. Combine the flour, baking soda, and cinnamon and add to the oat mixture. Knead to a smooth, stiff dough. Proceed as for version I.

YIELD: 1 9-INCH ROUND LOAF
(MAKES ABOUT 24 THIN SLICES)   62 CALORIES/SLICE

APPLE-OAT BRAN MUFFINS

4 egg whites, lightly beaten
¾ cup nonfat milk
½ cup nonfat yogurt
¼ cup frozen apple-juice concentrate
1 cup regular rolled oats
1 cup bran
2 apples, peeled and grated
½ cup raisins or chopped pitted dates (optional)
1½ cups whole-wheat pastry flour
1½ teaspoons baking soda
1 teaspoon cinnamon

Combine eggs, milk, yogurt, apple juice, oats, and bran, and stir to mix lightly. Stir in the apples and raisins or dates, if used. In a separate bowl, combine the flour, soda, and cinnamon, stirring to mix well. Add the dry ingredients to the fruit mixture, stirring lightly to combine well. Spoon into nonstick muffin pans and bake in a 425° oven for 25 minutes.

YIELD: ABOUT 24 MUFFINS   67 CALORIES/MUFFIN

BLUEBERRY MUFFINS

1 12-ounce package frozen unsweetened blueberries
(unthawed)
2½ cups whole-wheat pastry flour
½ cup bran
1 tablespoon baking powder
1½ teaspoons baking soda
⅔ cup nonfat milk
½ cup nonfat yogurt
¼ cup frozen apple-juice concentrate
1 tablespoon vanilla extract
4 egg whites, beaten until stiff

Toss the blueberries with ½ cup of the flour; set aside. Combine the remaining dry ingredients in a large bowl. Combine the milk, yogurt, apple juice, and vanilla and stir into the dry ingredients. Fold the egg whites into the batter; then fold in the floured blueberries. Pour the batter into nonstick muffin tins. Cover with a dome of aluminum foil. Bake at 425° for 25 minutes, removing the foil for the last 5 minutes. Cool the muffins, then remove from tins. Replace foil cover to keep them moist or store in an airtight container.

YIELD: 24 MUFFINS   63 CALORIES/MUFFIN

OAT-WHEAT-RICE PANCAKES

If you have a little leftover cooked rice, try making these easy-to-fix blender-mixed pancakes. The rice adds texture to the pancakes. You can also use the batter to make waffles using a nonstick waffle iron. (You may need to brush the grids with a very light coating of oil.)

2 cups water
1½ cups regular rolled oats
1 cup whole-wheat pastry flour
¼ cup frozen apple-juice concentrate
2 heaping tablespoons cooked brown rice
1 scant tablespoon baking powder
1½ teaspoons vanilla extract
2 egg whites, beaten until stiff

Combine all the ingredients except the egg whites in a blender; blend until smooth. Fold in the egg whites. Heat a nonstick skillet to a moderate temperature until a drop of water will "dance" over the surface. Pour the batter into the skillet to make pancakes of desired size. Bake until bubbles form on the top and the underside is browned; then flip over and bake until the other side is browned. Serve with a sprinkling of cinnamon and unsweetened applesauce or with other sweet toppings.

MAKES 2–4 SERVINGS   253 CALORIES/¼ RECIPE

VARIATION: OAT-WHEAT-RICE FRUIT PANCAKES

Add 1 small diced banana and ½ cup frozen unsweetened blueberries (separated and drained of ice) to the pancake batter.

CORN PANCAKES

⅓ cup sifted whole-grain yellow cornmeal
⅓ cup whole-wheat pastry flour
1 teaspoon baking powder
¼ teaspoon baking soda
½ cup water
1 tablespoon bottled white grape juice or frozen apple-juice concentrate
2 egg whites, beaten until stiff

Combine the dry ingredients in a mixing bowl. Stir in the water mixed with the fruit juice; then fold in the beaten egg whites. Heat a nonstick skillet over moderate heat until a drop of water steams or "dances" over the surface. Pour the batter into the skillet to make cakes of desired size. Bake until lightly browned on the underside; then turn and bake the other side until sufficiently browned.

MAKES 1–2 SERVINGS   165 CALORIES/½ RECIPE

FRENCH TOAST

You can make French toast in the conventional way, dipping the whole slice of bread in the egg-white–milk batter.

or you can break the bread into little pieces to expose more surface to the batter. Serve French toast with unsweetened applesauce or other sweet fruit toppings and a sprinkling of cinnamon. Nonfat yogurt or Mock Sour Cream (page 408) are also good accompaniments.

BATTER:

1 egg white, fork-beaten
1½ tablespoons nonfat milk or canned evaporated skim milk
½ tablespoon frozen apple-juice concentrate (optional)
½ teaspoon vanilla extract
½ teaspoon cinnamon

2 slices whole-wheat bread (acceptable kind), or 1½ slices broken into pieces

Beat together the batter ingredients. Dip the bread (or bread pieces) into the mixture, allowing it to soak briefly; then turn to soak the other side. Place a nonstick skillet over moderate heat until a few drops of water "dance" over the surface. Cook the bread on the skillet for about 2–3 minutes or until lightly browned; then turn and brown the other side.

MAKES 1–2 SERVINGS   108 CALORIES/½ SERVING

UNSCRAMBLED EGG

An enjoyable egg dish can be made with only the egg white and a few other ingredients. Serve it on top of toasted whole-grain bread.

1 egg white
1 tablespoon grated onion
1 teaspoon grated green pepper
1 teaspoon grated Sapsago cheese
Dash turmeric

Beat the egg white until soft peaks form. Fold in the other ingredients. Pour the egg mixture into a heated small non-stick skillet and lightly flatten to spread the mixture to a round about 6 inches in diameter. Cook over moderate heat, covered, for 2 minutes; then turn off heat, keep covered,

and let steam for 2 minutes. Remove the egg with a spatula
(the underside should be lightly browned); or if you prefer
both sides browned, flip over and quickly brown the other
side over moderate heat.

MAKES 1 SERVING   26 CALORIES/SERVING

BLUEBERRY JAM

*This jam thickens on standing, but if you like a thicker
jam, increase the gelatin, as indicated.*

> 1 teaspoon unflavored gelatin (or 1½ to 2 teaspoons, for a
>   thicker jam)
> ⅓ cup bottled white grape juice
> 1 tablespoon lemon juice
> 1 12-ounce package frozen unsweetened blueberries or 2¼
>   cups fresh blueberries

Sprinkle the gelatin over 2 tablespoons of the grape juice to
soften. Place the rest of the grape juice with the other ingre
dients in a saucepan. Stir and cook over moderate heat for
about 5 minutes until the berries are thick and crushed. Stir
in the softened gelatin and cook over low heat until dissolved. Cool, then store in a covered jar in the refrigerator
or freezer.

YIELD: ABOUT 1⅔ CUPS   44 CALORIES/¼ CUP

FRUIT JAM

*Prepare several containers of this wonderful spread when
summer fruits are plentiful, or use frozen unsweetened fruits
at other times. The jam is a delicious spread for bread and
can be served in many other ways—a teaspoonful on your
hot cooked cereal makes your everyday breakfast an occa
sion! Freeze extra amounts or put the jam up in Mason-type
jars for pantry storage, following proper home-canning procedures.*

> 4–5 pounds fully ripe peaches, nectarines, plums, or other
>   fruit, or 5 cups frozen unsweetened fruit, partially thawed

    ¼ cup pectin
    ¼ cup frozen apple-juice concentrate
    1 tablespoon date sugar (health-store item), optional
    1 tablespoon lemon juice
    1 teaspoon vanilla extract

If using fresh fruit, cook the fruit in boiling water for 3–4 minutes; then transfer to a pan of cold water to cool for handling. Remove peels and pits. Place the fruit in a colander and press lightly with a potato masher to break up the pulp coarsely (do not overprocess).

Place 5 cups of the fruit pulp (or partially thawed frozen fruit) in a pot and stir in the other ingredients, mixing thoroughly. Bring to a boil, lower the heat, and simmer for 5 minutes. To store in the refrigerator or freezer, cool first, then ladle into containers with tight-fitting lids.

YIELD: ABOUT
6 CUPS   APPROXIMATELY 30 CALORIES/¼ CUP

FRUIT-EGGPLANT SPREADS

This unlikely combination works surprisingly well—the eggplant provides a smooth, bland base, and the fruit takes over to lend color and flavor. Follow the recipe below to make an apple-eggplant spread and the instructions under "Variations" to combine other fruits with eggplant.

    1 large eggplant
    4 green apples, peeled, cored, and grated
    2 tablespoons lemon juice
    2 tablespoons frozen orange-juice concentrate
    2 tablespoons frozen apple-juice concentrate (optional)
    1 tablespoon pectin
    1 teaspoon cinnamon
    ½ teaspoon cloves

Pierce the eggplant with a fork in a few places, set on a cookie sheet, and bake in a 400° oven until soft (about 45 minutes). Cool and peel; cut away portions with seeds and chop the pulp. Place the eggplant pulp in a saucepan with all the other ingredients. Bring the mixture to a boil, reduce heat very low, and cook, stirring frequently, for about 15 minutes until sufficiently thick. At the end of the cooking period, use a potato masher to smooth the mixture, if necessary.

YIELD: ABOUT 3 CUPS   47 CALORIES/¼ CUP

VARIATIONS:

Substitute for the apples 2 cups fruit of your choice. Use hulled strawberries, sliced plums, sliced nectarines, etc (Plums, nectarines, peaches, and similar fruits are best peeled. Plunge them briefly into boiling water to loosen the skins, then peel.) More watery fruits, such as strawberries, will require slightly longer cooking time to achieve desired consistency

APPLE SYRUP

¼ cup frozen apple-juice concentrate
¾ cup water
2 tablespoons vanilla extract
½ teaspoon pumpkin-pie spice
1 tablespoon cornstarch

Place the apple juice, water, vanilla, and pumpkin-pie spice in a saucepan. Bring to a boil, reduce heat, and simmer, covered, for 5 minutes. Mix the cornstarch with 1½ tablespoons water until smooth. Stir the cornstarch paste into the juice mixture and continue to simmer, stirring constantly, until the syrup is thickened and clear. Serve hot over pancakes or French toast.

YIELD: ABOUT 1⅓ CUPS   74 CALORIES/¼ CUP

BLUEBERRY TOPPING

This rather thin spread is excellent for use on toasted bread or English muffins, French toast, or pancakes

2 cups fresh or frozen unsweetened blueberries
¼ cup frozen apple-juice concentrate
1½ tablespoons cornstarch
½ teaspoon vanilla extract or lemon juice

Place blueberries and apple juice in a blender; add the cornstarch and blend until smooth. Transfer to a saucepan and heat the mixture over moderate heat, stirring frequently, until thickened. Add vanilla or lemon juice and stir.

YIELD: ABOUT 1⅓ CUPS   65 CALORIES/¼ CUP

HOT BERRY SAUCE

This easily made sauce using frozen berries is wonderful over pancakes, but can also be used to top tapioca or rice pudding or fresh-fruit desserts. You can substitute frozen cherries or other fruits for the berries, or add more apple-juice concentrate if a sweeter sauce is desired.

2 cups frozen unsweetened berries (strawberries, blueberries, etc.)
3 tablespoons frozen apple-juice concentrate
1 teaspoon vanilla extract (or white wine)
1–2 tablespoons cornstarch
2–4 tablespoons water

Place the berries in a saucepan with the apple juice and vanilla or wine. Bring to a boil, cover, and cook over low heat for about 10 minutes, stirring occasionally, until the berries are soft and partially cooked. Combine the cornstarch with the water, using enough water to make a smooth paste. Stir the cornstarch mixture into the simmering berries and continue cooking over low heat, stirring constantly, until the mixture is thickened. Serve hot or chilled.

YIELD: ABOUT
1½ CUPS   APPROXIMATELY 53 CALORIES/¼ CUP

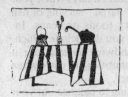

19
CHAPTER

Luncheon Dishes

This versatile array of recipes is suited to every luncheon purpose, from a quick bite on the run to a relaxed sit-down meal with friends. In addition, you'll find recipes in the dinner-menu section that are perfect for lunch as well—among them, *Quick Pita-Bread Pizza, Eggplant-Tomato Stew* or *Vegetable Stew, Tuna-Linguine Salad, Potato Salad Vinaigrette,* and, of course, the soups. Hearty, satisfying soups, teamed with a green salad and good bread or a sandwich, are a favorite lunch. Dieters can modify this plan easily by substituting a low-calorie soup brimming with vegetables and broth and an extra-large green salad, and skipping the bread or sandwich. A complete listing of soups, stews, and other luncheon dishes can be found under subject headings in the recipe index. Refer to Chapter 16, pages 204 to 206, for a more detailed discussion of lunch suggestions.

In planning your lunches, don't forget the guidelines for animal foods, dairy foods, and legumes (see pages 193 to 195). Too much of these foods could elevate your cholesterol and protein levels. The information provided beneath recipes that contain poultry, fish, or meat, or substantial amounts of dairy foods, will let you know when you should use certain recipes with discretion. You should avoid those and legume dishes at your luncheon meal on days when your dinner is built around a Pritikin-size "large" serving of fish or poultry, or on dishes high in dairy foods or beans. Instead, choose a low-protein lunch. If you do include a high-protein item like a cheese-based sandwich spread, use it sparingly. Treat yourself to larger quantities on days when you plan a relatively low-protein dinner.

You'll need to do a little bit of juggling to balance out your day's cholesterol and protein intakes to stay within the prescribed limits. It may take a little thought at first, but you'll soon find yourself making these adjustments almost automatically.

HOT DISHES

MILLET-APPLESAUCE ENCHILADAS

If you enjoy mystifying your guests with recipes that have them lining up for more but completely bewildered as to the ingredients, try this one on them! People love these unusual enchiladas.

FILLING:
½ cup whole millet
1½ cups canned or homemade unsweetened applesauce
1 cup cottage cheese, 1 percent fat (by weight) maximum
⅓ cup chopped red onions
1 tablespoon ground cumin

SAUCE:
1 15-ounce can tomato sauce
1 tablespoon chile powder

12 corn tortillas
3 tablespoons grated Sapsago cheese

Spread the millet in a baking pan and place in a 350° oven for 10 minutes or until lightly browned. Bring 1½ cups water to a boil in a saucepan; add the toasted millet, cover, and cook over low heat for 25 minutes. Combine the cooked millet and other filling ingredients in a bowl, mixing well. Mix the sauce ingredients in a separate bowl. Spread a thin layer of the sauce in a 10-by-14-inch nonstick baking pan.

Heat two tortillas in a 350° oven for about a minute, or until softened; remove them and heat another two while filling the first ones. Spoon about 2½ tablespoons filling into each softened tortilla, roll tortilla, and place seam side down in the pan. Repeat this procedure with the remaining tortillas and filling. Pour the sauce over the enchiladas and sprinkle with the cheese. Bake uncovered at 350° for 30 minutes. Serve with nonfat yogurt and additional applesauce, if desired.

YIELD: 12 ENCHILADAS   260 CALORIES/SERVING
(6 SERVINGS)   ¾ *DAIRY SERVING*/SERVING

THE PRITIKIN PROMISE
ZUCCHINI AND NOODLES

Corn noodles (wheat-free corn pasta available at many health stores) are especially delicious with this dish, but you could also use whole-wheat pasta.

> 4 zucchini, sliced 1 inch thick
> ½ teaspoon garlic powder
> 1 Spanish or white onion, chopped
> 1 red onion, cut in strips
> 2 cloves garlic, minced or crushed
> ½ cup canned green chile salsa
> 2 tablespoons chopped parsley
> 2 tablespoons sherry
> 1 teaspoon soy sauce
> 1 10-ounce package corn noodles (or whole-wheat pasta of
> choice)

Place the zucchini in a steamer basket and sprinkle with the garlic powder; set over boiling water and steam, covered, for about 3 minutes until tender-crisp. In a skillet, stir-fry the onions and garlic in ¼ cup water for a few minutes until the water has evaporated and the vegetables are partially cooked. Add the salsa, parsley, sherry, soy sauce, and zucchini and heat through. Cook the noodles according to package directions, but cut cooking time to only 2 minutes if using the corn noodles; rinse and drain. Toss the noodles with the hot vegetables and serve at once.

MAKES 8 SERVINGS   180 CALORIES/SERVING

CORNMEAL DUMPLINGS AND GREENS

This is "soul food" at its most divine. You can substitute other greens, alone or in any desired combination, for the collards. Good choices would be mustard and turnip greens and kale.

> 3 quarts chopped collard greens
> ½ cup chopped celery
> 2 cups defatted chicken or turkey stock or vegetable stock

½ cup canned green chile salsa
2 teaspoons lemon juice
1 teaspoon soy sauce
¼ teaspoon garlic powder

DUMPLINGS:
½ cup sifted whole-grain yellow cornmeal
⅓ cup whole-wheat pastry flour
2 tablespoons potato flour
1 teaspoon onion powder
1 teaspoon baking powder
½ teaspoon baking soda
Dash pepper
½ cup finely chopped green onions
⅓ cup skimmed buttermilk
1 tablespoon frozen apple-juice concentrate
1 egg white, beaten until soft peaks form

Place the collards and celery in a large pot with 5 cups water. Stir in the stock and seasonings. Bring to a boil, cover, and cook over medium-low heat for an hour before adding the dumplings.

To make the dumplings, combine the dry ingredients in a bowl, mixing well. Stir in the green onions. Combine the buttermilk and apple juice and stir into the dry ingredients. Fold in the beaten egg white. With your hands, form spoonfuls of batter into soft balls (there should be enough batter for 16 balls). Lower the balls, one by one, onto the simmering greens. Cover and cook over medium-low heat for 25 minutes, turning the balls once or twice. If the pot gets too dry, add a little hot water. Serve the dumplings and greens with the broth, and offer a spicy condiment such as Picante sauce on the side.

(If you prefer, you may remove the greens from the pot with a slotted spoon before adding the dumplings. Place the greens in the center of an ovenproof dish, allowing space for the dumplings to go around them. Cover and set the dish in a 200° oven. Form the batter into balls as directed above and gently drop the balls into the simmering liquid in the pot. Cook them as directed above; then arrange the finished dumplings around the greens to serve.)

MAKES 4–5 SERVINGS   245 CALORIES/¼ RECIPE

CAMPER'S CHILE

Backpack or pantry-shelf food items—grains, pasta, a small can of tomato paste, and seasonings—cook in a skillet or saucepan into a quick but satisfying hot meal. Embellish it, if you like, by adding a chopped onion and fresh minced garlic at the beginning of the cooking period, or some pre-cooked chopped vegetables about 5 minutes before serving.

> 1 6-ounce can tomato paste
> 1 teaspoon chile powder
> ½ teaspoon ground cumin
> ¼ teaspoon each: basil, oregano, onion powder, ana garlic powder
> 4 cups water
> 1 cup bulgur wheat
> ½ cup whole-wheat pasta (noodles, macaroni, etc.)

Place the tomato paste and spices in a pot. Add the water and stir to blend well. Stir in the bulgur wheat and pasta. Bring to a boil, reduce heat, and simmer, covered, for 15–20 minutes until sufficiently thick.

YIELD: 4 CUPS   160 CALORIES/CUP

SPICED TOASTED RICE

This good-tasting rice can be eaten hot or cold, by itself or in combination with sliced fresh fruit or cooked fruit, for breakfast, lunch, dinner, or a snack. That's versatility! Although the rice can be cooked in the usual manner (pages 219 to 221), it tastes especially good when it is first oven-toasted as in the recipe below.

> 1 cup long-grain brown rice
> 3 cups water

3 tablespoons frozen apple-juice concentrate
1 tablespoon cinnamon

Place the rice in a large baking dish with sides and set in a 350° oven for 20 minutes or until lightly browned. Combine the toasted rice and other ingredients in a skillet or pot and bring to a boil. (Avoid using a waterless cooker, which results in a gummy-textured product.) Reduce the heat, cover, and simmer for 40–45 minutes.

YIELD: 4½ CUPS   85 CALORIES/½ CUP

CREAMY CORN SOUP

You can concoct this creamy, satisfying corn soup in minutes with a few staple ingredients.

3 cups frozen corn kernels, divided
1 potato, peeled and sliced into ½-inch rounds
1 small onion, coarsely chopped
1½ cups nonfat milk
1 13-ounce can evaporated skim milk
1 2-ounce jar sliced pimiento, chopped
½ tablespoon dillweed
Dash cayenne pepper

Place 2 cups of the corn and the potatoes in a pot with 1 cup water. Bring to a boil and cook, covered, over medium heat for about 3–4 minutes. Transfer the corn mixture to a blender and add the onion and nonfat milk; blend until smooth. Return the mixture to the pot (or use a double boiler —excellent for this purpose) and stir in the evaporated milk. Bring to a boil slowly, stirring as needed; then reduce heat to very low and simmer, covered, about 5 minutes. Stir in the pimiento, seasonings, and remaining corn. Simmer for another 5 minutes, stirring occasionally.

YIELD: ABOUT 6½ CUPS   150 CALORIES/CUP
                                 ¾ *DAIRY SERVING*/CUP

THE PRITIKIN PROMISE
POTATO CAKES

    2 large boiling potatoes
    1 onion, chopped
    ⅓ cup chopped green pepper
    1 teaspoon garlic powder
    1 teaspoon caraway seed
    Dash pepper
    2 egg whites, whisked until frothy
    Paprika

Place the potatoes in a saucepan with water to cover and boil until almost done. Cool, peel, and grate coarsely. Combine potatoes with the other ingredients except the egg whites and paprika. Fold in the egg whites. Form cakes about ½ inch thick and place them on a nonstick baking sheet, flattening them, if necessary, to correct thickness. Sprinkle with paprika. Bake in a 500° oven until tops are crisp and lightly browned, about 20 minutes. Let cool briefly; then loosen cakes with a spatula. Serve with unsweetened applesauce and nonfat yogurt, if desired.

MAKES 2–3 SERVINGS   140 CALORIES/⅓ RECIPE
                          (WITHOUT ACCOMPANIMENTS)

"FRENCH FRIES"

Use leftover baked, boiled, or steamed potatoes to make these tasty mock fries.

    2 large cooked, peeled potatoes
    Onion powder (optional)
    Paprika (optional)

Slice potatoes and arrange slices, separated, on a nonstick baking sheet. Bake in a 400° oven, uncovered, for 12–15 minutes. Turn the potatoes with a spatula and bake the other sides for another 5 minutes, or until golden brown. Sprinkle with onion powder and/or paprika, if desired, a few minutes before the end of the baking period.

MAKES 1–2 SERVINGS   APPROXIMATELY 100
                                     CALORIES/POTATO

VARIATION: SKILLET FRIES

Cube 2 large cooked, peeled potatoes and add to a heated nonstick skillet with ¼ cup grated minced onions. Cook for 7–10 minutes over moderate heat, stirring as required. Sprinkle with garlic powder and paprika.

SANDWICH SPREADS

These spreads can double for dips. Simply thin the spread with a little nonfat yogurt, skimmed buttermilk, or other appropriate ingredient, and correct the seasoning, if needed. Most of the spread recipes use skim milk cottage cheese, which tends to vary as to density and water content. You may need to add a little more or less of the cheese to the blender to get the consistency you want, so add the cheese a little at a time as you blend—which will also make blending easier.

EGG-CHEESE PÂTÉ

4 hard-boiled eggs (discard yolks)
2 teaspoons lemon juice
¼ cup canned green chile salsa
2 teaspoons onion powder
1 teaspoon curry powder
1 teaspoon grated Sapsago cheese
½ teaspoon tarragon
Dash Tabasco
About 1 cup cottage cheese, 1 percent fat (by weight) maximum

Place all ingredients except the cottage cheese in a blender; blend until smooth. Add the cottage cheese and continue to blend, stirring as required, until the mixture is smooth.

YIELD: ABOUT 1⅓ CUPS   40 CALORIES/¼ CUP
                              ¾ DAIRY SERVING/¼ CUP

VARIATION: DEVILED EGGS

Hard-boil eggs, then cut in half lengthwise and discard yolks, taking care to keep egg whites intact. Fill each egg-white cavity with pâté mounded to look like a whole yolk. Sprinkle the "yolks" with paprika or, for a zestier accent, Schilling's Mexican Seasoning.

SALMON PÂTÉ

1 7¾-ounce can pink salmon, drained
½ cup canned water-packed artichoke hearts, drained
1 2-ounce jar pimiento
1 tablespoon onion powder
1 tablespoon garlic powder
1½ teaspoons chopped fresh dill or 1 teaspoon dried dillweed
1 teaspoon paprika
Dash Tabasco
2 cups cottage cheese, 1 percent fat (by weight) maximum

Remove skin and bones from salmon. Place salmon and the other ingredients, except the cheese, in a blender and blend well. Add the cheese, blending and stirring as required until the mixture is smooth and well blended. Chill.

YIELD: 2 CUPS

80 CALORIES/¼ CUP
⅔ OUNCE SALMON/¼ CUP
1 *DAIRY SERVING*/¼ CUP

PIMIENTO CHEESE

2 pepperoncini (bottled peppers in vinegar), seeds and stems removed
1 2-ounce jar pimiento
1 teaspoon onion powder
¼ teaspoon vinegar from pepperoncini jar
¼ teaspoon white wine
1 cup cottage cheese, 1 percent fat (by weight) maximum

Finely chop one pepperoncini and set aside. Place the other pepperoncini and the remaining ingredients, except the cheese, in a blender and puree. Add the cheese and blend until very smooth, stirring as required. Stir in the chopped pepperoncini. If desired, additional pimiento may be chopped and mixed in with the cheese or used as a garnish. Chill before serving.

YIELD: 1 CUP

50 CALORIES/⅓ CUP
1 *DAIRY SERVING*/⅓ CUP

BEAN SPREAD

1 cup cooked and drained pinto beans
¼ cup nonfat yogurt
¼ cup chopped green onions
1 tablespoon canned diced green chiles
1 tablespoon onion powder
Dash cayenne pepper or, for a zingier spread, 1 teaspoon
    Schilling's Mexican Seasoning

Place the beans in a bowl and mash them. Stir in the other ingredients and mash again to combine well.

YIELD: ABOUT 1 CUP

100 CALORIES/¼ CUP

GREEN PEPPER-CHEESE SPREAD

1 cup chopped green pepper
¼ cup chopped celery
1 tablespoon white tarragon vinegar
2 teaspoons onion powder
Dash cayenne pepper
1½ cups cottage cheese, 1 percent fat (by weight) maximum
1 tablespoon minced fresh or dried parsley

Place all ingredients except the cheese and parsley in a blender; puree. Add the cheese and blend until very smooth. stirring as required. Stir in the parsley.

YIELD: 1¼ CUPS

50 CALORIES/¼ CUP
1 *DAIRY SERVING*/¼ CUP

GREEN ONION-CHEESE SPREAD

½ cup chopped green onions
¼ cup skimmed buttermilk
2 pepperoncini (bottled peppers in vinegar), seeds and stems removed
1 teaspoon onion powder
½ teaspoon vinegar from pepperoncini jar
Dash cayenne pepper
1½ cups cottage cheese, 1 percent fat (by weight) maximum
2½ tablespoons canned green chile salsa

Place all ingredients except the cheese and salsa in a blender; puree. Add the cheese and blend until very smooth, stirring as required. Stir in the salsa. (For a zestier flavor, increase the chile salsa slightly.)

YIELD: 1¼ CUPS

50 CALORIES/¼ CUP
1 *DAIRY SERVING*/¼ CUP

COLD SALADS and RELISHES

Here is a wide variety of salads and relishes using grains, fruits, vegetables, occasional small amounts of fish or poultry, and pasta. Pasta salads, so popular now, are a fine Pritikin lunch: filling, tasty, and easily prepared. Leftover pasta stored in the refrigerator or freezer is perfectly suitable. Simply pour some boiling water over the pasta to separate the strands or pieces; then cool it before adding it to the salad. Vary pasta salads by using different dressings (you may be able to substitute leftover dressings which you had prepared for other salads), combinations of raw or cooked chilled vegetables, and flaked tuna or bits of chicken, if you wish. Toss gently, and your lunch is ready!

CORKSCREW-PASTA SALAD

3 cups cooked whole-wheat corkscrew noodles, drained
2 cups chopped tomatoes
1 cup thinly sliced zucchini

½ large red bell pepper, sliced in julienne strips
½ cup frozen green peas, thawed

DRESSING:
⅓ cup tarragon vinegar
2 tablespoons water
1 clove garlic, minced or crushed
1 teaspoon dillweed
1 teaspoon pectin
½ teaspoon soy sauce
½ teaspoon dry mustard (hot Chinese-type)
Dash cayenne pepper

Combine the salad ingredients. Mix the dressing ingredients in a small bowl and beat vigorously with a fork. Pour the dressing over the salad and toss well. Serve chilled in a lettuce-lined salad bowl.

MAKES 3 SERVINGS   190 CALORIES/SERVING

MACARONI SALAD VINAIGRETTE

2¼ cups whole-wheat elbow macaroni (about 4½ cups cooked)
¾ red bell pepper, diced
¾ small carrot, shredded
3 green onions, chopped

DRESSING:
¼ cup plus 2 tablespoons cider vinegar
¼ cup plus 2 tablespoons frozen apple-juice concentrate
3 cloves garlic, crushed
1½ tablespoons fresh lemon juice

Bring at least 4 cups water to a boil. Add the macaroni and cook for about 15 minutes or until tender yet firm; drain and cool. Combine the macaroni, bell pepper, carrot, and green onion and mix thoroughly. Place the vinegar, apple juice, garlic, and lemon juice in a small jar with a tight cover and shake vigorously to blend. Add the dressing to the salad ingredients and toss well. Chill.

MAKES 3 SERVINGS   116 CALORIES/SERVING

PASTA PRIMAVERA SALAD

Use lightly steamed or stir-fried vegetables of contrasting colors and textures; or, if you wish, just add leftover cooked vegetables from last night's dinner. Broccoli florets, red bell pepper, cauliflower, green beans, carrots, sliced mushrooms, snow peas, yellow crookneck squash, and red, white, or green onions are all good choices. For a special touch you can stir-fry the vegetables in a little vegetable or chicken stock with a hint of white wine, and serve your creation with a sprinkling of grated Sapsago cheese.

6 cups cooked vegetables, cut in small pieces
2 cups cooked whole-wheat pasta, drained

DRESSING:
½ cup *Sweet-Sour Vinaigrette Dressing* (page 404), or
Piquant Dressing:
¼ cup rice vinegar
¼ cup frozen apple-juice concentrate
2 cloves garlic, crushed
1 tablespoon lemon juice
1 teaspoon soy sauce
1 teaspoon onion powder
½ teaspoon basil, savory, or crushed rosemary
Dash cayenne pepper

Combine the vegetables and pasta, tossing gently. For the *Piquant Dressing,* place the dressing ingredients in a small jar with a tight-fitting lid and shake vigorously. Toss the pasta salad with the dressing; chill before serving.

MAKES 3 SERVINGS   180 CALORIES/SERVING

POTATO SALAD

The hard-boiled egg whites that are blended into the dressing give this potato salad a very authentic flavor.

5 russet or long white potatoes
3 pepperoncini (bottled peppers in vinegar), seeds and stems removed
⅔ cup chopped celery
½ cup finely chopped onions
⅓ cup chopped green onions
1 4-ounce jar sliced pimiento, chopped

DRESSING:

1½ cups nonfat yogurt, divided
⅓ cup cottage cheese, 1 percent fat (by weight) maximum
3 hard-boiled eggs (discard yolks), reserving 1 for garnish
2 tablespoons prepared mustard
2 teaspoons rice vinegar
2 teaspoons lemon juice
1½ teaspoons soy sauce
1½ teaspoons frozen apple-juice concentrate
1 teaspoon onion powder
⅛ teaspoon garlic powder
Dash cayenne pepper
1 scant teaspoon dillweed

Place the potatoes in a vegetable steamer set over boiling water, cover, and steam until potatoes are just tender when pierced with a fork. (Or cook potatoes in boiling water until tender.) Cool, peel, and place in refrigerator to chill while proceeding with the recipe. Finely chop 2 pepperoncini (reserve 1 for the dressing), and combine with the celery, onions, green onion, and pimiento in a large bowl. Place the reserved pepperoncini, ½ cup of the yogurt, and the remaining dressing ingredients, except 1 hard-boiled egg white and the dillweed, in a blender; blend until smooth. Stir in the dillweed and the remaining yogurt by hand. Slice the chilled potatoes; add them to the vegetables in the bowl, mixing gently. Add the dressing and toss well. Transfer the salad to a lettuce-lined serving bowl and garnish with slices of the reserved egg white and a sprinkling of paprika.

YIELD: ABOUT 7 CUPS

185 CALORIES/CUP
½ *DAIRY SERVING*/CUP

CHICKEN-SALAD-STUFFED TOMATOES

DRESSING:

1 cup nonfat yogurt
2 hard-boiled eggs (discard yolks)
2½ tablespoons wine vinegar
½–1 tablespoon soy sauce
1½ teaspoons curry powder
1½ teaspoons onion powder
1 teaspoon ground ginger
1 cup cottage cheese, 1 percent fat (by weight)
   maximum

STUFFING:

2 cups diced cooked chicken breast
1 cup sliced canned water chestnuts, drained
1 cup diced celery
1 cup green or red seedless grapes
½ cup finely chopped onions

6 large ripe whole tomatoes
6 large lettuce leaves

Place the dressing ingredients in a blender and blend until smooth. Combine the chicken, water chestnuts, celery, grapes, and onions in a bowl. Add 1 cup dressing and toss lightly to coat the salad well. Chill. Cut each tomato at the stem end into eight equal wedges, leaving the bottom quarter of the tomato intact; pull segments apart gently. Just before serving, fill the center of each tomato with the salad. Place each stuffed tomato on a lettuce leaf and garnish with additional grapes and parsley or watercress sprigs. Serve the remaining dressing on the side.

MAKES 6 SERVINGS

210 CALORIES/SERVING
2 OUNCES POULTRY/SERVING
¾ *DAIRY SERVING*/SERVING

CHEF'S SALAD WITH TUNA OR BEANS

This picture-pretty main-dish salad can be varied with other ingredients to suit your whims or the contents of your vegetable bin. Consider chopped watercress, bean or alfalfa sprouts, cooked green beans, quartered tomatoes, sliced jicama, or shredded carrots or red cabbage. Make garlic croutons, for a special addition, by baking cubes of sea-soned acceptable bread (use crushed garlic or garlic pow-der, herbs, perhaps grated Sapsago cheese) in a hot oven until lightly toasted.

SALAD:
8 cups torn lettuce (romaine combined with another variety such as butter or red-leaf)
1 cup shredded iceberg lettuce (optional)
1 cup drained and flaked canned tuna (water-packed), *or* cooked garbanzo or kidney beans, *or* a combination of tuna and beans
1 cup diced celery
½ cup sliced mushrooms
½ basket cherry tomatoes (halved, if large)
4 radishes, sliced
½ small cucumber, sliced (peeled, if waxed)
½ small red onion, thinly sliced

GARNISHES:
1 cup drained canned artichoke hearts (water-packed), quartered
1 cup sliced cooked beets
1 red or green bell pepper, sliced in rings
Hard-boiled eggs (discard yolks), sliced, or *Deviled Eggs* (page 374), optional

Chill ingredients well; combine salad ingredients in a large
serving bowl. Garnish the salad with the artichoke hearts,
beets, bell pepper rings, and sliced egg whites or *Deviled
Eggs*, if used. Serve with *French* or *Vinaigrette Dressing*
(page 403) or other dressing of choice.

MAKES 4 SERVINGS   145 CALORIES/SERVING
                              (WITHOUT DRESSING)
                              1¼ OUNCES TUNA/SERVING
                              (BASED ON 1 CUP TUNA IN RECIPE)

FRUITED RICE SALAD

*This festive-looking, delicious salad features luscious
summer fruits, but you can make it anytime with a few sub
stitutions. Use apples bananas, citrus fruits, winter pears
and pineapple chunks (fresh or unsweetened canned) in the
off-season months. Add an exotic touch with papaya or
mango, when available, and for special occasions you might
add a tablespoon of white wine or Grand Marnier to the
marinade*

    4 cups cold cooked long-grain brown rice
    1½ teaspoons chopped fresh mint
    3 nectarines
    3 plums
    2 peaches
    1 large orange, sectioned
    2 cups green or red seedless grapes

    MARINADE:
    ¼ cup orange juice
    3 tablespoons rice vinegar
    1 tablespoon plus ½ teaspoon frozen orange-juice concentrate
    ¼ teaspoon dry mustard

    GARNISH: whole or halved strawberries, fresh mint sprigs

Combine the rice and chopped mint in a large bowl, set
aside. Slice the nectarines, plums, and peaches (peel first, if
desired), varying the shapes of the fruit slices for maximum

eye appeal: try long, narrow slices for nectarines or chunks for peaches. Place the sliced fruit in a bowl. Add the orange sections, cut into halves or thirds, and the grapes. Stir together the marinade ingredients and combine with the fruit. Refrigerate for 15–20 minutes, stirring gently once or twice. Just before serving, toss the fruit and any marinade in the bowl with the rice, and transfer to a lettuce-lined bowl. Garnish with strawberries and mint sprigs. (The salad is most attractive when freshly tossed, so do not combine rice and fruit in advance.)

MAKES 8–10 SERVINGS   155 CALORIES/¹⁄₁₀ RECIPE

CREAMY FRUIT SALAD

If the cottage cheese you use for this delicious fruit salad is dense and crumbly (such as hoop cheese), you may need to add a little more yogurt and decrease the amount of cheese accordingly.

DRESSING:

1 cup cottage cheese, 1 percent fat (by weight) maximum
1 tablespoon vanilla extract
1 tablespoon date sugar (health-store item) or frozen apple-
   juice concentrate, optional
1 teaspoon lime juice
⅛–¼ teaspoon ground ginger
½ cup nonfat yogurt

2 oranges, cut into small chunks and drained
1 red apple, diced
½ papaya, diced
½ cup red grapes, seeded and halved
½ cup chopped dates (about 8 dates)
½ cup diced celery
½ cup diced jicama or water chestnuts
1 8-ounce can unsweetened crushed pineapple (juice-packed),
   drained, or 1 cup diced fresh pineapple
1 small banana

Place all the dressing ingredients except the yogurt in a blender; blend until smooth. Stir in the yogurt by hand.

Combine the salad ingredients, except the banana, in a large bowl. Add the dressing, tossing gently to coat the salad, and mix well. Slice the banana and stir it in.

YIELD: ABOUT 5½ CUPS   180 CALORIES/CUP
                              ¾ DAIRY SERVING/CUP

VEGETABLE MOUSSE

This is a good way to use up leftover vegetables. The recipe below uses zucchini, but you could substitute any cooked vegetable you like, alone or in combinations. Team the mousse with a grain dish, such as Tabbouli *(page 385), to make a fine lunch. If using a ring mold, put quartered tomatoes or other colorful fresh vegetables in the center*

> 3 cups cut-up cooked zucchini (or other vegetables of choice), drained
> 2 envelopes unflavored gelatin
> 1 teaspoon soy sauce
> ½ teaspoon each: onion powder, dillweed, and crushed tarragon
> Dash cayenne pepper
> ½ cup canned evaporated skim milk, well chilled

Puree the zucchini in a blender and set aside. Sprinkle the gelatin over ¼ cup cold water and let soak for a few minutes. Add ½ cup boiling water and stir until the gelatin is completely dissolved. Combine the zucchini puree, gelatin mixture, and other ingredients except the milk, mixing well. Refrigerate for ½ hour or until slightly thickened. Beat the cold milk until it is at least 4 times its original volume. Using an egg beater, beat the slightly thickened zucchini mixture to fluff it. Fold the whipped milk into the zucchini mixture until no streaks of milk show. Transfer to a 1½-quart mold and chill until set.

MAKES 4–6 SERVINGS   55 CALORIES/¼ RECIPE

TABBOULI

Bulgur wheat, fresh vegetables, and a tangy dressing go into this Lebanese salad—almost a meal in itself. Traditionally, the diner scoops up the salad on romaine lettuce leaves to eat it. It's also delicious served on a bed of vermicelli, a very fine pasta (usually refined); or you can cut up the cooked pasta and mix it into the Tabbouli. A finely milled bulgur is preferable to a coarser one for this recipe.

½ cup uncooked bulgur wheat
1 cup defatted chicken stock or vegetable stock, boiling hot
2 tablespoons lemon juice
½ teaspoon soy sauce
1 clove garlic, minced or crushed
Dash cayenne pepper
1 tomato, diced
½ cup chopped green onions
½ cup minced parsley
¼ cup finely chopped fresh mint
2 teaspoons dried chopped onions
Small romaine lettuce leaves (optional)

Soak the bulgur in the hot stock for 30 minutes. Combine the lemon juice, soy sauce, garlic, and cayenne in a small jar with a tight-fitting lid and shake vigorously to blend; set aside. Drain the bulgur and combine it with the tomato, green onions, parsley, mint, and dried onions. Add the dressing and toss thoroughly. Chill well. Serve on individual salad plates each garnished with 3–4 lettuce leaves, if desired.

MAKES 3–4 SERVINGS   **120 CALORIES/⅓ RECIPE**

TUNA SALAD

1 7-ounce can water-packed tuna, drained and flaked
2 cups bean sprouts, lightly steamed and chopped, or
    uncooked if preferred
1 cup chopped celery
½ cup chopped bell pepper

1 large green onion, chopped, or ½ cup finely chopped white
onion
2 hard-boiled eggs (discard yolks), chopped (optional)

DRESSING:

½ cup *Vinaigrette Dressing* (page 403), or use ⅓ cup herb- or
garlic-flavored red or white wine vinegar, plus 3 tablespoons
water
2 teaspoons prepared mustard (regular or Dijon)
1 large apple, peeled and grated

Combine all the salad ingredients in a bowl and chill well.
Mix the dressing ingredients thoroughly and pour over the
salad, tossing gently. Use as a sandwich filling or as a stuffing for a fresh tomato.

YIELD: ABOUT 4 CUPS

150 CALORIES/CUP
1⅓ OUNCES TUNA/CUP

TUNA-GREEN PEA SALAD

*Uncooked frozen green peas and leftover cooked brown
rice are surprise ingredients in this tasty tuna salad.*

1 cup frozen green peas
1 cup chopped celery
1 cup cold cooked brown rice
½ cup chopped bell pepper
1 large green onion, chopped, or ½ cup finely chopped white
onion
1 7-ounce can water-packed tuna, drained and flaked

DRESSING:

½ cup nonfat yogurt
1 tablespoon prepared mustard
1 teaspoon tarragon
1 teaspoon curry powder

Put the peas in a colander and rinse under lukewarm running
water; drain. Place the peas and other salad ingredients in a
bowl and toss to mix. Combine the dressing ingredients.

mixing well, and stir gently into the salad. Serve with lettuce and sliced tomatoes on salad plates or in sandwiches.

YIELD: ABOUT 4 CUPS   165 CALORIES/CUP
                                    1⅓ OUNCES TUNA/CUP

CARROT-FRUIT SALAD

1 8-ounce can unsweetened crushed pineapple, juice-packed
4 cups grated carrots
2 small oranges, cut in chunks
½ cup chopped dates (about 8 dates)

DRESSING:
1½ cups nonfat yogurt
¼ cup frozen orange-juice concentrate
2 teaspoons poppy seeds
1 teaspoon lemon juice
¼ teaspoon nutmeg

Drain the pineapple well, pressing with a fork to remove excess juice, and combine with the carrots, oranges, and dates in a large bowl. In a separate bowl, stir the dressing ingredients together; add to the carrots and fruits. Toss thoroughly to coat the salad ingredients with the dressing.

YIELD: ABOUT 5 CUPS   105 CALORIES/½ CUP
                                   ½ *DAIRY SERVING*/CUP

CARROT RELISH

Grated carrots, combined with fruit juice and seasonings, make a refreshing relish to accompany luncheon sandwiches or salads. You can also add other ingredients to vary the salad, as shown below.

2 cups grated carrots
1 tablespoon plus 1 teaspoon frozen apple-juice concentrate
1 tablespoon plus 1 teaspoon fresh lemon juice
⅛–¼ teaspoon cinnamon

Combine all ingredients. Chill at least four hours before serving to permit flavors to blend.

MAKES 2 CUPS   35 CALORIES/½ CUP

VARIATIONS:

I. Add ⅓ cup grated apple just before serving.
II. Omit the cinnamon and add ⅓ cup finely chopped pineapple and ⅓ cup thinly sliced celery.
III. Grate the carrots more finely; increase the lemon juice to 2 tablespoons, and substitute ⅔ cup fresh orange juice for the apple-juice concentrate and ½ teaspoon grated fresh ginger for the cinnamon.

EGGPLANT RELISH

1 eggplant
1 tart green apple, peeled and finely chopped
½ cup finely chopped onions
¼ cup canned tomato paste
1 clove garlic, crushed
Juice of ½ lemon
1 teaspoon chile powder
1 teaspoon ground coriander
½ teaspoon soy sauce
Dash cayenne pepper

Pierce the eggplant with a fork in a few places, set it on a cookie sheet, and bake in a 400° oven until soft, about 45 minutes. Remove eggplant from oven, cool, and peel. Mash the pulp; then stir in the other ingredients, mixing well. Serve chilled on lettuce with crackers, bread, or raw vegetables, or serve as a side dish.

MAKES ABOUT 3½ CUPS   50 CALORIES/½ CUP

PICKLE RELISH

Use this piquant relish as an ingredient in potato salads and fish or chicken salads; or add to Mustard-Yogurt Topping *(page 407) to make a "tartar sauce," or to* French

Dressing *(page 403) or* Creamy French Dressing *(page 405) to make a Thousand Island-type dressing. Like the* Pickled Cucumbers *(below), this relish will keep for weeks in the refrigerator and can also be put up for pantry-shelf storage following suitable procedures for home canning.*

2⅓ cups finely chopped pickling cucumbers
½ cup water
½ cup rice vinegar
¼ cup apple-cider vinegar
1 tablespoon pickling spices (in tea ball or tied in cheesecloth bag)
1 tablespoon chopped dried red pepper or 1 2-ounce jar pimiento, chopped
1 tablespoon pectin
1 teaspoon unflavored gelatin
1 teaspoon ground celery seed
½ teaspoon dry mustard
½ teaspoon garlic powder

Place all the ingredients in a saucepan, bring to a boil, and simmer over low heat, covered, for 25 minutes. (Add the pimiento, if used, about 5 minutes before end of cooking period.) Remove the container of pickling spices, pick out the bay leaves and cloves, and return the remaining spices to the relish mixture. Transfer to a container with a tight-fitting lid and refrigerate.

YIELD: 1 CUP   20 CALORIES/TABLESPOON

PICKLED CUCUMBERS

These excellent pickles will keep refrigerated for weeks. If desired, they may be put up in Mason-type jars for pantry-shelf storage following proper home-canning procedures.

1 cup rice vinegar
½ cup apple-cider vinegar
½ cup water
2 tablespoons frozen apple-juice concentrate
¼ cup pickling spices

4 whole cloves
1 clove garlic, chopped
1 teaspoon chopped dill or ¼ teaspoon dried dillweed
½ teaspoon dried minced garlic
4 small pickling cucumbers, quartered lengthwise

Combine the vinegars, water, apple juice, and seasonings in a saucepan and bring to a boil. Add the cucumbers and simmer over low heat for 15 minutes. Transfer the contents of the saucepan to a pint jar with a tight-fitting lid and refrigerate.

YIELD: 1 PINT
        5 CALORIES/¼ PICKLE

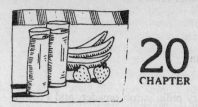

20
CHAPTER

Beverages and Snacks

These satisfying beverages and snacks, including nibbling foods, hot and cold drinks, smoothies, and "ice creams." should carry you happily through and beyond the 28-day program. If you are especially fond of some of these recipes that are made with milk products, save some of your dairy servings for snack time.

For additional ideas and discussion on beverages and snacks, be sure to see pages 210 to 213.

THE PRITIKIN PROMISE
HOT CAROB

¼ cup cold water
½ cup nonfat dry milk
¼ cup carob powder
2 teaspoons dry Postum
2 cups boiling water

Place the cold water, dry milk, carob powder, and Postum in a blender. Blend until the dry ingredients look wet. Add the boiling water and blend at high speed for about 30 seconds, or until mixture becomes frothy and all the ingredients are well blended. Serve immediately.

MAKES 2 SERVINGS   128 CALORIES/SERVING
                                  1 *DAIRY SERVING*/SERVING

HOT APPLE TODDY

Serve this marvelous and unusual beverage for breakfast or as a nightcap.

1 cup nonfat milk
1 cup unsweetened applesauce
½ teaspoon vanilla extract
¼ teaspoon cinnamon

GARNISH: stick cinnamon (optional)

Put all the ingredients in a blender and blend at high speed until smooth and frothy. Heat mixture, but don't boil. Serve immediately in mugs garnished with cinnamon sticks.

MAKES 2 SERVINGS   94 CALORIES/SERVING
                                 ½ *DAIRY SERVING*/SERVING

FROSTY BLENDER AND PROCESSOR CONCOCTIONS usually call for frozen ripe bananas because they add such smooth texture, body, and sweetness. So save your excess ripe bananas for the freezer, peeling first and storing them in a covered container or plastic bag. Freeze bananas overnight or longer for best results. Try them, too, "as is" from the freezer, sliced or whole, for a chilly treat. A blender works for the first two recipes that follow; others require a food processor.

SMOOTHIE

You can make smoothies so thick they are sherbetlike in consistency; or by adding more liquid (or yogurt), you can thin them down as much as you like.

½ cup, or more, liquid (nonfat milk, skimmed buttermilk, unsweetened fruit juice, or frozen unsweetened juice concentrate mixed with water), or nonfat yogurt
1 large frozen banana, cut into chunks
½ cup frozen unsweetened berries or other frozen unsweetened fruit
½–1 teaspoon vanilla extract (optional)

Put ½ cup liquid into a blender. Add the banana with the rest of the frozen fruit and the vanilla, if used. Blend until smooth, stirring as required, adding more liquid, if desired. Serve at once.

YIELD: ABOUT 1 CUP (USING ½ CUP LIQUID)	ABOUT 190 CALORIES AND ½ DAIRY SERVING/CUP (BASED ON USE OF ½ CUP NONFAT MILK)

BANANA-PINEAPPLE "ICE CREAM"

You'll need to freeze canned unsweetened crushed pineapple (do not drain) as well as a banana for this recipe. Just transfer the contents of the can to a plastic seal-top bag, freeze, and break off chunks as needed; or divide the contents of an 8-ounce can into 4 equal portions and freeze in separate plastic bags for making 4 individual servings.

1 large frozen banana, cut into chunks
About 2 ounces canned unsweetened crushed pineapple, frozen
½–1 teaspoon vanilla extract (optional)

Place the frozen fruit and vanilla, if used, in a blender. Blend, stopping the motor to stir frequently, until the mixture is smooth. Serve at once.

MAKES 1 SERVING   140 CALORIES/SERVING

PROCESSOR "ICE CREAM" WITH BANANAS

For each frozen banana—which provides the smooth-textured base for this "ice cream"—add ¼ cup thick liquidy ingredient of choice, such as nonfat yogurt, unsweetened applesauce, frozen unsweetened fruit that has been partially thawed, Blueberry Jam (page 361), Fruit Jam (page 361), or other suitable ingredient, and a small quantity of flavoring (vanilla extract, frozen apple-juice concentrate, cinnamon, carob powder, etc.).

    3 large frozen bananas, cut into chunks
    ¼ cup nonfat yogurt
    unsweetened applesauce, or other suitable ingredient (see
        above)
    2 teaspoons vanilla extract

Place the ingredients in a food processor and start blending, using pulse action. When almost smooth, process continuously for a few seconds longer until completely smooth. (Do not overprocess or "ice cream" will become too soft.) Serve at once.

MAKES 3 SERVINGS   144 CALORIES/SERVING
                                    ¼ DAIRY SERVING/SERVING

CARROT-BANANA-ORANGE AMBROSIA

Since carrots are the principal ingredient, it's important that they be sweet. If not sweet enough, add about 2 tablespoons frozen apple-juice concentrate to the food processor, along with the other ingredients.

    2 large frozen carrots, cut into chunks
    1 large frozen banana, cut into chunks
    1 small frozen seeded orange, cut into chunks

⅓ cup canned evaporated skim milk
½ teaspoon orange extract
1 drop coconut extract

Place all ingredients in the food processor. Start blending using a pulse action. When almost smooth, process continuously for a few seconds longer until completely smooth and well fluffed. Serve at once

MAKES 3 SERVINGS   106 CALORIES/SERVING

STRAWBERRY "ICE CREAM"

If you have a fabulous multipurpose machine called a Vita-Mix® (for everything from bread to ice cream) you'll be able to make this recipe one of many developed for the Pritikin diet by the Vita-Mix® people. This 'ice cream' is unique in that it uses no milk products and has rice as a chief ingredient. The rice should be soft-cooked, so add a little extra water in cooking it

2 cups soft-cooked brown rice
2 tablespoons frozen apple-juice concentrate plus water to
    make ½ cup
4 cups frozen unsweetened strawberries
Few drops each of almond and vanilla extracts

Process the rice and diluted juice in the Vita-Mix® on high speed forward until very smooth; add the strawberries and flavorings and continue to process until the strawberries are worked into the mixture. Serve immediately

MAKES 3 SERVINGS   275 CALORIES/SERVING

YOGURT PARFAIT

Borrow one of baby's jars of pureed fruit for this easy-to-make delicious parfait. You may substitute canned unsweetened crushed pineapple for the fresh fruit or use them together, if you wish. Other suggestions for combining yogurt with fruit appear on pages 202 to 203

THE PRITIKIN PROMISE

1 cup nonfat yogurt
1 7¾-ounce jar unsweetened baby-food peaches, or other fruit
   variety
Few drops almond or vanilla extract (optional)
½ cup packaged breakfast cold cereal (no-sugar-added,
   whole-grain variety)
1 cup sliced bananas or other fresh fruit, or a combination of
   fresh fruits

Combine the yogurt, baby food, and flavoring extract. Crush
the cereal or blend it briefly in a blender to make a medium-
fine crumb texture. Using parfait glasses or other suitable
glasses, alternate layers of the yogurt mixture, cereal, and
fresh fruit, beginning with the yogurt mixture and ending
with the fruit.

MAKES 2 SERVINGS   ABOUT 307 CALORIES/SERVING
                              (USING BANANAS)
                          ½ DAIRY SERVING/SERVING

MINERAL-WATER "MIXED DRINKS"

*A good choice (if you want something with more flavor
than water) for a nonalcoholic thirst quencher or as a substitute for an alcoholic beverage is plain or flavored mineral
water. Mineral waters vary greatly in sodium content, however: Vichy is unacceptably high in sodium, and Schweppes
is also too high, but you can use Perrier, Poland, and Mountain Valley, among others. Most club sodas are too high in
sodium.*

*To make a mineral-water "mixed drink," mix mineral
water with your choice of fruit or tomato-type juice (as directed below), then add a few drops of Angostura bitters, if
you like. The most authentic-tasting "mixed drink" is made
by combining mineral water, bottled white grape juice, and
the bitters. Some like the mineral water with the bitters
alone, without juice. Here are some combinations you may
wish to try.*

to 1 cup mineral water, chilled
   ADD:
   ⅓ cup bottled white grape juice, chilled, *or*

1–2 tablespoons lime or lemon juice, *or*

2 tablespoons orange juice, *or*

1 cup V-8 or tomato juice, chilled

AND:

A few drops Angostura bitters (optional)

Combine mineral water, juice of choice, and bitters, if used. If your drink needs a little sweetening, add a hint of apple-juice concentrate (or bottled white grape juice). Serve over ice.

MAKES 1 "MIXED DRINK"
5–50 CALORIES (DEPENDING UPON JUICE ADDED)

APPLE BUTTER

Apple Butter *spread on crackers or warm toast can make a lovely snack. You'll find other fruit-spread recipes in other sections; see "fruit spreads" in the recipe index.*

6 large or 8 medium apples
1 cup water
¼ cup plus 2 tablespoons frozen apple-juice concentrate, divided
1 tablespoon cinnamon
⅛ teaspoon cloves
1 tablespoon cornstarch

Peel, core, and thinly slice the apples. Place in a pot with the water, ¼ cup of the apple juice, cinnamon, and cloves. Bring to a boil, reduce heat, and simmer uncovered for an hour. Mix the cornstarch with the remaining 2 tablespoons apple juice until smooth. Add the cornstarch paste to the apples a few minutes before the end of the cooking period, stirring while the mixture thickens. Transfer to a blender and puree; continue to blend until smooth.

YIELD: 4 CUPS
14 CALORIES/TABLESPOON

CHIP 'N' DIP

Accompany your homemade Corn Chips *with any of these delicious dips.* Onion Dip *is a favorite, or try* Green Bean Guacamole *(page 281),* Salsa *(page 407), or any of the sandwich spreads (pages 373 to 375) thinned to dip consistency as directed in the recipes. You can also serve any dip with crackers or raw vegetables such as cut-up cauliflower or broccoli; celery, carrot, or zucchini sticks; or whole cherry tomatoes.*

CORN CHIPS:
6 packaged corn tortillas

Using the point of a sharp knife, score each tortilla into 8 equal wedges as you would a pie. Start each cut an inch or more from the edge, pass through the center, and finish an inch or so from the opposite side. The score marks will make it easy to break the tortillas, after baking, into neat wedge shaped chips. Lay the scored tortillas on an oven rack or baking pan, avoiding overlapping, and bake in a hot oven until crisp and lightly browned, turning once or twice to promote even crisping. Break the crisped tortillas at the score marks into wedge shapes.

YIELD: 48 CHIPS   ABOUT 7 CALORIES/CHIP

ONION DIP:
2 tablespoons skimmed buttermilk, or more, if required
2 teaspoons lemon juice
¼ small onion, coarsely chopped
1 cup cottage cheese, 1 percent fat (by weight) maximum
1 teaspoon dried minced onions
Pinch dillweed

Put the buttermilk, lemon juice, fresh onion, and cheese in a blender and blend until completely smooth. Add the dried onions and dillweed; blend for a few seconds longer. If the dip consistency is too thick, add a little more buttermilk

YIELD: 1 CUP   ABOUT 10 CALORIES/TABLESPOON

GARBANZO "NUTS"

Snack on these "beanuts" or add them to dishes like "Fried" Rice or Couscous to provide a nutty quality. If the cooked beans are frozen for a day or more before baking, they will have an even better consistency when finished.

> 2 cups dried garbanzo beans (chick-peas)
> About 1 tablespoon each: onion powder and garlic powder

Place the beans in a pot and cover with water to about 3–4 inches above the beans. Soak overnight; or bring to a boil and simmer about 10 minutes, then turn off heat and soak for about an hour. Discard the water and replace with fresh water, again to about 3–4 inches above the beans. Bring to a boil, reduce heat to moderate, and cook the beans uncovered for about 1½ hours; cover and cook over low heat another ½ hour or until tender, stirring occasionally to prevent sticking. Drain well. (See note in introduction about freezing the beans.)

Place the beans in a single layer on a nonstick baking pan and, while still damp, sprinkle with the onion and garlic powders. Bake in a 350° oven for about 45 minutes, or until the beans are quite dry and browned. From time to time during the baking period, loosen the beans from the pan with a spatula and turn them by shaking the pan, to brown more evenly.

YIELD: ABOUT 5⅓ CUPS   93 CALORIES/⅓ CUP

POTATO CHIPS

These salt- and fat-free chips are fun to make and are surprisingly good. The key to success in making them is to slice the potatoes ultra-thin with a food processor. (Some ovens do better than others, too.) If you like, sprinkle a seasoning over the finished chips, such as onion powder, chile powder, or garlic powder.

> 2 medium baking potatoes, peeled
> Ice water, as required

Using a food processor with the thinnest slicing setting, slice the potatoes into "potato chips" (approximately 55 chips per potato). Place the chips in a bowl of ice water for about 20 minutes. Drain thoroughly and pat dry with paper towels. Without overlapping them, lay the chips on nonstick baking sheets. Bake in a 425° oven for about 12 minutes, or until golden brown.

YIELD: ABOUT 110 CHIPS   ABOUT 2 CALORIES/CHIP

VEGETABLE FINGER FOODS are fine snacks, but if you've been stuck on carrot and celery sticks, it's time to expand your vegetable vistas and include others. Try cut-up broccoli, cauliflower, zucchini, cabbage, and that delicious Mexican root vegetable, jicama. In the warmer months, freeze jicama slices and carrot sticks, or whole baby carrots, placing them side by side on a sheet of foil and covering them with plastic wrap. You'll find the frozen vegetable morsels make good nibbling right from the freezer. These are ideal snacks, especially suited to dieters.

If you are not watching your calories, try breading and baking raw vegetables cut finger-food size for an unusual treat. Children who balk at vegetables have been known to consume these by the plateful.

BREADED VEGETABLES

Vegetables of choice: zucchini, eggplant, onion, russet or Idaho potatoes, or yams or sweet potatoes

BREADING (sufficient to bread "sticks" from about 3 zucchini
    or ½ eggplant *or* 2 potatoes; *or* slices from about 2 onions *or*
    1 large sweet potato or yam):
¼ cup whole-wheat pastry flour
¼ cup canned evaporated skim milk
2 egg whites, fork-beaten
1 teaspoon lemon juice
1 teaspoon onion powder
1⅓ cups fine whole-wheat bread crumbs (from acceptable
    bread), sprinkled with 1 teaspoon onion powder

Peel the vegetables, if needed (zucchini and eggplant do not require peeling), and cut into crosswise slices about ½ inch thick, or French-fry–shaped sticks about ½ inch thick and measuring about ½ inch by 5 inches. Combine breading ingredients, except the bread crumbs, in a bowl; mix well. Place the bread crumbs in a separate bowl. Coat the vegetables by dipping them, one by one, in the wet flour mixture, then in the bread crumbs. Lay the vegetables on a nonstick baking sheet. Bake in a 350° oven for about 35 minutes. Serve warm. (If you like a softer breading, wrap the pan with aluminum foil for about 10 minutes just after removing it from the oven.)

MAKES 2–4 SERVINGS   ABOUT 100 CALORIES FOR BREADING
AND ABOUT 25–75 CALORIES FOR
VEGETABLES (DEPENDING UPON
VEGETABLES USED)/¼ RECIPE

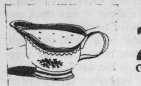

21
CHAPTER

Salad Dressings and Other Toppings

With these diversified recipes you will be able to complement any salad and many side dishes and entrées with a delicious dressing or topping. You will be especially delighted with the dressings that have a consistency and appealing glossiness to rival the best commercial or restaurant dressings. The secret is the use of two thickening agents, pectin and arrowroot, as well as a short cooking period. You'll find it is well worth the little extra trouble. In addition to using these dressings for salads, they work well as marinades for raw or cooked vegetables, chicken, or fish.

The topping recipes include spicy *Salsa*, a tomato-chile relish; *Mock Sour Cream*, which tastes like sour cream but is made from skim-milk products; and *Nonfat Yogurt*, a simple preparation you may wish to make if you are unable to buy *nonfat* yogurt in your area. All three toppings are excellent with baked potatoes, bean and Mexican dishes, some vegetable dishes, and even with salads, as a change from dressings.

FRENCH DRESSING

2 cloves garlic, coarsely chopped
½ cup rice vinegar
⅓ cup water
⅓ cup canned tomato sauce
3½ tablespoons frozen apple-juice concentrate
1 teaspoon pectin
1 teaspoon arrowroot
1 teaspoon dry mustard
1 teaspoon onion powder
½ teaspoon oregano
½ teaspoon ground thyme
⅛ teaspoon paprika

Place the garlic, vinegar, water, tomato sauce, and apple juice in a blender; blend thoroughly. Transfer the blender contents to a saucepan and add the remaining ingredients, stirring to mix well. Bring to a boil; then lower heat and simmer, stirring constantly, until thickened (about 4–5 minutes). Serve chilled.

YIELD: 1 CUP   12 CALORIES/TABLESPOON

VINAIGRETTE DRESSING

¾ cup bottled white grape juice
½ cup tarragon white-wine vinegar
2 cloves garlic, crushed
2 tablespoons water

403

THE PRITIKIN PROMISE

1 tablespoon lemon juice
2 teaspoons soy sauce
1 teaspoon Dijon mustard
1 tablespoon pectin
2 teaspoons arrowroot
½ teaspoon each: onion powder and garlic powder
¼ teaspoon each: crushed rosemary, dillweed, and thyme
Dash cayenne pepper

In a small saucepan, combine all ingredients; stir to mix well. Bring to a boil, reduce heat, and simmer, stirring constantly, until thickened (about 4–5 minutes). Transfer to a blender and blend briefly. Serve chilled.

YIELD: 1½ CUPS   8 CALORIES/TABLESPOON

SWEET-SOUR VINAIGRETTE DRESSING

Try this dressing warmed for a change, on top of a Pritikin spinach salad made of romaine lettuce mixed with a few fresh spinach leaves, garnished with chopped hard-boiled egg whites, sliced tomato, and sliced red onion.

¾ cup water
¼ cup frozen apple-juice concentrate
3 tablespoons rice vinegar
1 tablespoon cider vinegar
1 tablespoon lemon juice
2 teaspoons soy sauce
2 cloves garlic, crushed
1 tablespoon pectin
1½ teaspoons arrowroot
1 teaspoon oregano
1 teaspoon onion powder
½ teaspoon each: garlic powder, savory, paprika, and dry mustard
Dash cayenne pepper

In a small saucepan, combine all ingredients and stir to blend well. Bring to a boil; then reduce heat and simmer,

stirring constantly, until thickened (about 4–5 minutes).
Serve chilled or warmed (see above).

YIELD: 1½ CUPS   8 CALORIES/TABLESPOON

ZESTY TOMATO DRESSING

Try this easy variation of French Dressing *(page 403) or*
Vinaigrette Dressing *(page 403).*

 1 cup canned tomato sauce
 ¼ cup canned green chile salsa
 ¼ cup frozen apple-juice concentrate
 ¼ cup *French Dressing* or *Vinaigrette Dressing*
 ¼ cup lemon juice
 3 cloves garlic, coarsely chopped
 ⅛–¼ teaspoon cayenne pepper

Place all the ingredients in a blender; blend well. Chill before
serving.

YIELD: 2 CUPS   9 CALORIES/TABLESPOON

CREAMY FRENCH DRESSING

*Mashed yams are the surprise ingredient that gives this
delicious French dressing its characteristic color and texture.*

 1 cup peeled and mashed baked yams
 ¾ cup water
 ½ cup rice vinegar
 3 tablespoons lemon juice
 2 tablespoons canned tomato paste
 1 tablespoon frozen apple-juice concentrate
 1 tablespoon soy sauce
 ½ teaspoon dry mustard
 ¼ teaspoon each: onion powder, garlic powder, and allspice
 Dash cayenne pepper

THE PRITIKIN PROMISE

Combine all ingredients in a blender; blend until smooth. Chill.

YIELD: 2 CUPS   12 CALORIES/TABLESPOON

ITALIAN DRESSING

- ½ cup freshly squeezed lemon juice
- ½ cup salad vinegar
- ¼ cup frozen apple-juice concentrate
- ¼ cup water
- 2 green onions, chopped
- ¼ teaspoon sage
- ¼ teaspoon garlic powder

Combine all ingredients in a blender; blend well. Chill and serve.

YIELD: 1⅔ CUPS   7 CALORIES/TABLESPOON

CUCUMBER-YOGURT DRESSING

- ½ large or 1 small cucumber, peeled, seeded, and grated
- 1 cup nonfat yogurt
- 2 teaspoons dillweed
- 1½ teaspoons garlic powder

Combine all ingredients, mixing well. Serve chilled.

YIELD: ABOUT   8 CALORIES/TABLESPOON
1½ CUPS   APPROXIMATELY ¼ *DAIRY SERVING*/½ CUP

BUTTERMILK-MUSTARD DRESSING

It is best to make this delicious dressing with a no-salt-added-type prepared mustard (available in health stores), since it uses such a large quantity of mustard.

- 1¼ cups skimmed buttermilk
- ½ cup plus 2 tablespoons prepared mustard
- 2 tablespoons frozen apple-juice concentrate

Combine all ingredients, mixing well. Chill.

YIELD: 2 CUPS   10 CALORIES/TABLESPOON
APPROXIMATELY ¼ *DAIRY SERVING*/½ CUP

MUSTARD-YOGURT TOPPING

Use this simple topping for baked potatoes or fish, over cooked vegetables such as broccoli, or as a sandwich spread.

1 cup nonfat yogurt
2 teaspoons Dijon mustard
½ teaspoon rice vinegar (optional)
½ teaspoon garlic powder
¼ teaspoon dillweed

Combine ingredients, mixing well. Chill.

YIELD: ABOUT   8 CALORIES/TABLESPOON
1 CUP   APPROXIMATELY ½ *DAIRY SERVING*/½ CUP

SALSA

This Mexican-inspired spicy relish can be used as a dip or as a topping for salads, baked potatoes, hot vegetables, and rice, as well as for Mexican or bean dishes. It's also excellent with fish and chicken. Nonfat yogurt or Mock Sour Cream *(page 408) team nicely with* Salsa *for any of these uses, adding another flavor and texture accent.*

4 cups canned tomatoes
1 cup chopped onions
½ cup chopped cilantro (Mexican or Chinese parsley)
2 tablespoons canned tomato paste
1 tablespoon red-wine vinegar
1 tablespoon lemon juice
1 teaspoon garlic powder
¼ teaspoon cayenne pepper
4 cloves garlic, minced or crushed
½ cup diced fresh green chiles

407

Place all the ingredients except the fresh garlic and chile in a bowl. Place the garlic and chile in a small saucepan with about ⅓ cup water. Bring to a boil, reduce heat, and stir-fry over moderate heat for about 4 minutes or until pan becomes dry. Add the cooked garlic and chile to the bowl and mix well. Chill and serve.

YIELD: ABOUT 5 CUPS   4 CALORIES/TABLESPOON

VARIATION: Use 4 cups diced fresh tomatoes instead of canned. Add tomatoes to the saucepan with the garlic and chile, increasing water to about 1 cup and cooking time to 6–7 minutes. Transfer to a blender and blend at low speed for about 15 seconds; mix with other ingredients and chill.

MOCK SOUR CREAM

This topping has countless uses, much like a conventional sour cream. It is creamy and cool—decorative, too—a complement to many dishes, from baked potatoes, salads, and Mexican- or Indian-style concoctions to fresh or cooked fruit, pancakes, and desserts. It also makes a versatile base for dips, spreads, and salad dressings, and may often be used in place of yogurt. If you wish, make it up in larger quantities for freezing. To use after freezing, thaw and stir vigorously.

¼ cup skimmed buttermilk, or more, as required
1 cup cottage cheese, 1 percent fat (by weight) maximum
½ teaspoon lemon juice or vinegar, or more, to taste
   (optional)

Pour the buttermilk into a blender and add the cheese, blending and stirring as required to mix well. Add more buttermilk, if necessary, to obtain a smooth consistency and desired thickness, and blend again. Blend in the lemon juice or vinegar, if used.

YIELD: ABOUT 1 CUP   9 CALORIES/TABLESPOON
                                   1 *DAIRY SERVING*/¼ CUP

NONFAT YOGURT

Yogurt has become increasingly popular and is assumed to provide good nutrition—though in fact it is a high-fat item in its whole-milk form. Fortunately, in many areas a nonfat yogurt is now being sold; but if you haven't yet found a source, or prefer to make your own, this recipe is for you. Use the agar if you can get it—it adds body and smoothness to the yogurt; you'll find it in health stores and some supermarkets.

Nonfat yogurt is a wonderfully versatile food, and is usually interchangeable with Mock Sour Cream (page 408).

    1 quart nonfat milk
    ⅓ cup nonfat dry milk
    3 tablespoons low-fat yogurt, or nonfat yogurt from previous
        batch
    1½ teaspoons agar (optional)

Combine the milks, stirring to dissolve the dry milk thoroughly. Heat the mixture in a saucepan until almost boiling; it should just start to bubble slightly. Pour the hot milk into a container (glass, crockery, or stainless steel) and let it cool to about room temperature. Remove ½ cup of the cooled milk and stir into it the low-fat or nonfat yogurt and agar, if used. Stir the mixture back into the milk in the container. Place the container inside a larger vessel filled with warm water and cover with a towel. Set in a warm oven (preheat to 150°, then turn off before placing yogurt assembly inside) for at least 8 hours or overnight. If you have an electric oven, turn the light on to provide continued warmth; in a gas oven, the pilot light is sufficient.

YIELD: 4 CUPS   7 CALORIES/TABLESPOON
                 ½ *DAIRY SERVING*/6 TABLESPOONS

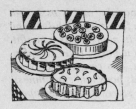

22

CHAPTER

Desserts

When a piece of fresh fruit, fruit cup, baked yam or sweet potato, or other simple sweet is not quite enough to end your meal, try one of the recipes below or look for other dessert-type recipes in the chapters on *Breakfast Fare* (Chapter 18) and *Beverages and Snacks* (Chapter 20). You'll also find good ideas for simple desserts in the dessert discussion in Chapter 16, pages 202 to 203.

Some of these desserts contain quite a bit of dairy food. We have indicated beneath the recipe when the amounts are substantial, so that you can keep track of your dairy-food servings.

BANANAS IN BERRY SAUCE

A simple but elegant fruit finale. Fresh fruit may be substituted for the frozen, if preferred.

1½ cups frozen unsweetened berries, partially thawed
    (strawberries, blueberries, boysenberries, raspberries)
1 to 1½ tablespoons frozen apple-juice concentrate (optional)
2 to 4 tablespoons white wine
3 bananas, halved lengthwise

Puree the berries in a blender, adding apple juice if more sweetness is desired. Pick out any large seeds. Heat the wine in a nonstick sauté pan or skillet, add the bananas, and sauté for about 3 minutes. (The bananas may be halved again, crosswise, for convenience in sautéing.) Pour the fruit puree over the bananas and heat thoroughly. Serve immediately

MAKES 3–4 SERVINGS   105 CALORIES/¼ RECIPE

BAKED APPLES

6 small green cooking apples, cored
1½ cups water
¼ cup frozen apple-juice concentrate
2 teaspoons vanilla extract
1 teaspoon cinnamon
1 teaspoon arrowroot

Remove the peel from the top third of each apple. Arrange the apples in a baking dish just large enough to hold them snugly. In a saucepan, combine the other ingredients and bring to a boil, stirring frequently; reduce heat and simmer for 2–3 minutes until slightly thickened. Pour the sauce over the apples. Bake uncovered in a 350° oven, basting occasionally, for 1 to 1½ hours until apples are easily pierced with a fork. Remove dish from oven and let apples cool in the sauce. Serve hot or cold, plain or with a whipped topping (pages 430–32).

MAKES 6 SERVINGS   83 CALORIES/SERVING

MARINATED MANDARIN ORANGES

If you don't have fresh mandarin oranges available, use tangerines or tangelos.

3 mandarin oranges
1 tablespoon frozen apple-juice concentrate
1 teaspoon grated fresh ginger
Drop almond extract

Separate the oranges into segments, removing any surrounding membrane. Clip the inside edge of each segment with a scissors to remove seeds, if any. Combine the other ingredients in a bowl and add the orange segments, stirring to coat well. Marinate oranges for several hours in the refrigerator. Serve chilled.

MAKES 3 SERVINGS   APPROXIMATELY 60 CALORIES/SERVING

FRUIT MERINGUE

Vary this delicious dessert by substituting other fruit combinations, selecting from fresh, frozen unsweetened (partially thawed), or canned juice-packed fruits (drained).

    3 cups strawberries, sliced
    2 cups frozen cherries, partially thawed and halved
    ¼ cup frozen apple-juice concentrate
    1 tablespoon lemon juice
    1 tablespoon pectin
    1 teaspoon each: vanilla extract and lemon extract
    6 egg whites

Combine all the ingredients except the egg whites in a pot. Stir and bring to a boil, then reduce heat and simmer, stirring constantly, for 3–5 minutes until slightly thickened. Pour the fruit mixture into a bowl to cool briefly. Beat the egg whites until stiff peaks form and fold into the fruit. Transfer the mixture to a 9-by-13-inch glass or nonstick baking dish. Set the dish into a larger ovenproof pan filled with enough boiling water to reach about halfway up the sides of the baking dish. Bake uncovered in a 375° oven for 20 minutes. Remove the baking dish from the water 2–3 minutes before the end of the baking period, placing it directly on the oven rack to finish baking. The meringue should brown only slightly. Remove from oven and let set for about 10 minutes or longer before serving, or serve chilled.

MAKES 10 SERVINGS   50 CALORIES/SERVING

APRICOT MOUSSE

    2 cups bottled white grape juice, divided
    3 tablespoons white wine
    1 tablespoon vanilla extract
    1 teaspoon orange extract
    2 envelopes plus 1½ teaspoons unflavored gelatin
    1 16-ounce can whole apricots (juice-packed), undrained
    ¾ cup diced fresh peaches or drained canned peaches (water-
       or juice-packed), mixed with ½ teaspoon lemon juice

½ cup nonfat dry milk
Nutmeg

Combine 1 cup of the grape juice, the wine, and the flavor extracts in a saucepan. Sprinkle the gelatin over the liquid, let soak briefly, and stir continuously over low heat to dissolve. Place the apricots and juice into a blender; add the peaches and gelatin mixture. Blend at low speed, then at high speed until frothy. Refrigerate the blender container until the fruit mixture begins to set (about 15 minutes). Blend again at high speed for 1–2 minutes, then transfer to a bowl. Add the remaining cup of grape juice to the blender with the dry milk and blend well; stir into the fruit mixture Pour into individual dessert dishes and sprinkle with a little nutmeg. Chill until set

MAKES 8 SERVINGS   85 CALORIES/SERVING

VARIATION: Substitute canned plums for the apricots, and pitted fresh, frozen, or canned cherries for the peaches (using juice- or water-packed canned fruit).

PINEAPPLE BAVARIAN CREAM

2½ tablespoons unflavored gelatin
¼ cup frozen apple-juice concentrate plus 2 tablespoons water
2 cups canned unsweetened pineapple juice
1 20-ounce can crushed pineapple (juice-packed), undrained
3 tablespoons grated orange rind
2 tablespoons lemon juice
½ teaspoon almond extract
1 cup canned evaporated skim milk

GARNISH: fresh mint

Sprinkle the gelatin over the diluted apple juice in a mixing bowl: let soak briefly In a saucepan, bring the pineapple juice to a boil and pour over the softened gelatin. stirring continuously until gelatin dissolves. Stir in the crushed pineapple, orange rind. lemon juice, and almond extract. Chill until partially set Meanwhile, pour the milk into a mixing bowl and place in the freezer; chill the rotary beater or beaters for an electric mixer in the freezer as well. When an icy glaze forms on the milk surface, remove from freezer and beat immediately until fluffy. Fold the whipped milk into the partially set gelatin mixture. Transfer to individual dessert dishes and chill until set. Garnish with mint. (If desired, the mixture may be put into a mold to set, then unmolded onto a serving plate and garnished with mint.)

MAKES 8 SERVINGS   125 CALORIES/SERVING
                          ¼ DAIRY SERVING/SERVING

CREAMY TAPIOCA PUDDING

⅓ cup quick-cooking small-pearl tapioca
3 cups canned evaporated skim milk
½ cup frozen apple-juice concentrate
1 tablespoon vanilla extract
1 teaspoon rum (optional)
Dash nutmeg
3 egg whites, beaten until stiff peaks form

Cover the tapioca with hot water and soak for 15–20 minutes; drain. Place the tapioca in a blender with 1 cup of the milk and the apple juice and blend well. Heat the remaining 2 cups milk in the top of a large double boiler (you can set a large stainless-steel bowl over a large pot of boiling water). When the milk is very hot, stir in the tapioca mixture, vanilla, rum (if used), and nutmeg. Vigorously stir in the beaten egg whites with a wire whisk and cook, stirring constantly, for about 3 minutes longer. Pour into individual serving dishes and chill.

MAKES 8–10 SERVINGS   135 CALORIES/¹⁄₁₀ RECIPE
                        ¾ DAIRY SERVING/¹⁄₁₀ RECIPE

VARIATION: CAROB TAPIOCA PUDDING
Follow the above directions but increase the vanilla to 2 tablespoons and add 3 tablespoons carob powder to the blender ingredients before blending.

RICE PUDDING

Use leftover brown rice, short- or long-grain, to make this satisfying dessert or snack. Serve it plain or, for a special treat, with a colorful fruit sauce such as Hot Berry Sauce (page 364).

3 egg whites, fork-beaten
1⅓ cups canned evaporated skim milk
⅓ cup frozen apple-juice concentrate
1 tablespoon orange juice
⅓ cup currants
1 teaspoon grated orange rind
1 teaspoon vanilla extract
1 teaspoon cinnamon
¼ teaspoon nutmeg
2 cups cooked brown rice

Put all the ingredients except the rice into a bowl and stir to combine well. Mix in the rice. Transfer to a lightly oiled 1½-quart ovenproof dish (a soufflé dish, if you have one) or a nonstick baking pan and bake in a 375° oven for 45 minutes, or until set and browned. Cool for 10 minutes or longer before serving, or serve chilled.

MAKES 4–6 SERVINGS   169 CALORIES/⅙ RECIPE
                            ½ DAIRY SERVING/⅙ RECIPE

NOODLE PUDDINGS fall somewhere between side dish and dessert and make any meal more special. Try one of the two recipes that follow—*Noodle Kugel* or *Fruit-Glazed Noodle Pudding*—at a company brunch, luncheon, or dinner. Since they are as good served cold, the puddings can be prepared well in advance to be reheated or not, as desired.

Though these dishes are traditionally made with noodles and so named, we opted for macaroni in the form of whole-wheat macaroni or corn macaroni, a wheat-free pasta, because of the somewhat better results. Both forms of macaroni and another ingredient in one of the puddings—four-grain cereal—are available at health-food stores and some supermarkets. Four-grain cereal is a commercial blend of wheat, oats, rye, and barley, sometimes with added apple bits, raisins, and cinnamon. (Look for Stone-Buhr "4-Grain Cereal Mates" and "Hot Apple Granola," or other brands.) If you can't find this product, substitute a cup of mixed cereal flakes, using individually packaged flakes of wheat, barley, oats, or rye, in roughly equal amounts; or you could use just regular rolled oats.

NOODLE KUGEL

5 cups slightly undercooked whole-wheat or corn macaroni, drained
1 cup four-grain cereal (see note above)
¾ cup raisins
1 20-ounce can crushed pineapple (juice-packed), undrained
½ cup canned unsweetened pineapple juice
¼ cup frozen apple-juice concentrate
2 cups cottage cheese, 1 percent fat (by weight) maximum
1 cup canned evaporated skim milk
2 tablespoons cinnamon
1 tablespoon vanilla extract (optional)
¼ teaspoon lemon extract (optional)
4 egg whites, beaten until soft peaks form

Place the macaroni in a large bowl. In a smaller bowl, place the cereal, raisins, pineapple, juices, and extracts, if used; stir well and let soak for about 5 minutes. Stir together the cheese, milk, and cinnamon and add to the macaroni. Add the cereal-fruit mixture and toss gently to mix all ingredients. Fold in the beaten egg whites. Transfer the mixture to a 9-by-13-inch glass or nonstick baking dish and bake in a 400° oven for 40 minutes, or until the top is lightly browned. Cut into squares when cooled. Serve at room temperature or chilled. If desired, serve with nonfat yogurt, plain or flavored with a little vanilla extract, cinnamon, and frozen apple-juice concentrate; or with *Cranberry-Apple Compote* (page 321).

MAKES 12 SERVINGS   187 CALORIES/SERVING
                          ¾ *DAIRY SERVING*/SERVING

THE PRITIKIN PROMISE
FRUIT-GLAZED NOODLE PUDDING

GLAZE:

1 20-ounce can crushed pineapple (juice-packed), undrained
½ cup frozen apple-juice concentrate
2 tablespoons date sugar (health-store item)
1 tablespoon vanilla extract
2 teaspoons brandy (optional)
1 teaspoon lemon extract
2 teaspoons arrowroot
1 large apple, peeled, quartered, and sliced
⅓ cup raisins, soaked in warm water and drained well

PUDDING:

¼ cup canned evaporated skim milk
1 tablespoon vanilla extract
2 cups cottage cheese (crumbly variety such as hoop cheese),
    1 percent fat (by weight) maximum
2 teaspoons pumpkin-pie spice
4 egg whites, beaten until stiff peaks form
2 cups slightly undercooked whole-wheat or corn macaroni,
    drained
½ cup regular rolled oats

Combine all the glaze ingredients except the apple and raisins in a saucepan. Bring to a boil, reduce heat, and simmer until thickened, stirring constantly, for about 2 minutes. Remove from heat and place apples and raisins on top. Set aside to cool.

Put milk, vanilla, cheese, and pumpkin-pie spice in a food processor (a blender can also be used, but you will have to stop the motor frequently to stir); blend until smooth. Transfer to a bowl and fold in the beaten egg whites, then stir in the macaroni. Line a 9-by-13-inch glass or nonstick baking pan with a thin layer of oats; stir the remaining oats into the noodle-cheese batter. Carefully spoon the batter over the oats layer, using a spatula to smooth the surface. Stir the apples and raisins into the glaze; then spoon the glaze over the batter layer, spreading it evenly. Bake at 400° for 25–30 minutes. Remove the pudding from the oven and cover loosely with aluminum foil

Let cool for about 10 minutes before cutting to serve. Serve warm or chilled.

MAKES 10–12 SERVINGS   140 CALORIES/¹⁄₁₂ RECIPE
                                                 ¾ *DAIRY SERVING*/¹⁄₁₂ RECIPE

SWEET POTATO FORK BREAD

If there is spoon bread, why not "fork bread," which seems a good name for this firm pudding. Serve it as a side dish with holiday meals, or as a dessert at any time. Yams can be substituted for sweet potatoes.

    4 cups mashed cooked sweet potatoes
    ½ cup frozen apple-juice concentrate
    1½ tablespoons vanilla extract
    1 teaspoon lemon extract
    1 tablespoon pumpkin-pie spice
    ¼ teaspoon cloves
    1 cup whole-wheat pastry flour
    ½ cup raisins
    4 egg whites

    TOPPING:
    ½ cup bran
    1 tablespoon cinnamon
    1 tablespoon frozen apple-juice concentrate

Combine the mashed sweet potatoes, apple juice, flavor extracts, and spices in a bowl and beat with an electric beater at low speed for 2–3 minutes. Mix in the flour gradually; then stir in the raisins. Beat the egg whites until soft peaks form; fold into the potato mixture. Combine the topping ingredients and sprinkle a small amount in a 9-by-9-inch nonstick baking pan. Spoon the potato mixture into the pan. Sprinkle with the remaining topping, pressing it in lightly with the back of a large spoon. Cover with aluminum foil and bake at 400° for 30 minutes; remove foil and bake another 15 minutes. Serve warm or at room temperature.

MAKES 10–12 SERVINGS   185 CALORIES/¹⁄₁₂ RECIPE

You'll enjoy the delicious crumb-crust open-faced pies with a variety of tasty fillings that follow. The unusual crust is made from fine whole-wheat bread crumbs (processed in a blender), sweetened slightly. Different quantities are given for the bread crumbs, allowing for a thinner or thicker crust depending on what best suits a particular pie. Each pie recipe will indicate the size of the pie pan and the amount of bread crumbs required, as well as any additions to the *Basic Crumb Crust* recipe below.

BASIC CRUMB CRUST
(for a 9- or 10-inch nonstick pie pan, as specified in the pie recipe)

1¼ to 1⅔ cups fine whole-wheat bread crumbs from
acceptable bread (amount specified in each recipe)
2 tablespoons frozen apple-juice concentrate

Place the ingredients in a bowl, mixing well. Using a rubber spatula, press the mixture firmly into the nonstick pie pan (bottom and sides) to form an even crust. Bake the crust in a 350° oven for 15 minutes until lightly browned. Remove from oven and allow to cool. Fill as directed.

NOTE: In the following pie recipes, using only the 2 tablespoons apple juice to moisten gives the best results, unless otherwise noted. However, if you prefer a moister crust, add up to 4 tablespoons water with the apple juice.

CRUMB-TOPPED FRUIT PIE

When summer fruits—peaches, apricots, nectarines, plums, and such—are abundant, this pie is a natural. But you needn't wait for these fruits to be in season; the pie is also delicious made with canned (drained) or frozen unsweetened fruits.

CRUST (for a 9-inch pie pan):
Follow the recipe for *Basic Crumb Crust* (above) using 1⅓ cups bread crumbs mixed with ⅓ cup bran.

FILLING:

3 cups sliced fruit or berries of choice (such as 1 cup each:
  sliced peaches, sliced apricots, and sliced strawberries)
⅓ cup frozen apple-juice concentrate
1 tablespoon each: arrowroot and pectin
1 tablespoon vanilla extract
1 teaspoon ground coriander
½ teaspoon lemon extract

TOPPING:

1 cup fine whole-wheat bread crumbs (from acceptable bread)
1 tablespoon cinnamon
1 teaspoon vanilla extract

Make the piecrust as directed. Place the filling ingredients in
a saucepan. Bring to a boil; then lower the heat and simmer
for a few minutes, stirring frequently, until the mixture is
thickened. Pour the fruit filling into the prepared crust.
Combine the topping ingredients, mixing well. Sprinkle the
topping over the filling, lightly pressing it into the fruit with
a spatula. Bake for 15 minutes at 375°. Let the pie cool; then
slice to serve.

MAKES 6–8 SERVINGS   155 CALORIES/⅙ PIE

APPLE-RAISIN PIE

CRUST (for a 10-inch pie pan):
Follow the recipe for *Basic Crumb Crust* (page 420) using 1½
  cups bread crumbs; add 4 tablespoons water to the
  ingredients.

FILLING:

4–5 pippin apples, peeled and cored
⅓ cup frozen apple-juice concentrate
⅓ cup raisins
1 teaspoon cinnamon
1 teaspoon grated lemon rind
1 tablespoon cornstarch

Make the piecrust as directed. Thinly slice the apples and combine with the apple juice, raisins, cinnamon, and lemon rind in a saucepan. Bring to a boil, reduce the heat, and simmer uncovered for about 15 minutes until the apples are tender. Mix the cornstarch with ½ cup cold water; stir into the simmering apples a few minutes before the end of the cooking period, stirring constantly until thickened. Pour the apple filling into the prepared crust and allow to cool. Serve warm or cold.

MAKES 8 SERVINGS   112 CALORIES/⅛ PIE

CAROB "CREAM" PIE

A rich-tasting, luscious chocolaty pie.

CRUST (for a 10-inch pie pan):
Follow the recipe for *Basic Crumb Crust* (page 420) using 1⅓ cups bread crumbs; add 1½ teaspoons vanilla extract to the frozen apple-juice concentrate.

FILLING:
3 tablespoons date sugar (health-store item)
3 cups canned evaporated skim milk
¾ cup mashed ripe banana with ¼ teaspoon lemon juice
½ cup frozen apple-juice concentrate
3½ tablespoons carob powder
1½ envelopes unflavored gelatin
1½ tablespoons arrowroot
1 teaspoon dry Postum
1 teaspoon cinnamon
1½ tablespoons vanilla extract
½ teaspoon almond extract
1 teaspoon brandy
3 egg whites, beaten until stiff peaks form

Make the piecrust as directed. Spread the date sugar in a small aluminum tin and place in a moderate oven for a few minutes to brown lightly. In a blender, combine 2 cups of the milk, the date sugar, and the other filling ingredients except the flavor extracts, brandy, and egg whites. Blend until smooth; then transfer part of the blender contents to another container. Add the rest of the milk and blend again until smooth. (Blending is done in two stages to avoid over-filling the blender.) Blend each batch again at high speed for several minutes.

Pour both batches into a large double-boiler arrangement (you can set a large stainless-steel bowl over a large pot of boiling water); cook for about 3 minutes, stirring with a wire whisk, until mixture is very hot. Add the extracts and brandy. Vigorously stir in the beaten egg whites with the whisk and cook, stirring constantly, for about 2 minutes longer. (Total cooking time is about 5 minutes.) Pour the filling into the prepared crust. (Any remaining filling can be put in small custard cups for an extra dessert.) Chill the pie several hours or overnight until firm.

MAKES 8 SERVINGS 170 CALORIES/⅛ PIE
¾ *DAIRY SERVING*/⅛ PIE

BANANA "CREAM" PIE

CRUST (for a 10-inch pie pan):
Follow the recipe for *Basic Crumb Crust* (page 420) using 1⅓ cups bread crumbs; add 1½ teaspoons vanilla extract to the frozen apple-juice concentrate.

FILLING:
3 tablespoons date sugar (health-store item)
3 cups canned evaporated skim milk
¾ cup mashed ripe banana with 1 teaspoon lemon juice
½ cup frozen apple-juice concentrate
1½ envelopes unflavored gelatin
1½ tablespoons arrowroot
1 tablespoon frozen orange-juice concentrate
Slight dash turmeric, for color (optional)
1½ tablespoons vanilla extract
¼ to ½ teaspoon banana extract
1 teaspoon brandy (optional)
1 egg white, beaten until soft peaks form

½ banana
Nutmeg

Make the piecrust as directed. Spread the date sugar in a small aluminum tin and place in a moderate oven for a few minutes to brown lightly. In a blender, combine 2 cups of the milk, the date sugar, the mashed banana with lemon juice, apple juice, gelatin, arrowroot, orange juice, and turmeric, if used. Blend until smooth; then transfer part of the blender contents to another container. Add the rest of the milk and blend again until smooth. (Blending is done in two stages to avoid overfilling the blender.) Blend each batch again at high speed for several minutes.

Pour both batches into a large double-boiler arrangement (you can set a large stainless-steel bowl over a large pot of boiling water); cook for about 3 minutes, stirring with a wire whisk, until mixture is very hot. Add the extracts and brandy, if used. Vigorously stir in the beaten egg white with the whisk and cook, stirring constantly, for about 2 minutes longer; remove from heat. (Total cooking time is about 5 minutes.) Slice the half-banana crosswise and arrange slices in a single layer in the prepared crust. Stir the filling once more, if needed, and pour into the crust. (Any remaining filling can be put in small custard cups for an extra dessert.) Garnish pie and cups with a very light sprinkling of nutmeg. Chill the pie several hours or overnight until firm.

MAKES 8 SERVINGS   145 CALORIES/⅛ PIE
                          ¾ DAIRY SERVING/⅛ PIE

PINEAPPLE-LEMON MERINGUE PIE

CRUST (for a 9-inch pie pan):
Follow the recipe for *Basic Crumb Crust* (page 420) using 1¼ cups bread crumbs, but increase the frozen apple-juice concentrate to 2 tablespoons plus 2 teaspoons, and add to it 1 teaspoon vanilla extract and ⅛ teaspoon lemon extract.

FILLING:
1 20-ounce can unsweetened crushed pineapple, juice-packed
1⅓ cups canned evaporated skim milk

½ cup frozen apple-juice concentrate

3 tablespoons lemon juice

2 tablespoons frozen orange-juice concentrate

1 envelope plus 2 teaspoons unflavored gelatin

2 teaspoons arrowroot

Dash turmeric (for color)

1½ teaspoons lemon extract

1 teaspoon vanilla extract

3 egg whites

Make the piecrust as directed. Place the filling ingredients, except the flavor extracts and egg whites, into a blender. Blend at high speed for about 5 minutes. Set a large strainer over a mixing bowl. Pour the blender contents through the strainer, stirring to help strain mixture; discard residue in strainer (to ensure a very smooth pie filling). Transfer the filling mixture to a double boiler (you can set a large stainless-steel bowl over a large pot of boiling water); cook for about 5 minutes, stirring with a wire whisk, until mixture is very hot. Stir in the flavor extracts. Let the filling cool briefly; then pour it into the prepared crust.

Beat the egg whites until stiff peaks form. Swirl the beaten egg whites gently over the pie. Place the pie in the oven on a middle rack under a hot broiler. Watch the meringue carefully, permitting it to brown just lightly; then remove from oven. Chill the pie for several hours or overnight until firm.

MAKES 6–8 SERVINGS   130 CALORIES/⅛ PIE
                                      ⅓ DAIRY SERVING/⅛ PIE

PUMPKIN PIE

CRUST (for a 10-inch pie pan):

Follow the recipe for *Basic Crumb Crust* (page 420) using 1⅔ cups bread crumbs mixed with 1 teaspoon cinnamon, and increasing frozen apple-juice concentrate to 2 tablespoons plus 2 teaspoons.

FILLING:

3 cups canned pumpkin

¾ cup canned evaporated skim milk

¾ cup frozen apple-juice concentrate
1½ teaspoons vanilla extract
1½ teaspoons cinnamon
¾ teaspoon each: ground ginger and nutmeg
⅛ teaspoon ground cloves
4 egg whites

Make the piecrust as directed. Combine all the filling ingredients except the egg whites in a bowl and mix well. Beat the egg whites until soft peaks form and fold into the filling mixture. Pour the filling into the prepared crust and bake at 350° for 1¼ hours or until a toothpick inserted in the center comes out "clean." Allow pie to cool and set. Serve warm or cold, plain or with a whipped topping (pages 430–32).

MAKES 8 SERVINGS   140 CALORIES/⅛ PIE

PUMPKIN CHIFFON PIE

CRUST (for a 10-inch pie pan):
Follow the recipe for *Basic Crumb Crust* (page 420) using 1⅓
  cups bread crumbs mixed with 1 tablespoon cinnamon; add
  1 teaspoon vanilla extract to the frozen apple-juice
  concentrate.

FILLING:
1 cup canned pumpkin
1 cup mashed ripe bananas, mixed with
  1 teaspoon lemon juice
½ cup canned evaporated skim milk
½ cup frozen apple-juice concentrate
1 envelope unflavored gelatin
1 teaspoon each: pumpkin-pie spice and cinnamon
⅛ teaspoon each: nutmeg and ground ginger
2 teaspoons vanilla extract
1 teaspoon rum (optional)
3 egg whites, beaten until stiff peaks form

Make the piecrust as directed. Place the filling ingredients, except the vanilla, rum (if used), and egg whites, in a blender. Blend at low speed until smooth, then at high speed for a few minutes. Transfer the mixture to a double boiler (you can set a large stainless-steel bowl over a large pot of boiling water); cook for about 3 minutes, stirring with a wire whisk, until mixture is very hot. Add the vanilla, and rum (if used). Vigorously stir in the beaten egg whites with the whisk and cook, stirring constantly, for about 2 minutes longer. (Total cooking time is about 5 minutes.) Pour the filling into the prepared crust. Chill until firm.

MAKES 8 SERVINGS   **120 CALORIES/⅛ PIE**

FRUITED "CHOCOLATE" CAKE

2 cups whole-wheat pastry flour
7 tablespoons carob powder
1½ teaspoons dry Postum
1 teaspoon baking powder
1 teaspoon baking soda
1 cup skimmed buttermilk
3 tablespoons frozen apple-juice concentrate
1 tablespoon vanilla extract
1 tablespoon rum or brandy
¾ cup raisins
½ cup frozen, unsweetened cherries, finely chopped
2 egg whites, beaten until stiff peaks form

In a large bowl, mix together the dry ingredients. Combine the rest of the ingredients except the egg whites; stir into the dry ingredients, beating the mixture with a large spoon for a few minutes to smooth the batter. Fold in the beaten egg whites. Turn the batter into a 9-inch round cake pan that has been lightly oiled and dusted with a little flour. Bake in a 350° oven uncovered for 30 minutes. Remove from oven and cover with aluminum foil. When cool, remove cake from pan with a spatula and slice. Store wrapped to keep moist

MAKES ABOUT 10 SERVINGS   **150 CALORIES/1/10 RECIPE**

THE PRITIKIN PROMISE
SPICE CAKE

This excellent cake isn't hard to make, so don't be put off by the number of ingredients and the fact that some have to be marinated in advance. For special occasions, bake it in a bundt pan and frost with Banana-Cherry Frosting *(page 432).*

2 cups finely grated apples
1 cup finely grated carrots
¾ cup raisins
¾ cup frozen apple-juice concentrate
2 tablespoons vanilla extract
2¾ cups whole-wheat pastry flour
½ cup bran
3 tablespoons date sugar (health-store item)
2 tablespoons cinnamon
1 tablespoon baking powder
1 teaspoon baking soda
1 teaspoon ground coriander
¼ teaspoon each: allspice, cloves, and cardamom
½ cup skimmed buttermilk
3 egg whites, beaten until stiff peaks form

Combine the apples, carrots, raisins, apple juice, and vanilla in a bowl and refrigerate, covered, to marinate for several hours or up to 2 days. (The cake flavor seems to improve with longer marinating.) Combine the dry ingredients in a large bowl. Mix the buttermilk into the marinated mixture and gradually add to the dry ingredients, stirring to mix well. Fold in the beaten egg whites. Lightly oil a 9-by-5-inch non-stick loaf pan and dust it with a little flour. Pour the batter into the pan, cover with aluminum foil, and bake in a 350° oven for 50 minutes. Remove foil and continue baking for 10 minutes, until cake is done. Remove from oven and re-cover with foil. When cool, remove cake from pan and slice. Store covered to keep moist.

YIELD: ABOUT 18 SLICES   130 CALORIES/SLICE

APPLE CAKE

This easy-to-make moist cake is not too sweet and keeps well for up to two weeks when covered and refrigerated.

  1 20-ounce can unsweetened peeled, sliced apples
  ½ cup raisins
  ½ cup frozen apple-juice concentrate
  1¼ cups whole-wheat pastry flour
  ¾ cup regular rolled oats
  1 teaspoon baking soda
  1 teaspoon cinnamon
  ¼ teaspoon cloves
  2 egg whites, beaten until stiff peaks form

Stir together the apples, raisins, and apple juice in a large bowl. Combine the dry ingredients and stir them into the apple mixture. Fold in the beaten egg whites. Turn the batter into a 9-inch round nonstick cake pan and bake uncovered in a 350° oven for 1¼ hours. Cover with aluminum foil and cool for about 10 minutes before removing from pan.

MAKES 10–12 SERVINGS   140 CALORIES/¹⁄₁₀ RECIPE

OATMEAL-APPLE-RAISIN COOKIES

  3 cups regular rolled oats
  1 cup whole-wheat pastry flour
  1 tablespoon plus 1 teaspoon cinnamon
  2 teaspoons baking powder
  1 teaspoon baking soda
  ¼ teaspoon nutmeg
  ⅔ cup frozen apple-juice concentrate plus ¼ cup water
  2 tablespoons vanilla extract
  1 cup grated apple
  ¾ cup raisins
  3 egg whites, beaten until stiff peaks form

Place the dry ingredients in a large bowl and mix well. Combine the diluted apple juice, vanilla, apple, and raisins; stir into the dry ingredients, blending well. Fold in the beaten egg whites. Drop by heaping tablespoons onto a nonstick cookie sheet. patting down each mound of batter to flatten slightly. Bake in a 400° oven for about 12 minutes. Allow the cookies to cool for several minutes; then loosen from sheet with a spatula.

YIELD: ABOUT 24 COOKIES   92 CALORIES/COOKIE

CEREAL-RAISIN COOKIES

These raisin cookies have special flavor and texture because of the packaged four-grain cereal—blended flakes of wheat, oats, rye, and barley (see discussion on pages 416 to 417).

> 2 cups regular rolled oats
> 1 cup four-grain cereal (see above)
> 1 cup whole-wheat pastry flour
> 1 tablespoon cinnamon
> 1 teaspoon baking powder
> 1 teaspoon baking soda
> ¼ cup frozen apple-juice concentrate
> ½ cup canned evaporated skim milk, or skimmed buttermilk
> 1 tablespoon vanilla extract
> 1 teaspoon lemon extract
> ¾ cup raisins
> 3 egg whites, beaten until stiff peaks form

Place the dry ingredients in a large bowl and mix well. Combine the apple juice. milk, extracts, and raisins, and stir into the dry ingredients, blending well. Fold in the beaten egg whites. Drop by heaping tablespoons onto a nonstick cookie sheet, patting down each mound of batter to flatten slightly. Bake in a 400° oven for about 12 minutes. Let the cookies cool for a few minutes; then loosen from sheet with a spatula.

YIELD: ABOUT 24 COOKIES   90 CALORIES/COOKIE

WHIPPED TOPPINGS

You don't require whipping cream to make whipped toppings. Skim milk—in the form of canned evaporated skim

milk or instant nonfat dry milk—*can be made into delightful dessert toppings to imbue even a simple baked apple with a certain glamour. To whip successfully, it is essential that you thoroughly chill the mixing bowl, rotary beater or beaters for an electric mixer, and milk or other liquids used. Place the liquids in a small mixer bowl and set the bowl in the freezer alongside the beater or beaters. Chill until an icy glaze forms over the liquid. Remove bowl and beater(s) and whip immediately at highest speed until thickened. (If you have a food processor, you can also whip fluid nonfat milk into a fluffy topping, using the chopper blade. Leave the plunger out of the feed tube.)*

I
(with evaporated skim milk)

½ cup canned evaporated skim milk
1 tablespoon frozen apple-juice concentrate
½ teaspoon vanilla extract

Combine the ingredients in a small mixer bowl; chill according to directions above; then beat at highest speed for about 5 minutes until thick. Serve at once.

MAKES 4 SERVINGS   30 CALORIES/SERVING
                                    ¼ *DAIRY SERVING*/SERVING

II
(with evaporated skim milk and gelatin)

Unflavored gelatin adds body to a whipped topping. Serve the topping immediately after beating it for a fluffy texture, or refrigerate it for an hour or longer for a more gelatinous texture—ideal for making fruit parfaits (alternating fruit with the topping) and other creations.

¼ cup canned evaporated skim milk
1 teaspoon vanilla extract
3 tablespoons frozen apple-juice concentrate plus water to make ½ cup
1½ teaspoons unflavored gelatin

Combine the milk and vanilla in a small mixer bowl; chill according to directions in introduction to *Whipped Toppings* (page 430). Meanwhile, place the diluted apple juice in a small saucepan and sprinkle with the gelatin; let soak briefly. Heat slowly, stirring continuously, until the gelatin dissolves. Cool the gelatin mixture but do not let it thicken. Remove bowl and beaters from freezer; immediately add the gelatin to the milk mixture and beat at highest speed for about 5–6 minutes until thick. Serve at once, or refrigerate if a stiffer texture is preferred.

MAKES 4 SERVINGS   40 CALORIES/SERVING
                           ¼ *DAIRY SERVING*/2 SERVINGS

III
(with nonfat dry milk)

When appropriate, try fruit juice in place of the ½ cup "flavored" water in this recipe, but keep the amount of liquid constant. Use unsweetened pineapple juice for a pine-apple-flavored whipped topping, or orange juice, sweetened with a little apple-juice concentrate, for an orange-flavored topping.

  1 tablespoon frozen apple-juice concentrate plus 1 teaspoon
    vanilla extract plus water to equal ½ cup
  ½ cup instant nonfat dry milk

Place the liquid ingredients in a small mixer bowl; chill according to directions in introduction to *Whipped Toppings* (page 430). Remove from freezer and immediately add the milk, beating at highest speed for 3–5 minutes until stiff. Serve at once.

MAKES 4 SERVINGS   38 CALORIES/SERVING
                        ALMOST ½ *DAIRY SERVING*/SERVING

BANANA-CHERRY FROSTING

  1 ripe banana, in chunks
  ½ cup frozen unsweetened cherries

432

1 cup cottage cheese, 1 percent fat (by weight) maximum
2 tablespoons nonfat dry milk
2 tablespoons carob powder
1 teaspoon vanilla extract

Place the banana chunks and cherries in a blender; add the other ingredients. Blend, stirring as required, until the mixture is smooth. Keep refrigerated.

YIELD: SCANT 2 CUPS   175 CALORIES/CUP

PUMPKIN FROSTING

½ cup canned pumpkin
⅔ cup nonfat dry milk
2 tablespoons frozen orange-juice concentrate
1 teaspoon cinnamon
¼ teaspoon nutmeg

Place the pumpkin in a blender. Add the other ingredients and blend until smooth.

YIELD: ¾ CUP   295 CALORIES/¾ CUP

LIME-YOGURT SAUCE

Use this simple and refreshing sauce to top fruit chunks (especially nice served in a pineapple boat). Grate only the outer green peel of the lime, as the white pith can impart a bitter taste.

1½ cups nonfat yogurt
2 tablespoons frozen apple-juice concentrate
1½ teaspoons grated lime rind
1 teaspoon fresh lime juice

Combine all ingredients, mixing well. Chill.

YIELD: ABOUT 1½ CUPS   38 CALORIES/¼ CUP
                                ⅓ DAIRY SERVING/¼ CUP

PART FIVE

THE RESEARCH EVIDENCE

23
CHAPTER

Nutritional Evaluation:
Why the Pritikin Diet Is Best

The nutritional content of the Pritikin diet, particularly with respect to its low fat content and restricted intake of meat, is quite similar to the diets people had before the Agricultural Revolution of the 1800s.[100]* At that time, the advent of more efficient agricultural methods greatly increased the availability of meat and dairy products. Then, in 1870, the roller mill was invented for the high-speed separation of bran from the starch and protein of grains. In this process, large quantities of vitamins, minerals, fiber, and essential fatty acids are lost; and so bread, the "staff of life" for millennia, no longer provided these essential nutrients. With increasing prosperity, the American middle class, and eventually almost the entire population, had access to types of food that in earlier times were available only to royalty and the rich. Thus, for more than a century, Americans have been drifting steadily and insidiously into a higher consumption of meat and dairy products, without realizing that they were also eating a great excess of saturated fat, total fat, and cholesterol, which are so bad for the arteries.

* See references at end of chapter, pages 470 to 477.

Meanwhile, primitive people in various parts of the world never made this change, and many epidemiological studies have shown that they do not suffer from the degenerative diseases so common in the Western world of today.

A varied diet, made up for the most part of unrefined foods, will quite adequately meet your nutritional needs. On the Pritikin diet you will have as much fat, carbohydrate, and protein as you need, as well as generous quantities of vitamins, minerals, trace elements, and fiber. Such a diet also guards against overdoing cholesterol, fats, sugars, and salt, which are the main culprits in several degenerative disease processes.

The regular, or maintenance, Pritikin diet allows for 8–12 percent of calories as fat, 12–15 percent as protein, 80 percent as carbohydrate, and no more than 100 mg cholesterol daily. You will eat primarily complex carbohydrate: there is very little simple carbohydrate in the diet, and most of it derives from unprocessed fruits, vegetables, grains, legumes, and nonfat dairy products. A small amount of sugar in the form of apple juice is used as a sweetening agent in some of the recipes. In addition, a maximum of 3½ oz of lean, low-to-moderate-cholesterol meat, fish, or chicken is permitted daily.

At the Pritikin Centers, the special therapeutic Pritikin diet is employed in the treatment of patients with degenerative diseases—mainly cardiovascular disease, diabetes, and hypertension.[3,4,36] This diet is much the same as the regular Pritikin diet, except that less than 3 oz of meat, fish, or chicken is permitted per week in order to keep cholesterol intake at less than 25 mg a day. The proportion of carbohydrate, fat, and protein remains the same. In addition to the therapeutic diet, you can find 700-, 850-, 1000-, and 1200-calorie versions of the diet outlined in *The Pritikin Permanent Weight-Loss Manual*.[82] In this present book, the Pritikin diet refers to the regular, or maintenance, Pritikin diet.

Because of its composition, you will actually require less of some nutrients on the Pritikin diet than recommended by the National Research Council's Food and Nutrition Board,[72] which has established guidelines for the daily intake of each nutrient to ensure adequate nutrition for men, women, and children of various ages and degrees of activity. These advised daily intakes are referred to as the RDAs, or recommended dietary allowances. The Pritikin diet is much lower in nonessential fat than the average American diet; lower in protein; and because of the high fiber and water content of foods as grown, lower in calories. Excessive fat. protein, and/or calories increase the need for several vitamins and minerals, including calcium, vitamin E, and some of the B vitamins.[72] For these reasons, you actually need less of these nutrients, although the Pritikin diet still provides you with some nutrients in excess of the RDA.

As you can see from the analysis of foods in the menu plans (pages 468–69), the Pritikin diet easily meets the RDA guidelines. In spite of this, however, a few issues do need to be addressed. Some question whether the fiber content of a diet consisting mainly of unrefined foods interferes with mineral or vitamin nutriture.

MINERAL AND VITAMIN NUTRITURE

Effect of Fiber on Vitamin Nutriture

It has been suggested that even though the Pritikin diet, as analyzed, more than meets the RDA for minerals and trace elements, it might be possible for a deficiency in one or more micronutrients to occur as a result of the relatively high fiber content of the diet. This premise is based on speculation. The diet really is not extraordinarily high in fiber (60–70 g dietary fiber per day),* although it is high in comparison with the diets of most Americans (19 g dietary fiber

---

* Most American tables of food composition give values for crude fiber only, which is the residue remaining after extraction with dilute acid and alkali. This old technique of analysis, originating in the textile industry, results in the loss of large fractions of dietary fiber Crude-fiber values represent a small but variable percentage of true dietary fiber content—on the average, 20 percent of the hemicellulose, 10–50 percent of the lignin, and 50–80 percent of the cellulose.[103] Dietary fiber values given in this chapter are calculated according to the modern values obtained by Southgate.[97]

per day),[7] who eat large amounts of processed foods, or foods from which the fiber has been removed, such as extracted oils and sugars, and refined flour. The Pritikin diet is composed mainly of foods as grown, intact with their natural fiber. Our increased consumption of refined foods since the turn of the century and the resulting decrease of fiber in our diet is quite dismaying. The total fiber intake of our diet in 1970 was 37 percent less than it was in 1880.

For many years it was thought that diets high in fiber might have the effect of inhibiting the absorption of minerals from the intestinal tract and compromising mineral nutriture. However, the consensus of recent studies, which I will outline for you, is that a varied diet containing large amounts of unrefined carbohydrate foods, although relatively high in fiber, does not compromise mineral nutriture. I have tried to make the scientific studies as clear as possible, and even though the information can be rather technical, I urge you to read this section carefully, for your peace of mind and to help you answer those who may criticize your diet plan unfairly.

Following a sudden change from a diet quite low in fiber to one that contains larger amounts, there is a tendency toward a small but temporary drop in the serum levels of certain minerals, such as calcium and iron; but this phenomenon is transient. After a period of a few weeks, the system adapts to the increase in dietary fiber, and serum levels of minerals rapidly normalize. This adaptive response was demonstrated 35 years ago in a study of people on a high-phytate, or bran-fiber, diet, in whom calcium absorption was initially inhibited, but which after a few weeks improved and regained equilibrium.[106]

Phytates in the bran layers have repeatedly been implicated as that fraction of grains responsible for the initial inhibitory effect on mineral availability. Recently, however, a study conducted by the Nutrition Institute of the U.S. Department of Agriculture demonstrated that the phytates have no effect on mineral absorption.[70]

In this study, dephytinized bran was prepared by incubation in water at 37°C. for 16 hours, permitting phytase, an enzyme in bran, to break down the phytate. Ten healthy adult men ate muffins containing 36 g of dephytinized bran for 15 days, and then ate muffins containing phytate bran for another 15 days. When dephytinized bran was consumed, mean apparent absorption of iron, zinc, manganese, and copper, as measured by intake/fecal excretion, tended to be lower, but positive, for the initial 5 days than for the concluding 10 days. When whole bran was consumed, the 5-day mean absorption for copper was higher, and for iron, zinc, and manganese, mean absorption was negative, but the 10-day mean was more positive than when dephytinized bran was consumed. This demonstrates that some type of adaptation in absorption resulted from the consumption of bran, and that the phytate did not compromise mineral nutriture.

Shortly thereafter, this study was confirmed.[94] Sixty men and women ate both phytate-containing and dephytinized bran, and the absorption of nonheme iron was measured. As the study involved only 2 test meals, there was not time for adaptation and the regaining of equilibrium demonstrated in longer-term studies. It was shown, however, that the phytate fraction of bran was not responsible for the inhibition of iron absorption.

In another study, when 24 g/day of wheat bran was added to the diet of 40 patients with diverticular disease for a minimum of 60 months, there were no significant changes in serum calcium, phosphorus, iron, or hemoglobin.[11]

Dr. James W. Anderson, Chief of Endocrinology at the University of Kentucky Medical Center, conducted a recent study of the effects of a diet of unrefined foods—that is, containing their original fiber—such as fresh or water-packed fruit and vegetables, whole-grain products, legumes, and small amounts of animal products, and supplemented with ⅔ cup bran each day.[2] He sought to determine whether a diet relatively high in fiber content would compromise mineral nutriture.

No evidence of deficiency was observed in diabetics who remained on diets containing 50–70 g dietary fiber per day, for an average of 21 months (some of them for as long as 51 months). Average values for serum, calcium, phosphorus, iron, total iron-binding capacity, and hemoglobin were normal. In addition, although Anderson found diabetics are commonly deficient in magnesium, on the high-fiber diet their serum levels of this mineral were normal. By indirect assessment, Anderson also found no evidence that fat-soluble-vitamin nutriture was compromised on this high-fiber regimen. Levels of serum calcium, phosphorus, and alkaline phosphatase indicated adequate availability of vitamin D. Serum calcium indicated normal to high levels of vitamin A. The ability of the blood to clot, as determined by the measurement of prothrombin and partial thromboplastin times, indicated vitamin K availability. Folic acid and vitamin B_{12} concentrations in the serum were also normal.

Studies using both animals and humans indicate that there are no *non*phytate factors in bran that affect the availability of iron. Bran seemed to have no inhibitory effect on iron absorption, even when 20 percent bran was included in the diet.[32a] For 7 weeks, newborn pigs were suckled and fed an iron-depleted diet. For the next 2 weeks they were not suckled but received only the low-iron diet. Twenty of the anemic animals were in experiments in which iron-rich diets (about 100 mg iron/kg fodder) were fed. In the first experiment, one group ($N = 7$) received a diet containing 7 percent bran. About 60 percent of the iron derived from the bran and 40 percent from ferrous sulfate. The other group ($N = 6$) received no bran, and 80 percent of the iron came from ferrous sulfate (Diet III). There were no differences in the increases of serum iron or of hemoglobin, as determined by the cyanmethhemoglobin method.

In the second experiment, one group ($N = 3$) again received no bran, with 80 percent of the iron coming from ferrous sulfate (Diet III). The other group ($N = 4$) received a diet containing 20 percent bran. All the iron was derived from bran and cereals. The hemoglobin test indicated no significant difference in the availability of the iron present in the diets containing no bran and 20 percent bran.

These 6 studies[2,11,70,94,106,32a] demonstrate that mineral balances remain positive even when relatively large amounts of fiber supplements are taken. After 51 months, not one of Anderson's patients showed any signs of deficiency. The Pritikin diet contains approximately the same amount of fiber consumed by these patients, and it also does not cause mineral deficiency.

Effect of Fat Content of the Diet

The average amount of fat consumed by Americans accounts for 42 percent of their total caloric intake,[102] while the Pritikin diet contains only 8–12 percent of total calories as fat. One of the reasons the Pritikin diet has been called "radical" is that it is so much lower in fat than the diet of most Americans. The Pritikin diet may seem radical to many Americans, but it would seem extremely rich to the natives of New Guinea, whose diet contains enough fat to meet the current essential-fatty-acid recommendations,[72] although it makes up only 3 percent of the total calories.

Dr. Victor Herbert, a hematologist with the Veterans Administration Hospital in the Bronx, New York, has expressed concern about whether a diet limited in animal products and refined foods contains enough fat for our bodies to absorb and utilize. One of the reasons nutritionists feel we might need more dietary fat than is contained in the Pritikin diet is to enable adequate absorption and utilization of the fat-soluble vitamins. vitamins A, D, E, and K.

Vitamin A was discovered in 1913. when McCollum *et al.*, at the University of Wisconsin. and Osborne and Mendel[76] at Yale, learned that in order to grow, rats needed a substance found in milk fat and egg yolk. Shortly thereafter, the substance was isolated, and became the first vitamin to be discovered, vitamin A, or retinol. At the same time that we learned that milk and eggs contained a nutrient essential for growth, Russian researchers found that these same foods caused hardening of the arteries in rabbits. Unfortunately, we overemphasized the importance of dairy products in our effort to prevent vitamin A deficiency Today, nearly a million Americans die every year of heart disease, as a result of eating excessive amounts of high-fat. high-cholesterol foods. Yet diseases due to vitamin deficiencies in 1977 killed fewer than 30 people.[37]

Vitamin A in its finished form as used by the body is found only in animal products. However, you do not have to eat dairy foods or other animal products to obtain vitamin A, as the body will make it from forms of provitamin A such as carotenes. These are found in large amounts in plant foods. and converted by your body into vitamin A in ample but not toxic amounts. One medium-sized carrot, for instance, contains 7930 IU (International Units) of vitamin A—80 percent of the Recommended Dietary Allowance.

The Tarahumara Indians of the Creel area of Chihuahua, Mexico, subsist on a diet of mainly corn, pinto beans, and other plant foods, with only 9–12 percent of calories coming from fat.[16] They exceed the Food and Agriculture Organization/World Health Organization recommendations for vitamin A by 2½ times, and only 3 percent of the vitamin A in their diet comes from animal products. Corn provides 56 percent of the vitamin A intake, and 35 percent comes from greens.

You will meet the RDA of 1000 retinol equivalents (RE) when you eat 10,000 IU of carotene, or one large carrot, daily. The menu plans in this book provide 4 times this amount.

We must also address the question of whether there is sufficient fat in the Pritikin diet to facilitate the absorption of carotene and other forms of provitamin A. Studies have, in fact, demonstrated that rats, even when fed an artificial diet containing *no* fat, do absorb carotene.[60] When 80 µg of carotene in the form of raw carrots was added to their diet, rats absorbed 13 percent of the carotene, and 37 percent of that was utilized. When fat was added to their diets, accounting for 2.7 percent of their total calories, the rats absorbed only an additional 1.5 percent. The following chart illustrates quite dramatically how little fat does to enable our bodies to absorb carotene.

	% calories from fat			
	0	2.7	19.3	40.0
% carotene absorbed from raw carrots	12.9	14.4	19.4	19.6

Human studies are equally impressive. In a recent controlled study[54] of 70 indigent preschool children, 1½ oz of spinach, providing about 1200 µg beta-carotene after cooking losses, was added to their diet. The children were divided into 3 groups. No supplemental oil was added to the diet of Group I; 5 g (1 teaspoon) of peanut oil was added for Group II; and 10 g was added for Group III. After 4 weeks, there was a significant increase in serum vitamin A *in all 3 groups*. In those children whose initial serum vitamin A levels were less than 20 μg/100 ml, the addition of leafy greens to the diet for 4 weeks resulted in raising the level of serum vitamin A when no fat was added to the diet, and only marginally more when fat was added to the diet.

Serum vitamin A (μg/100 ml)

Added Fat	% of total calories as added fat *	Before adding spinach to diet	After adding spinach to diet
None	0	13.1	22.7
5 g	4.5	16.1	25.4
10 g	9.0	12.4	25.7

* Assuming these 2- to 6-year-old children were consuming 1000 calories/day, the addition of 5 g fat/day was equivalent to 4.5% of total calories and 10 g/day equivalent to 9.0% of calories.

The beta-carotene was not only absorbed but converted to vitamin A on a low-fat diet, and there were no significant differences in absorption of carotene and conversion to vitamin A when fat was added. These serum levels were maintained for 6 weeks after discontinuation of the spinach.

The above study confirms prior research [61] demonstrating that vitamin A nutriture is adequate when carotenoid-containing vegetables are included in the diet, even when the diet is deficient in fat, protein, and calories. In this study, when 1½ oz of a leafy green vegetable, amaranth, was added to the diet of children with a mild degree of protein-calorie malnutrition, and serum vitamin A levels were below 25 μg/100 ml, there was 86-percent absorption of beta-carotene which was converted into vitamin A, raising serum levels after 10 days from 15 to 28 μg/100 ml. Levels below 20 μg/100 ml are considered subnormal, yet in only 10 days these children on an otherwise inadequate diet were able to raise their vitamin A level to a reasonably normal range. [66] In children with serum levels above 25 μg/100 ml, serum levels increased from 31 to 38 μg.

Eating a diet that includes ample quantities of carotene-containing fruits and vegetables, as recommended in the Pritikin dietary guidelines (see page 194), not only provides for optimal vitamin A nutriture, but has recently been shown to protect against some kinds of cancer. Preformed vitamin A was found not to have this protective effect.[93]

Vitamin D is not a true vitamin, but a steroid with hormonal activity which is not found to a great extent in food It is not a dietary requirement when we have enough exposure to sunlight. Rickets, the symptom of deficiency, occurs in children with a genetic error resulting in defective phosphate transport.[12] In spite of this defect, many of the children would not have had symptoms had it not been for adverse environmental factors. They lived in extremely polluted industrial areas where the sun's rays were deflected, or their cultures dictated that they wear clothing that would prevent the few minutes' daily exposure of small areas of the skin to the ultraviolet light necessary for vitamin D synthesis. In the absence of ultraviolet exposure, an average daily intake of 1.0 μg of vitamin D daily prevents rickets in normal growing children.[12] One glass of skim milk contains 1.25 μg. Since fortified milk is one of the few dietary sources of vitamin D, the Pritikin diet contains neither more nor less than other diets

Because vitamins A and D are readily stored in body tissues, taking vitamin supplements as well as eating foods fortified with these vitamins can result in overdoses of these vitamins and produce symptoms of toxicity.[99] Toxicity is seen more frequently in children. Excessive amounts of vitamins A or D interfere with bone growth, and malformation can occur in infants whose mothers took too much A or D during the first 3 months of pregnancy, or who, in a misguided attempt to do well by their children, overdosed them with vitamin preparations [77]

Vitamin D toxicity is exacerbated by high calcium intake.[31] Since milk has been fortified with vitamins A and D, we have seen many more cases of toxicity in youngsters who drink large quantities of milk.[92] Chronic vitamin A intoxication is also often seen in adults. Among the earliest symptoms are dry, scaly, and itchy skin and cracked lips Other symptoms may include headache, hair loss, visual disturbances, dizziness, loss of bone minerals, bone and joint pains, and liver damage.[25 41] While these symptoms quickly disappear after withdrawal of vitamin A supple ments, some of the more severe side effects, which include stammering and loss of memory, coordination, balance, and sexuality, are sometimes irreversible. Vitamin D does not act like a vitamin in the body, but as a potent steroid hormone. Excessive amounts of D or of vitamin A can cause an increase in serum cholesterol, hardening of the aorta, and loss of bone minerals.[27,38]

The RDA for vitamin E in adult man is 10 mg. Plant foods are rich sources of vitamin E: one cup of collards contains 10 mg; a cup of cole slaw, 7; and a cup of summer squash, 5.[79] Vitamin E deficiency will occur only in premature infants, or persons with malabsorption problems. You will often read, however, that vitamin E will increase physical endurance and sexual potency, prevent heart attacks, protect against the effects of air pollution, and slow the aging process. It is supposed to cure heart disease, sterility, muscular weakness, cancer, ulcers, skin problems, burns, and shortness of breath. These claims are unscientific and untrue.

Although it may have psychological benefits, vitamin E in the form of supplements is an expensive placebo. The more you take, the less efficiently it is absorbed. In fact, if you consume large amounts, more than 80 percent may pass unchanged through the intestine. In spite of the fact that so little is absorbed, and vitamin E appears to be the least toxic of the fat-soluble vitamins, side effects have been associated with its use.

In a recent study, 13 adult males and 5 young boys took 300 mg of vitamin E as *dl*-α-tocopheryl acetate daily for 3 weeks. The dosage produced significant depression in the ability of their white cells to destroy bacteria in the system.[80]

In a controlled double-blind study of 202 adults, the experimental group received 600 IU *dl*-α-tocopheryl acetate for 4 weeks.[101] It caused a significant reduction of serum thyroid-hormone levels and also an elevation of serum triglycerides in women.

Vitamin E supplementation has been reported to cause muscle weakness accompanied by an undesirable increase of creatinine and creatinine phosphokinase activity in the urine.[10,17,45] Daily ingestion of 800 IU of vitamin E has caused excessive prolongation of blood-clotting time [18,48] due to interference with vitamin K activity. Animal experiments indicate that excessive vitamin E interferes with calcium and phosphorus metabolism and vitamin D utilization.

Vitamin K is necessary for the formation of prothrombin and other clotting factors, and is found in abundance in many foods, especially leafy green vegetables. It was the last of the vitamins to be discovered, probably because a primary deficiency has never been demonstrated in healthy adults.[104] Once intestinal flora are established in the newborn, there is bacterial synthesis of the vitamin, and as long as bile salts are present, adequate amounts will be absorbed. Deficiency is seen only in persons with biliary obstruction, sprue, steatorrhea, or other conditions in which fat and fat-soluble vitamins are poorly absorbed; those on warfarin anticoagulation or oral antibiotic therapy; and in persons on prolonged fasts. Deficiency could also be caused by supplementation with excessive amounts of vitamin E.[19]

Dr. Herbert has been outspoken in stating that a diet of 8–10 percent fat is unsafe in regard to vitamin and mineral absorption.[43] He says he knows of no evidence that vitamin K can be adequately absorbed on a diet of 8–12 percent fat.[42] However well meant, this type of unsubstantiated criticism can delay for years people's willingness to change to a healthful low-fat diet.

As a hematologist, Dr. Herbert certainly is aware that decreased sensitivity to oral anticoagulants can be caused by increased absorption of vitamin K. However, people on low-fat diets who eat large amounts of green vegetables, the primary source of vitamin K, can also show this decreased sensitivity, demonstrating that vitamin K can be absorbed when dietary fat is low.[30]

Deficiency of vitamin K is associated with an increase in clotting time. The New Guinea highlanders are probably on one of the lowest-fat diets in the world, with only 3 percent of total calories from fat. On only a third of the fat contained in the Pritikin diet, the New Guineans apparently have no problem absorbing vitamin K: their clotting times were 50 percent faster than those of Australians.[35] In a study of a

New Guinean tribal community of 1489 people, there was no clinical evidence of vitamin deficiencies.[96]

Fat-soluble vitamins are stored in body tissues that store fat, such as the liver, and the level of these vitamins can become toxic if you take vitamin pills or eat excessive quantities of foods fortified with vitamins. In extreme cases, people have evidenced toxicity from eating too much liver from fish or other animals containing high amounts of vitamin A. Eating a diet composed mainly of unrefined plant foods provides *optimal* fat-soluble vitamin nutriture, and obviates the purported need for vitamin supplements or fortified foods.

FATTY-ACID REQUIREMENTS

Our bodies require certain fatty acids (linoleic and linolenic acids) for growth, maintenance, and proper functioning of many physiological processes, and people have been concerned whether the Pritikin diet contains sufficient fat to meet the requirements for these essential fatty acids (EFA). The EFA make up almost all of the polyunsaturated fatty acids (PUFA) in common foods.

Fifteen volunteers in a penal institution were fed Vivonex,* containing a balanced proportion of l-amino acids, the required vitamins, mineral salts, glucose or other simple sugars, and less than 1 percent of calories in the form of fat (ethyl linoleate) for 6 months.[108] Extensive and frequent blood-chemistry, hematology, urinalysis, and physical, neurological, and psychological examinations indicated the diet was nutritionally adequate.

These findings confirmed data obtained from another study in which Vivonex was fed to 5 children institutionalized for phenylketonuria, a genetic disorder in which the amino acid phenylalanine cannot be properly metabolized and which results in severe mental retardation.[69] Over a period of 30 months, the children grew rapidly on the diet.

New Guineans, who consume 0.7 percent of calories as EFA, exhibit none of the symptoms of EFA deficiency, which include scaly skin, unusual pigmentation, and inabil-

---

* Supplied by Vivonex Corporation, 867 West Dana Street, Mountain View, California 94040.

ity of the skin to heal.[96] Hair loss, one of the first symptoms of EFA deficiency, was not observed. Blood in the urine was not mentioned in the urinalysis reports, although it is also a symptom of deficiency. Further, problems of sensory and motor deficits and neurological abnormalities were also uncommon among the New Guineans.

In patients with severe intestinal malabsorption and EFA deficiency, the problem was corrected by application of only 2–3 mg of linoleic acid/kg body weight per day to the skin in the form of a drop of sunflower oil[81]—the amount of linoleic acid in ½ ear of sweet corn.[107] However, there were only 3 subjects in this experiment, and other researchers were unable to confirm the results. To ensure an adequate supply of linoleic acid, the Food and Nutrition Board recommends that EFA represent 1 percent of caloric intake.

The linoleic acid (LC) and linolenic acid (LN) content of the diet are also of interest, because of recent research on the fatty acid/prostaglandin relationship and its effect on cardiovascular disease.

A diet low in total fat—low in both animal fats and extracted vegetable oils—has, in fact, a *positive* effect on EFA nutriture. Because of competition for the enzymes that me tabolize fats, an excess of either saturated or monounsaturated fat in the diet suppresses the ability of the body to metabolize polyunsaturated fatty acids (PUFA),[46] which are mostly LC and LN.[46,95] Some researchers believe that not only LC but also LN, and perhaps small quantities of eicosapentanoic acid and docosahexanoic acid and other EFA derivatives, are essential. They believe the optimal LC/LN *ratio* of 5:1 to 10:1 for the adult is, therefore, more important than the absolute *amount* of these fatty acids obtained in the diet.[20]

Some researchers have raised the question as to whether a tendency toward absolute or relative EFA deficiency may be caused by the American diet. On the one hand, the utilization of both LC and LN is suppressed by the high amount of saturated fat in animal products; and on the other hand, the high concentration of LC as compared with LN in margarines and many extracted vegetable oils may suppress the utilization of LN.

Any interference with the utilization of LN could ad

versely involve the synthesis of prostaglandins. These hormonelike substances affect cardiovascular health by influencing the amount and type of cholesterol-carrying lipoproteins in the blood; the clumping of platelets, which control blood clotting; and the degree to which the small arteries are constricted.

In the early 1960s the AHA (American Heart Association) was concerned about the association between heart disease and the low ratio of dietary polyunsaturated fats to saturated fats (P/S ratio) in our diet. They thought the P/S ratio should be at least 1. They didn't realize that the important thing is to have a low intake of fat, such as you would have if all or most of the fat you consumed derived from whole plant foods. When this is the case, the P/S ratio is automatically high. For instance, the P/S ratio of the average American diet is 0.3,[62] but the ratio of the Tarahumara[16] and the Pritikin diets, both of which consist mainly of unrefined plant foods, is 2.

The AHA erroneously believed it could prevent the harmful effects of the high-fat (40 percent of calories) diet by increasing the P/S ratio of our dietary fat. It attempted to do this by substituting vegetable oils in the diet for some of the saturated fat.

Unfortunately, the dietary recommendations of the AHA, when first made to the nation in 1961, had not been adequately tested. Pearce and Dayton, who directed the 8-year Wadsworth VA Hospital AHA diet trial with 846 men, warned that no population under study had been consuming a diet high in polyunsaturated fats over long periods of time. After the Wadsworth study, Dayton said not only that he would not recommend a high-PUFA diet to most of his patients, but that a diet of 10 percent fat would be his choice. In the official report, Dayton wrote, "The diet tested in this program was selected for purely pragmatic reasons: we did not believe we could mount and sustain a trial of any other type of lipid-lowering diet in this institution. Epidemiological studies favor the conclusion that a low-fat diet is perhaps the promising path to longevity."[24] Results from the Wadsworth study indicated that those on PUFA had 3 times the incidence of gallstones, and over 50 percent more cancer. No significant difference in total deaths occurred.

Though high-PUFA diets fail to reduce the risk of heart disease, they apparently *enhance* the risk of cancer—particularly breast, colon, ovarian, uterine, and prostate cancer. The 1982 National Academy of Sciences report *Diet, Nutrition, and Cancer* concluded that a relationship between fat and cancer was most persuasive, especially for polyunsaturated fats.[73] Dr. T. C. Campbell, one of the authors of the report, stated that if a diet is high in PUFA, total fat should be less than 20 percent of total calories because of the possible increased cancer risk. So convinced is Campbell of the danger of excess fat that he stated, "The relationship between diet and cancer, in my opinion, is now more persuasively established than the one between diet and heart disease."[14]

Some vegetable oils have a high ratio of LC to LN, and as so often occurs when we eat food extracts rather than whole foods, an imbalance may be created. Again, another alternative has been offered to solve the problem. Instead of cutting down on the high amount of total fat in the diet, an excess of which tends to suppress the utilization of essential fatty acids and their long-chain derivatives made in the body, some scientists are recommending supplementing the diet with fish oils which contain these derivatives.

But Hornstra and colleagues caution that a large intake of such long-chain derivatives of the LN family has had harmful effects on the heart muscle and other organs of animals.[47] This is probably due to the high degree of unsaturation of these derivatives.

A diet need not be high in fat to effect adequate EFA nutriture. This was demonstrated in a 1969 study of Japanese and American men.[51] The Japanese eat a low-fat diet with a linoleic acid intake of 8.9 g. The linoleic acid intake of Americans was estimated at 10.5 to 12.5 g. (The intake *per unit of body weight* of the two groups is probably the same, since Japanese weigh about 20 percent less than Americans of comparable height.) However, the adipose tissue, which reflects the fat content of the diet,[23] of the Americans contained 10.2 percent linoleic acid, compared with the adipose tissue of the Japanese, which contained 16.5 percent linoleic acid. Since the adipose tissues are the source of free fatty acid for cell requirements, the cells of the Japanese were far better nourished with EFA than the cells of the Americans.

One could hypothesize that the adipose tissues of the Japanese contained a higher percentage of linoleic acid (60 percent more) than the adipose tissue of Americans because of genetic differences. However, a study in 1962 demonstrated in human subjects that dietary manipulation effects a change in adipose-tissue composition:[23] the adding of PUFA to the diet increased PUFA in the adipose tissue. The results were confirmed in a 1968 study of Cleveland men in which dietary changes resulted in a decrease in adipose oleic acid from 50.1 to 48.5 percent and an increase of adipose-tissue linoleic acid from 8.6 to 10.2 percent.

If marginal EFA deficiency exists to any significant extent in this country, it is a result of a malnutrition of imbalance due to overconsumption of saturated fats and those extracted oils which are disproportionally high in linoleic and linolenic acids. We could try to effect a cure by overcompensating with other nutrients. For instance, we could consume fish oils with a high LN-to-LC ratio. Or we could take supplements of vitamins or minerals with antioxidant properties in order to prevent the excessive formation of free radicals or cross-linked proteins caused by a high PUFA intake. The result, in all probability, would be an onslaught of new complications or diseases. There is no need for experimentation to find a way to adapt man to a high-fat diet.

We can meet the EFA requirement when 1 percent of our calories are derived from EFA.[72] As earlier described, this requirement may be related to the effect of different intakes of non-EFA fats on the utilization of EFA. Because of competition for fat-metabolizing enzymes, an increase in unsaturated fats in the diet may increase the requirement for LC and LN. In other words, a low intake of total fat is likely to improve the utilization of EFA and lower their requirement.

As you can see from the menu-plan analysis on pages 468 to 469, the Pritikin diet supplies adequate EFA (1 percent of calories); LC and LN occur in the diet in optimal ratio to each other; and the P/S ratio of more than 2.0 is most satisfactory.

PROTEIN REQUIREMENTS

The idea that we must eat plenty of protein is one of the biggest nutritional myths in America, and one that is perpetuated by government agencies and health associations. For example, the Los Angeles District of the California Dietetic Association recently said that the Pritikin diet could promote a deficiency of essential amino acids because of the very limited quantities of animal protein and the possibility that at any one meal vegetables and grains wouldn't be eaten in the proper combinations.[98]

Such misinformation is confusing to the public. Even the 700-calorie-per-day version of the Pritikin weight-reduction diet contains 56 g of protein,[82] the RDA for men and 20 percent above the RDA for women.

How much protein humans actually require is still uncertain. Americans routinely eat 100 g or more per day, although people of undeveloped countries do well on less than 50 g per day of protein derived primarily from plants.

Historically, athletes have eaten muscle meats to improve their muscular performance. Dr. Carl von Voit, a German physiologist of the 19th century, surveyed 1000 German laborers and found that they were consuming about 118 g of protein per day.[105] This recommendation persisted for many years as the necessary protein requirement for steady muscle use.

By 1946, however, Bricker[9] and Hegsted[39] had demonstrated that man required only about 30 g of protein per day. After reviewing hundreds of studies done during the past 40 years,[52] Irwin found that 35 g for a 154-lb man with a ±15-percent variation for individual difference would be quite adequate. That 35 g would constitute only 5 percent of total calories for protein. The average U.S. adult male, if he can afford it, eats closer to 20 percent of the total calories as protein.

In 1941, the RDA for protein for men 18–35 years old was 70 g. In 1968 it was reduced to 65 g, and in 1980, to 56 g. West Germany still recommends 115 g of protein per day; Rumania, 110 g per day; the Netherlands and Poland, 90 g per day.[110]

Studies on protein requirements started on rats, and the

work of Osborne and Mendel[76] helped develop the recommendations for protein quality and quantity. They found vegetable proteins to be inferior for rats to animal proteins, resulting in poor growth and low protein-efficiency ratio (PER) in rat studies. Later work confirmed that the ratio of lysine to other essential amino acids was lower in wheat and many plant proteins, and compared with whole egg, as a result, rats on plant-food diets grew less rapidly. Supplementation of lysine increased the PER of wheat, and produced faster growth in rats. Almost all the studies of protein quality have been performed on rats; and unfortunately, this work has been the basis for human protein recommendations.

The term "incomplete protein" refers almost exclusively to plant proteins. It means that the percentages of amino acids in the food vary enough from those in egg protein, which has a PER of 94 percent, to cause slower growth in rats.

You should be aware, however, that rat studies are not always directly applicable to humans, and food that will not promote growth in rats may promote good growth in humans. Adding lysine to wheat to raise it to levels found in eggs improved the PER of wheat for rats and improved their growth. But Reddy could not confirm this finding in humans.[83] Six children 2–5 years old were hospitalized and studied on two diets. They were fed a diet in which wheat provided 2 g protein/100 calories/kg body weight. The remaining calories were provided by sugar and safflower oil. On the first diet, the wheat was supplemented by added lysine to bring this amino acid to the level of egg, and on the other diet, the wheat was unsupplemented. The children ate the unsupplemented wheat for 10 days, the supplemented wheat for 10 days, and the unsupplemented wheat again for the final 10-day period. Twenty-four-hour samples of urine and feces were collected the last 3 days of each period. These samples and the diet were analyzed for total nitrogen by the Kjeldahl method. The results of this balance study showed that the amounts of nitrogen retained during the unsupplemented periods were at least as high as during periods of lysine supplementation (see chart on page 456).

	Nitrogen retention percentage		
	1st 10 days	2nd 10 days	3rd 10 days
Unsupplemented	14.4		
Lysine-supplemented		13.9	
Unsupplemented			16.3

The data suggest that the lower lysine in wheat may, in fact, be better for humans than the higher lysine in eggs, in spite of the studies with rats suggesting that low lysine will inhibit growth.

The amino acids lysine and threonine occur at lower levels in rice.[78] Rosenberg, in his rat studies, reported that both these amino acids must be added simultaneously to the diet, in proper proportions, to promote satisfactory growth.[89] In young rats, Kik found that when he replaced an all-rice diet with 99 percent rice and just 1 percent chicken, PER was significantly improved.[57]

This improvement was *not* confirmed in a study by Lee on human adults.[63] In a 59-day experiment, normal young men 20–27 years old were fed diets of equal caloric value. On the first diet, rice provided 100 percent of the protein, and on the other, rice provided 85 percent of the protein and chicken 15 percent. In both diets, protein accounted for 6.5 percent of total calories. Nitrogen-balance studies showed that *for humans* the essential amino acid pattern in rice is equal, if not superior, to that of a chicken-and-rice diet. In fact, those on all-rice protein had a positive nitrogen balance 20 percent *higher* than those on 85 percent rice and 15 percent chicken.

Kofranyi demonstrated the same type of improvement with young adults on two isocaloric diets: one with egg as the protein, and the other with egg plus potato as the protein sources.[59] Those on the egg-and-potato diet required 36 percent *less* protein to achieve positive nitrogen balance than those on egg alone. Yet egg has a PER of 94 percent and potato only 67 percent in rat studies.

On the basis of Kofranyi's studies with egg and potato, the requirements for the essential amino acids are as low as 40–50 percent of Rose's values.[88] Rose used the egg as the ideal protein, and the results of his studies on rats were used to establish the generally accepted standards for essential amino acid requirements for men.

I believe the subsequent studies are more than conclusive in demonstrating that amino acid metabolism in rats is significantly different from that of humans, and that Rose erred in his assumptions. In another project, college women aged 17–21 years were studied by Fisher at Rutgers University [29] They required only 5 g of nitrogen, or 31 g of protein, per day to maintain their nitrogen balance. The amino acid pattern in their diet was deliberately modified so as not to be equivalent to that of whole-egg protein. Requirements for the amino acids leucine, methionine, and valine were reassessed on this low-protein diet. In the case of leucine, it was found that the 40 mg per day required was only ¼ to ¹/₁₀ the amount established by Rose. Rose's study had used twice as much protein, and the amino acid pattern of whole egg was used as a standard. Earlier studies by Fisher had also demonstrated that people have lower requirements for the amino acids lysine and tryptophan when on a diet of only 5 g of nitrogen daily.[28]

These observations by Fisher do not support the prevailing notion of an absolute amino acid requirement for man. In fact, Fisher's observations indicate that on low-protein diets we require less nitrogen and amino acids than when we have a diet high in protein. Hegsted also warned against accepting high amino acid requirements based on high-protein diets when we are on low- but adequate-protein diets.[40] Yet scientists have declared vegetable proteins incomplete principally *because* they contain 30–60 percent of the lysine in egg when in fact, low-protein diets are quite adequate for humans. Although they may cause problems for rats.

Plant protein should not be considered inferior in meeting our protein needs. In long-term studies of 102 infants between the ages of 5 and 14 months, Knapp found no difference in growth rate between babies fed milk proteins and babies fed vegetable proteins.[68]

The consensus of nutritional authorities is that our bodies must have a positive nitrogen balance—that is, we must consume more nitrogen than we excrete. In human studies, 6–8 percent of total calories of plant protein has been found adequate to maintain positive nitrogen balance. The Pritikin diet, which provides 13 percent of total calories from protein —mostly from plants—has twice the requirement.

Another myth, based on false reasoning in the past, is that humans require large amounts of total protein. Although there is much discussion of a worldwide protein shortage, the fact is that a true protein shortage hardly exists.[6] The problem is a *food* shortage. When your calorie intake does not meet your energy demands, your body will use dietary protein first for calories before supplying protein for the tissues. If children do not have enough calories, the protein will not promote growth, regardless of its source.

Kwashiorkor, a starvation disease of young children in Africa and other Third World countries, is believed to result from protein deficiency. Yet Golden reported in a study of 103 children, all suffering from the edema of kwashiorkor, that feeding them adequate calories resolves their edema, even if the diet contains only 2.5 percent of total calories in protein.[33] Golden wrote, "It is suggested that protein deficiency is not the cause of the edema of kwashiorkor."

In human milk only 6 percent of the total calories comes from protein; in rat milk, 20–25 percent. Furthermore, human milk is more dilute. If we were to base our recommendations for feeding human babies on rat studies, human milk would be found so inadequate nutritionally that we would not allow it to be fed to our infants. But our babies thrive on breast milk!

One of the longest studies testing low protein intake in humans was done by Walter Kempner, M.D., of Duke University. In 1949, he presented the findings of his rice-fruit diet at the American College of Physicians 30th Annual Session.[56] He defined his diet as having 2000 calories, consisting of 4 percent protein all from plant sources, 2.3 percent fat, and 93 percent carbohydrates, both complex and simple, and no cholesterol. Only 20 g of protein was provided, and this was adequate to maintain adults in positive nitrogen balance.

It is important to be aware that the studies documenting these results[22,55] established that positive nitrogen balance was sometimes not achieved for 2 or 3 months. Almost all the experimental protein-feeding studies on humans to establish protein requirements have been very short in comparison, as little as 3-7 days Therefore, the results are misleading, and the conclusion could be drawn that more protein is required to maintain positive nitrogen balance than is the case.

Besides doing nitrogen-balance studies to confirm the adequacy of 20 g of plant protein for adults, Kempner made other important observations. A small amount of nitrogen is also excreted through the bowels; a comparison of the daily nitrogen intake with the daily nitrogen output by stool and urine shows that the nitrogen equilibrium can easily be maintained.

"There are other indications that, because of the protein sparing action of the carbohydrates, the protein part of the rice diet is adequate and that there is no lack of essential amino acids; e.g., the fact that the production of hemoglobin is normal and that anemia does not develop. Also, the fact that blood urea and non-protein nitrogen decrease on the rice diet whereas in starvation and in protein deficiency, the body uses its own protein, and the non-protein nitrogen and the urea nitrogen in the blood increase."[56]

The concept of carbohydrates' sparing protein was tested[84] in healthy young men on two diets, both using milk as the only protein at approximately 5 percent of total calories (0.57 g protein per kg body weight). In one diet the fat carbohydrate ratio was 1:1 (F = 47 percent, C = 47 percent), and in the other it was 1:2 (F = 32 percent, C = 63 percent). While on the 1:1-ratio, 47 percent carbohydrate diet, the men maintained a negative nitrogen balance of 0.25 g N 24 hrs. On the 63-percent-carbohydrate, 1:2 diet, they were in positive nitrogen balance, +0.23 g N/24 hrs. Kempner demonstrated that a 93-percent carbohydrate diet is the ultimate for protein-sparing. Richardson wrote, "In these subjects, the efficiency of utilization of milk protein was raised by as much as 50% as a result of the protein-sparing action of the carbohydrate in diet B [ratio 1:2, fat = 32 percent, carbohydrate = 63 percent, protein = 5 percent]."[84]

Many nutritionists forget that the 6 percent of total calories in protein present in breast milk is adequate for the fastest growth in humans; babies double their birth weight in the first 6 months of life. During no other growth period is there as great a protein requirement. The young men in Richardson's study did well on a 5-percent-protein diet; Kempner's patients, on a 4-percent plant-protein diet. But how about a lifetime on a 4-percent primarily plant protein diet?

Highlanders in Papua New Guinea have been studied extensively because of their very-low-protein diet (4.4 percent) which by Western standards would seem to guarantee malnutrition, ill health, and protein deficiency. But the New Guineans have none of these conditions, and in fact not only are healthy and muscular and do heavy work, but are free of heart disease, diabetes, hypertension, and breast and colon cancer.[34,67,96]

For generations their diet has been limited to sweet potatoes, sweet-potato leaves, and a pig feast every 2 or 3 years.[67] The adult male eats 2300 calories per day—three meals of 2 kg of sweet potatoes and 200 g of sweet-potato leaves. Nutritional analysis,[96] which includes an average of the 14 types of sweet potatoes eaten, showed: carbohydrates, 93 percent of total calories; protein, 4.4 percent; fat, 2.6 percent, and essentially no cholesterol.

The amino acid pattern, as compared with the FAO recommended pattern, was grossly inadequate.[67] Only phenylalanine and tyrosine met the standards. Isoleucine and lysine were at 50 percent of standard, and methionine and cystine were less than 25 percent of the recommended standard.

They eat only 25 g of protein—all of it derived from plants —per day. No clinical evidence of malnutrition[34] has been noted since these New Guineans were first studied in the 1930s. Hemoglobin and serum albumin levels are normal, and even by European standards, both men and women are at just about their ideal weight in their early 20s. Obesity is practically nonexistent.

Physical-fitness testing, using the Harvard Pack Test, demonstrated the New Guineans to be measurably superior in fitness to the people of Australia, whose male adults consume 100 g of mainly animal protein per day.

Unlike more developed populations, New Guineans show no rise in either systolic or diastolic blood pressure with age. Neither cholesterol levels (adult males and females average

150 mg/dl) nor fasting glucose levels change with age. A total of 777 New Guineans from 15 to 65 years old were tested with 100 g of glucose in a standard glucose-tolerance test, and no cases of diabetes were found. None of the more developed nations in the world that have high-protein and high-fat diets can even approach these standards.

No children were found who had kwashiorkor, or nutritional marasmus,[96] and no cases of vitamin deficiency or nutritional edema could be found in the entire tribal community of 1489 people, of whom only 2 persons did not wish to be examined. In addition, serum albumin levels were within normal limits, and hemoglobin values were normal for that altitude.

Cardiovascular disease, the principal killer in developed countries, was almost nonexistent, even though 21 percent of the population was over 40 years old. Only 2 gave a history compatible with the possibility of angina pectoris, and no hypertensive disease, cerebrovascular disease, or peripheral vascular disease was seen. No evidence of a previous cerebrovascular accident or Parkinson's disease was found.

Yet 70 percent of the adult males and 20 percent of the females smoke home-grown tobacco. Apparently the smoking risk factor will not increase the danger of atherosclerosis on a low-fat, low-cholesterol diet. The smoking, plus the fact that people spend up to 12 hours in smoke-filled houses, does, however, present a major health problem. Respiratory disease in 1960–62 accounted for 29.2 percent of 2000 hospital admissions and is a major cause of morbidity and mortality.

In the United States, pregnant women are believed to require 74 g of protein per day—30 g per day *more* than nonpregnant women—even though only 4 g per day would satisfy the total known needs for the 9-month growth of the fetus.[72] This excessive protein intake bears some responsibility for the toxemia and kidney problems so common among pregnant American women.

New Guinean women between the ages of 14 and 45 are either pregnant or nursing babies—or both—for that 30-year span. In one study, 83 percent of the women between 20 and 39 years old were either lactating or pregnant, yet their average protein intake was 20 g of plant protein per day, and they consumed *no* dairy products for calcium.

Studies of monkeys[44,85] confirm that diets even lower in protein (3.35 percent protein) than the New Guinean diet have no deleterious effect on the offspring of primate mothers. Birth weights were no different for monkeys on 3.35 percent protein diets or on 13.4 percent protein diets No difference in physical or mental ability could be found among any of the monkey youngsters. The authors state. "Accordingly, our finding of no behavioral deficit in offspring of deprived mothers is exactly what we should expect, because the infant itself is not deprived despite the mother's low-protein diet. Because of this fact, we should expect no loss on any test, whether already invented or yet to be devised."[44]

In spite of scientific evidence to the contrary, many nutritionists continue to believe that a high-protein diet is necessary for optimal health. Puzzled as to how the New Guineans could appear so healthy and muscular on their sweet-potato diet, one researcher, Dr. Oomen, believed that the sweet potatoes or their leaves must be protein-rich.[49] The tubers analyzed were found to contain only 1.0–1.1 percent crude protein, and protein from leaves was negligible. He then did nitrogen-balance studies and found New Guineans of all ages to be in negative nitrogen balance Rather than question the unwritten law of positive nitrogen balance, he theorized that the New Guineans may be capable of having their intestinal bacteria fix atmospheric nitrogen and make protein like a legume.

Walking human legumes! Dr. Oomen admits that there are few facts on which to base his theory, but he can't imagine how the New Guineans could otherwise survive on so little protein.

Why do we have such a love affair with protein?

Some typical reactions to the New Guinean data: "A prime characteristic of much of the world's malnutrition is a shortage of proteins; high-carbohydrate, low-protein diets are the affliction of much of the third world. Scientists [Dr. F. J. Bergersen and others] had observed several times in the past decade that certain sweet-potato-eating people in the New Guinea highlands were far healthier than they should be, given their high-carbohydrate diet. . . . 'It could be,' says Dr. Bergersen, 'that there is something magic about the sweet potatoes.' "[75]

Kempner required no magic to maintain his patients on 4 percent protein, less than eaten by the New Guineans. Golden used only 2.5 percent protein, but adequate calories, to cure kwashiorkor.

Another example: "Despite the frequency of protein deficiency [among the New Guineans] in childhood, the area is densely populated, and the adults are able to do heavy work. This is possible *only* [my emphasis] when these subjects retain sufficient nitrogen either from the sweet-potato diet alone or from the sweet-potato diet and some *still unknown supplement* [my emphasis]."[67]

And again, "Certain groups of people in developing countries, despite consuming what appear to be extremely poor diets over long periods of time, appear to be relatively well grown and to be leading productive lives. Many nutritionists and physicians noting this phenomenon have expressed cautious bewilderment but have generally not challenged the 'laws' on which nutritional science is based."[49]

I am not arguing for a 4-percent-protein diet. But I have no reason to quarrel with the findings of the studies done on the New Guineans. They stay very healthy on a high-carbohydrate diet, and there's no magic in that! Still, I recommend adequate calories and that 12–13 percent of total calories should come primarily from plant protein; this will more than meet the needs of healthy, active people.

Several animal studies demonstrate increased life expectancies of 25–100 percent when the total caloric quantity of the diet is reduced throughout the lifetime, or the diet is low in protein (8 percent) and high in carbohydrate (83 percent) with no caloric restriction.[53,64,90]

In Leto's study with mice[64] reducing protein from 26 percent to 4 percent protein increased life-span from 840 days to 1167 days. Barrows[5] observed a 25-percent increase in life-span when protein was reduced from 24 percent to 12 percent, even though the experiment was done with rats already 16 months old.

An unexpected finding with rats on a low-protein (5 percent) diet when compared with rats on an isocaloric high-protein (25 percent) diet had to do with excess fat deposited.[26] In only 8 weeks, 23.9 percent of the body mass of the high-protein group was fat, compared with only 15.8 percent fat on the 5-percent-protein group.

At least 30 million adults in the United States are obese— 20 percent or more over their ideal body weight; and yet most weight-reduction programs are based on high-protein diets and encourage lifetime diets high in animal protein However, Carroll found that *even on a cholesterol-free diet*, the animal protein casein can produce atherosclerosis, but the disease can be prevented by substitution of plant protein for animal protein.[15]

Diets high in animal protein, so universally recommended by nutritionists, can produce negative mineral balance of calcium, magnesium, and zinc.[50,68,91] A 16-percent-protein diet can produce negative calcium balance even in young men who take 1400-mg calcium supplements each day.[65] In the same study, a diet of 24 percent protein created a sub stantial negative balance. In 1974, the Food and Nutrition Board not only set an unnecessarily high RDA for protein, but encouraged 30-percent-protein diets and stressed the use of animal protein for "palatability."[71] Diets high in animal protein are high in cholesterol, although the Food and Nu trition Board set no limit on cholesterol intake. The 1980 RDA for protein was not lowered, nor were cholesterol guidelines provided,[72] although the Food and Nutrition Board has the data that diets high in animal protein *guaran tee* epidemics of cardiovascular disease and osteoporosis. In addition, a relationship has been observed between the increased incidence of calcium and oxalate kidney stones and diets high in animal protein.[87]

Kidney-function decline in developed populations begins in people about 30 years old and continues so that by the age of 70 or 80, function has dropped as much as 50 percent This is in "normal" people. Those with diabetes, hypertension, or heart disease can totally lose function and go into kidney failure

Is this an inevitable effect of aging? I believe that this decline takes place only on the high-fat and high-cholesterol "Western" diet.

GLOMERULAR
SCLEROSIS

EFFERENT
ARTERIOLE

AFFERENT
ARTERIOLE
(CUTAWAY)

TUBULE

GLOMERULUS

MALPIGHIAN CORPUSCLE

The nephron is the basic functional unit of the kidney. About 1 million of these nephrons in each kidney filter the protein waste products out of the blood and return the cleansed blood to the circulation. Part of each nephron has a structure called the renal, or Malpighian, corpuscle (see illustration). The blood to be filtered enters a small artery, the afferent arteriole, which branches into about 50 capillary loops, collectively called the glomerulus. Each loop is about $\frac{1}{50}$ inch long, and they do not short-circuit into each other. As the blood flows through these glomerular capillaries, the waste products filter, or perfuse, through the capillary walls, drain down the tubule, and eventually become part of the urine and are excreted. After the blood has passed through the glomerulus, it goes to the exit artery, the efferent arteriole, and returns to the circulation.

The decline in kidney function is due to a progressive glomerular sclerosis, which is a thickening of the wall of the afferent arteriole. The thicker the vessel becomes, the smaller the opening, until it can completely close and cut off the blood supply to the glomerulus, leading to failure.

The flow through the glomeruli each day is enormous.

Every 24 hours, 55 gallons of fluid are filtered. Yet the filtration, or perfusion, cannot be carried out at full capacity continuously without damaging the glomeruli from overwork—no more than one can run at top speed indefinitely.

Brenner[8] links the high protein in the U.S. diet to this problem. He writes, "Unlimited intake of protein-rich food, now generally regarded as 'normal,' may be responsible for dramatic differences in renal function between modern human beings and their remote predecessors who hunted and scavenged for meat."

In intermittently fed animals and man, perfusion of superficial (reserve) glomeruli is minimal between meals. The deeper glomeruli are usually well perfused at all times. Thus, in the periods between feedings a low level of glomerular filtration rate is found, since the reserves (superficial glomeruli) are not used. With the next meal, especially if high in protein, the large superficial-nephron population provides a reserve capacity to handle the protein waste products.

Animal studies demonstrate that changing the diet of dogs from carbohydrates to meat increased renal flow and glomerular filtration flow by as much as 100 percent. In rats, a 35-percent-protein diet increased the glomerular filtration rate by 70 percent over that on a 6-percent-protein diet.

Kidney mass increases with long-term high-protein feeding. Sustained elevated glomerular filtration rates are responsible for the increase of kidney mass seen in animals maintained on high-protein diets. Ralph Nelson, M.D., of the Mayo Clinic has reported[74] increase of kidney mass in 20-year-old football players on high-protein diets.

Chronic elevated glomerular filtration rates are the result of a diet consistently high in protein. Chronic elevation of kidney flow and filtration rates takes place only with continuous perfusion of both deep and superficial nephrons. This appears to be the precursor of glomerular sclerosis.

When a kidney is removed, the blood flow and glomerular filtration rates increase about 40 percent in the surviving kidney and lead to moderate acceleration of glomerular sclerosis. High pressure and flows of blood are seen not only in a surviving kidney after one has been removed, but in hypertension, glomerulonephritis following acute strep infections, and other causes of kidney damage.

Nutritionists base recommendations for protein consumption upon the amount of protein required to maintain positive nitrogen balance as determined from nitrogen-balance studies. Such studies by several investigators, however, consistently found New Guinean subjects, ranging from young boys to adults, to be remarkably healthy although they were in negative nitrogen balance.[49,67,96] These findings challenge the accepted axiom that humans cannot grow unless they are in positive nitrogen balance.

It may be that the investigators who determine the RDA recommend excessive protein consumption because they themselves are on diets high in animal protein. In the 8th Revised Edition, 1974, of the *Recommended Dietary Allowance,* one finds: "... nor is there evidence that intakes double or triple the recommended allowances [of protein] are harmful. In fact, protein intakes that exceed RDA are often desirable, since low-protein diets usually contain only small amounts of animal products and thus tend to be unpalatable and low in important trace nutrients."[71] In fact, as you are now well aware, grains, which are generally eaten in large amounts on low-protein diets, are rich sources of trace elements if the grains are unrefined.

One of the major penalties of a diet high in animal protein and the accompanying cholesterol is the premature death of 1 million U.S. citizens each year from avoidable atherosclerosis.

On the basis of the research evidence I have cited, I am convinced that the optimal requirement not only for total protein, but also for amino acids is lower than those recommended by the Food and Nutrition Board. Contrary to the prevailing notion, there may not be absolute amino acid requirements for man. Hegsted warned about accepting the recommendation that we need the same amount of amino acids on high-protein diets as we do on low- but adequate-protein diets.[40]

Brenner writes: "Recent studies suggest that high protein intake in the presence of renal [kidney] injury contributes to the increased perfusion of remnant glomeruli and thus to their eventual destruction. A reduction of dietary protein content from 24 percent to 6 percent has been shown to

Nutritional Analysis of

Menu Plan	kcal	Protein			Fat		Carbohydrate		Minerals				
		g	kcal	% kcal	g	% kcal	g	% kcal	Ca	P	Fe	Na	K
									mg	mg	mg	mg	mg
Sample Day I	2014	75.6	260	13	17.4	7	416	80	790	1577	25.0	1424	6470
Sample Day II	1957	78.6	271	14	17.0	7	401	79	803	1709	26.0	1505	6923
Sample Day III	1897	71.9	245	13	11.0	5	406	82	1016	1716	23.9	2506	6695
Average	1956	75.4	259	13	15.1	6	408	80	870	1667	24.6	1812	6696
RDA*		56.0							800	800	18.0		

* RDA used are the highest for nonpregnant, nonlactating adults between the ages of 23 and 50.

blunt the hemodynamic changes associated with ablation of 90% of renal mass."[8]

Kidney function was nearly normalized by protein restriction which stopped excretion of protein in the urine and preserved glomerular structure. In diabetes mellitus, glomerular hyperfiltration precedes loss of nephron units, and is probably the initial step in the progression of this disease of the glomeruli.

In humans and animals, the findings are consistent with the concept that sustained hyperfiltration is ultimately detrimental to glomerular function and structure, and eventually leads to glomerular sclerosis.

Brenner speculates: ". . . the possibility [should be considered] of a fundamental mismatch between the evolutionary design characteristics of the human kidney and the functional burden imposed by modern *ad libitum* eating habits. Sustained rather than intermittent excesses of protein (and perhaps other solutes) in the diet impose similarly sustained increases in renal [kidney] blood flow and glomerular filtration rates, which require that the 'reserve' glomeruli of the outer cortex be in use more or less continuously. Consequently, time-averaged pressures and flows in the outer cortical glomeruli contribute to unrelenting 'intrarenal hypertension' and predispose even healthy people to progressive glomerular sclerosis and deterioration of renal function. . . . An obvious first step, as suggested by Addis, might be a reduction of protein intake."[8]

Three Sample Day Menu Plans

Vitamins					Fatty-Acid Analysis							
A	B₁	B₂	Niacin	C	Total sat.	18:2		18:3	18:2/18:3	Other polys.	Total polys.	P/S
IU	mg	mg	mg	mg	g	g	% kcal	g		g	g	
40968	1.95	1.74	30.3	429	1.4	2.2	0.9	.5	4	1.1	2.6	1.9
18380	2.40	1.80	27.6	525	1.2	2.6	1.1	.6	4	.4	3.3	2.8
46752	2.20	2.09	20.2	338	1.8	3.6	1.6	.9	4	0	4.6	2.6
35367	2.2	1.9	26.0	431	1.5	2.8	1.2	.7	4	.5	3.5	2.4
5000	1.4	1.6	16.0	60								

Little is known about human adaptation to different diets and to plant-protein intake. Even when new data accumulate, there is reluctance to challenge the established "laws" of nutrition.[49]

The diet eaten by most people in modern industrialized nations differs tremendously from that eaten two centuries ago. We now consume much less of unrefined plant foods and vast quantities of refined foods and animal products. We eat much less of complex carbohydrates and much more protein, fat, and cholesterol. Yet Dr. Annemarie Crocetti, Doctor of Public Health, and Dr. Helen Guthrie found that today fewer than 20 percent of Americans achieve a desirable balance of dietary protein, fats, and carbohydrates: "The significance of the findings for fat imbalances, alone or in combination with carbohydrates, is of enormous interest in the light of the relationships of some prevalent chronic conditions and some nutritional factors which are held to be implicated in their etiology. These conditions are some forms of cancers, obesity, some acquired heart disease and hypertension."[21]

The researchers explain that subsequent to the identification of vitamins in the early 1900s, food guides from the National Dairy Council, The American Meat Institute, and the USDA promoted dietary patterns based on nutrient-dense foods they thought would provide the necessary vitamins and minerals. However, as the researchers point out, "Today the major nutritionally related problems in the

United States are not nutrient deficiencies, but obesity and weight control, hypertension, coronary heart disease and dental caries."[21]

The prejudices in government agencies against the high-carbohydrate diet and in favor of a diet high in protein, fat, and cholesterol are still strong. The RDA as established by the nutritionists on the Food and Nutrition Board of the National Academy of Sciences are unrealistic, and their recommendations for some minerals are so high that you would have to eat excessive amounts of animal products to meet the requirements, if indeed they can be met at all.

I hope you will listen carefully to the advice of Dr. Catherine Woteki of the USDA Human Nutrition Information Service. "Forcing diets to meet RDA leads to imbalances in proportion of energy from protein, fat, and carbohydrate, and high levels of cholesterol in diets," she says.[109] "For the food plans of teenage girls and women, attempting to meet the RDA for iron and the RDA for zinc forces the proportion of energy derived from protein up to 20 percent or more." Dr. Woteki says the RDA for pregnant and lactating women cannot be achieved at all through food.

The varied, balanced, and scientifically formulated Pritikin diet, composed in the main of unrefined plant foods, meets nutritional needs with no problems. The diet not only prevents the overconsumption of foods implicated in the etiology of several degenerative disease processes, but also ensures meeting the requirements for the whole spectrum of macro- and micro-nutrients. On the Pritikin diet you will eat wisely, eat well, and be very healthy for a very long time.

REFERENCES

1. Alfin-Slater, R. B., and Aftergood, L. Lipids. In *Modern Nutrition in Health and Disease*, 6th ed., Goodhart, R. S., and Shils, M. E., eds. Philadelphia: Lea & Febiger, 1980, p. 128.

2. Anderson, J. R., *et al.* Mineral and vitamin status on high-fiber diets: Long-term studies of diabetic patients. *Diab. Care,* 1980, 3:38–40.

3. Barnard, R. J., *et al.* Effects of an intensive, short-term exer-

cise and nutrition program on patients with coronary heart disease. *J. Cardiac Rehab.*, 1981, *1*:99–105.

4. Barnard, R. J., *et al*. Response of non-insulin-dependent diabetic patients to an intensive program of diet and exercise. *Diab. Care*, 1982, *5*:370–74.

5. Barrows, C. H., and Kokkonen, G. Protein synthesis, development, growth and life span. *Growth*, 1975, *39*:525–33.

6. Beaton, G. H., and Swiss, L. D. Evaluation of the nutritional quality of food supplies: Prediction of "desirable" or "safe" protein: Calorie ratios. *Am. J. Clin. Nutr.*, 1974, *27*:485–504.

7. Bingham, S., and Cummings, J. H. Sources and intakes of dietary fiber in man. In *Medical Aspects of Dietary Fiber*, Spiller and Kay, eds. New York: Plenum, 1980, pp. 261–84.

8. Brenner, B. M., *et al*. Dietary protein intake and the progressive nature of kidney disease: The role of hemodynamically mediated glomerular injury in the pathogenesis of progressive glomerular sclerosis in aging, renal ablation, and intrinsic renal disease. *N. Eng. J. Med.*, 1982, *307*:652–69.

9. Bricker, M., *et al*. The protein requirements of adult human subjects in terms of the protein contained in individual foods and food combinations. *J. Nutr.*, 1945, *30*:269–84.

10. Briggs, M. Vitamin E supplements and fatigue. *N. Eng. J. Med.*, 1974, *290*:579–80.

11. Brodribb, A. J. M., and Humphreys, D. M. Diverticular disease: Three studies. Pt. I—Relation to other disorders and fibre intake; Pt. II—Treatment with bran; Pt. III—Metabolic effect of bran in patients with diverticular disease. *Brit. Med. J.*, 1976, *1*:424–30.

12. Bronner, F. Vitamin D deficiency and rickets. *Am. J. Clin. Nutr.*, 1976, *29*:1307–14.

13. Burkitt, D. P., *et al*. Effect of dietary fibre on stools and transit-times, and its role in the causation of disease. *Lancet*, 1972, *2*:1408–12.

14. Campbell, T. C. Quoted in "In the war against cancer, the latest weapons are fruits and vegetables." *People*, 1982 (July 12):65–68.

15. Carroll, K. K. The role of dietary protein in hypercholesterolemia and atherosclerosis. *Lipids*, 1978, *13*:360–65.

16. Cerqueira, M. T., *et al*. The food and nutrient intakes of the Tarahumara Indians of Mexico. *Am. J. Clin. Nutr.*, 1979, *32*:905–15.

17. Cohen, H. M. Fatigue caused by vitamin E? *Calif. Med.*, 1973, *119*:72.

18. Corrigan, J. J., and Marcus, F. I. Coagulopathy associated with vitamin E ingestion. *JAMA*, 1974, *230*:1300–1301.

19. Corrigan, J. J., and Ulfers, L. L. Effect of vitamin E on prothrombin levels in warfarin-induced vitamin K deficiency. *Am. J. Clin. Nutr.*, 1981, *34*:1701–5.

20. Crawford, M. A., personal communication.

21. Crocetti, A. F., and Guthrie, H. A. *Eating Behavior and Associated Nutrient Quality of Diets*. New York: Anarem System Res. Corp., 1982.

22. Currens, J. H., *et al.* Metabolic effects of rice diet in treatment of hypertension. *N. Eng. J. Med.*, 1951, *245*:354–59.

23. Dayton, S., *et al.* A controlled clinical trial of a diet high in unsaturated fat. *N. Eng. J. Med.*, 1962, *266*:1017–23.

24. Dayton, S., *et al.* A controlled clinical trial of a diet high in unsaturated fat in preventing complications of atherosclerosis. *Circ.*, 1969, *40*, Suppl. II:1–63.

25. Di Bendetto, R. J. Chronic hypervitaminosis A in an adult. *JAMA*, 1967, *201*:700–702.

26. Donald, P., *et al.* Body weight and composition in laboratory rats: Effects of diets with high or low protein concentrations. *Sci.*, 1981, *211*:185–86.

27. Eisenstein, R., and Zeruolis, L. Vitamin D–induced aortic calcification. *Arch. Path.*, 1964, *77*:27. [Abstract in *JAMA*, 1964; *187*:186]

28. Fisher, H., *et al.* Reassessment of amino acid requirements of young women on low nitrogen diets. I. Lysine and tryptophan. *Am. J. Clin. Nutr.*, 1969, *22*:1190–96.

29. Fisher, H., *et al.* Reassessment of animo acid requirement of young women on low nitrogen diets. II. Leucine, methionine, and valine. *Am. J. Clin. Nutr.*, 1971, *24*:1216–23.

30. Flute, P. T. Acquired disorders of blood coagulation. In: *Blood and Its Disorders*, Hardisty, R. M., and Weatherall, D. J., eds. Oxford: Blackwell Scient. Pub., 1974, p. 1081.

31. Forbes, G. B. Present knowledge of vitamin D. *Nutr. Rev.*, 1967, *25*:225–28.

32. Fraser, D., and Scriver, C. R. Familial forms of vitamin D–resistant rickets revisited. X-linked hypophosphatemia and autosomal recessive vitamin D dependency. *Am. J. Clin. Nutr.*, 1976, *29*: 1315–29.

32a. Frølich, W., and Lysø, A. Bioavailability of iron from wheat bran in pigs. *Am. J. Clin. Nutr.*, 1983, *37*:31–36.

33. Golden, M. H. N. Protein deficiency, energy deficiency and the oedema of malnutrition. *Lancet*, 1982, *1*: 1261–65.

34. Goldrick, R. B. *et al.* An assessment of coronary heart disease and coronary risk factors in a New Guinea highland population. In *Atherosclerosis: Proceedings of the Second International Symposium*, Jones, R. J., ed. Berlin: Springer-Verlag, 1970, pp. 366–68.

35. Grace, C. S., *et al.* Blood fibrinolysis and coagulation in New Guineans and Australians. *Aust. Ann. Med.*, 1970, *4*:328–33.

36. Hall, J. A., *et al.* Effects of diet and exercise on peripheral vascular disease (case report). *Phys. and Sportsmed.*, 1982, *10*:90–101.

37. Hausman, P. *Jack Sprat's Legacy: The Science and Politics of Fat & Cholesterol.* New York: Richard Marek, 1981, p. 29.

38. Hazards of overuse of vitamin D. *Nutr. Rev.*, 1974, *33*:61–62.

39. Hegsted, D. M., *et al.* Protein requirements of adults. *J. Lab. Clin. Med.*, 1946, *31*:261–84.

40. Hegsted, D. M. Minimum protein requirements of adults. *Am. J. Clin. Nutr.*, 1968, *21*:352–57.

41. Herbert, V Toxicity of 25,000 IU vitamin A supplements in "health" food users. *Am. J Clin. Nutr.*, 1982, *36*:185–86.

42. Herbert, V., personal communication.

43. Herbert, V. Quoted in "The Pritikin Program: Claims vs Facts." *Consumer Repts.*, 1982, *47*:513–18.

44. Hillman, N. M., *et al.* Protein deprivation in primates. X. Test performance of juveniles born of deprived mothers. *Am. J Clin. Nutr.*, 1978, *31*:388–93.

45. Hillman, R. W. Tocopherol excess in man: Creatinuria associated with prolonged ingestion. *Am. J. Clin. Nutr.*, 1958, *5*:597–600.

46. Holman, R. T. How essential are essential fatty acids? *J. Am. Oil Chem. Soc.*, 1978, *55*:774a–82a.

47. Hornstra, G., *et al.* Fish oils, prostaglandins, and arterial thrombosis. *Lancet*, 1979, *2*:1080.

48. Hypervitaminosis E and coagulation. *Nutr. Rev.*, 1975, *33*:269–70.

49. Humans as walking legumes. *Nutr. Rev.*, 1971, *29*:223–26.

50. Hunt, S. M., and Schofield, F. A. Magnesium balance and protein intake level in adult human females. *Am. J. Clin Nutr.*, 1969, *22*:367–73.

51. Insull, W., *et al.* Studies of arteriosclerosis in Japanese and American men. I. Comparison of fatty acid composition of adipose tissue. *J. Clin. Invest.*, 1969, *48*:1313–27.

52. Irwin, M. I., and Hegsted, D. M. A conspectus of research on protein requirements of man. *J. Nutr.*, 1971, *101*:385–430.

53. Jakubczak, L. F. Behavioral aspects of nutrition and longevity in animals. In *Nutrition, Longevity, and Aging*, Rockstein, M., and Sussman, M. L., eds. New York: Academic Press, 1976, pp. 103–22.

54. Jayarajan, P., *et al.* Effect of dietary fat on absorption of β-carotene from green leafy vegetables in children. *Indian J. Med. Res.*, 1980, *71*:53–56.

55. Kempner, W. Compensation of renal metabolic dysfunction; Treatment of kidney disease and hypertensive vascular disease with rice diet. *N. Carolina Med. J.*, 1945, *6*:61 (pt. 1), 117 (pt. 2).

56. Kempner, W. Treatment of heart and kidney disease and of hypertensive and arteriosclerotic vascular disease with the rice diet. *Ann. Int. Med.*, 1949, *31*:821–56.

57. Kik, M. D. Nutritive value of chicken meat and its value in supplementing rice protein. *J. Agr. Food Chem.*, 1962, *10*:59–61.

58. Knapp, J., *et al.* Growth and nitrogen balance in infants fed cereal proteins. *Am. J. Clin. Nutr.*, 1973, *26*:586–90.

59. Kofranyi, E., and Jekat, J. Zur Bestimmung der biologischen Wertigkeit von Nahrungsproteinen, XI. Die Wirkung von Methionin auf den Stickstoffbedarf. "The determination of the biological value of dietary protein, XI. The effect of methionine on nitrogen requirement." *Z. Physiol. Chem.*, 1965, *342*:248.

60. Korycka, M., *et al.* Influence of fat level in the diet on carotene and vitamin A utilization. *Acta Physiol. Pol.*, 1969, *20*:662–67.

61. Lala, V. R., and Reddy, V. Absorption of β-carotene from green leafy vegetables in undernourished children. *Am. J. Clin. Nutr.*, 1970, *23*:110–13.

62. Lampman, R. M., *et al.* Type IV hyperlipoproteinemia: Effects of a caloric restricted type IV diet versus physical training plus isocaloric type IV diet. *Am. J. Clin. Nutr.*, 1980, *33*:1233–43.

63. Lee, C. J., *et al.* Nitrogen retention of young men fed rice with or without supplementary chicken. *Am. J. Clin. Nutr.*, 1971, *24*:318–23.

64. Leto, S., *et al.* Dietary protein, life-span, and physiological variables in female mice. *J. Geront.*, 1976, *31*:149–54.

65. Linkswiler, H. M., *et al.* Calcium retention of young adult

males as affected by level of protein and of calcium intake. *Trans N.Y. Acad. Sci.*, 1974, Ser. II, 36:333–40.

66. Lui, N. S. T., and Roels, O. A. The vitamins: A. Vitamin A and carotene. In *Modern Nutrition in Health and Disease*, 6th ed., Goodhart, R. S., and Shils. M. E., eds. Philadelphia: Lea & Febiger, 1980, p. 156.

67 Luyken, R., *et al.* Nutrition studies in New Guinea. *Am J Clin. Nutr.*, 1964, *14*: 13–27

68. Mahalko, J. R., *et al.* Effect of a moderate increase in dietary protein on the retention and excretion of Ca, Cu, Fe, Mg, P, and Zn by adult males. *Am. J. Clin. Nutr.* 1983, *37*:8–14.

69. McKean, C. M. Growth of phenylketonuric children on chemically defined diets. *Lancet*, 1970, *1*:148.

70. Morris, E. R., *et al.* Trace element nutriture response of adult men consuming dephytinized or non-dephytinized wheat bran. In *Trace Substances in Environmental Health—XIV*. Columbia: Univ. of Missouri Press, 1980, pp. 103–9.

71. National Research Council, Food and Nutrition Board, Committee on Dietary Allowances. *Recommended Dietary Allowances* 8th rev. ed., Washington. DC: Natl. Acad. Sci., 1974.

72. National Research Council, Food and Nutrition Board, Committee on Dietary Allowances. *Recommended Dietary Allowances* 9th rev ed. Washington, DC: Natl. Acad. Sci., 1980.

73. National Research Council, Committee on Diet, Nutrition, and Cancer. *Diet. Nutrition, and Cancer.* Washington, DC: Natl Acad. Sci., 1982, pp. 1–5, 5–20, 5–21

74. Nelson, R. A. Quoted in "Are we eating too much protein?" *Med. World News*, November 8, 1974, p. 106.

75 New Guinea natives: More on nitrogen fixing. *Sci. News*, 1970, *98*:161

76. Osborne, T. B., and Mendel, L. B. Amino-acids in nutrition and growth. *J Biol. Chem* 1914, *17*:325–49.

77 Pease, C. N. Focal retardation and arrestment of growth of bones due to vitamin A intoxication. *JAMA*, 1962, *182*:980–85

78. Pecora, L. J and Hundley, J. M. Nutritional improvement of white polished rice by the addition of lysine and threonine *J Nutr*, 1951, *44*:101–12

79. Pennington, J A T *Dietary Nutrient Guide* Westport, CT: Avi, 1976

80. Prasad, J. S. Effect of vitamin E supplementation on leukocyte function. *Am J Clin Nutr* 1980, *33*:606–8

81. Press, M., et al. Correction of essential fatty-acid deficiency in man by the cutaneous application of sunflower-seed oil. *Lancet,* 1974, *1*:597–99.

82. Pritikin, N. *The Pritikin Permanent Weight-Loss Manual.* New York: Grosset & Dunlap, 1981, 399 pp.

83. Reddy, V. Lysine supplementation of wheat and nitrogen retention in children. *Am. J. Clin. Nutr.,* 1971, *24*:1246–49.

84. Richardson, D. P., et al. Quantitative effect of an isoenergetic exchange of fat for carbohydrate on dietary protein utilization in healthy young men. *Am. J. Clin. Nutr.,* 1979, *32*:2217–26.

85. Riopelle, A. M., and Shell, W. F. Protein deprivation in primates. XI. Determinants of weight change during and after pregnancy. *Am. J. Clin. Nutr.,* 1978, *31*:394–400.

86. Rizek, R. L., and Jackson, E. M. *Current Food Consumption Practices and Nutrient Sources in the American Diet.* Hyattsville, MD: USDA, 1980.

87. Robertson, W. G., et al. Should recurrent calcium oxalate stone formers become vegetarians? *Brit. J. Urol.,* 1979, *51*:427–31.

88. Rose, W. C. The amino acid requirements of adult man. *Nutr. Abstr. Rev.,* 1957, *27*:631–47.

89. Rosenberg, H. R., et al. Lysine and threonine supplementation of rice. *J. Nutr.,* 1959, *69*:217–28.

90. Ross, M. H. Protein, calories and life expectancy. *Fed. Proc.,* 1959, *18*:1190–1207.

91. Schuette, S. A., et al. Studies on the mechanism of protein-induced hypercalciuria in older men and women. *J. Nutr.,* 1980, *110*:305–15.

92. Seelig, M. S. Are American children still getting an excess of vitamin D? Hyperreactive children at risk. *Clin. Pedia.,* 1970, *9*:380–83.

93. Shekelle, R. B., et al. Dietary vitamin A and risk of cancer in the Western Electric Study. *Lancet,* 1981, *2*:1186–90.

94. Simpson, K. M., et al. The inhibitory effect of bran on iron absorption in man. *Am. J. Clin. Nutr.,* 1981, *34*:1469–78.

95. Sinclair, H. M. Prevention of coronary heart disease: The role of essential fatty acids. *Postgrad. Med. J.,* 1980, *56*:579–84.

96. Sinnett, P. R., and Whyte, H. M. Epidemiological studies in a highland population of New Guinea: Environment, culture, and health status. *Human Ecol.,* 1973, *1*:245–77.

97. Southgate, D. A. T., et al. A guide to calculating intakes of dietary fibre. *J. Human Nutr.,* 1976, *30*:303–13

98. Storey, R., *et al. Popular Diets: How They Rate.* Los Angeles District, California Dietetic Assoc., 1982.

99. Toxic reactions of vitamin A. *Nutr. Rev.*, 1964, *22*:109–11.

100. Trowell, H. Dietary changes in modern times. In *Refined Carbohydrate Foods and Disease.* Burkitt, D. P., and Trowell, H. C., eds. London: Academic Press, 1975, p. 53.

101. Tsai, A. C., *et al.* Study on the effect of megavitamin E supplementation in man. *Am. J. Clin. Nutr.*, 1978, *31*:831–37.

102. U.S. Senate, Select Committee on Nutrition and Human Needs. *Dietary Goals for the United States,* 2d ed. Washington, DC: U.S. Govt. Print. Off., 1977, p. 41.

103. Van Soest, P. M., and McQueen, R. W. The chemistry and estimation of fibre. *Proc. Nutr. Soc.*, 1973, *32*:123.

104. Vitamin K: Deficiencies and interactions with vitamin E. *Nutr. & the M.D.*, 1982, *8*:1.

105. Voit, C. Ueber die Entwicklung der Lehre von der Quelle der Muskelkraft und einiger Theile der Ernahrung seit 25 Jahren. "On the development in the past 25 years of the theory of the source of muscle strength, and some aspects of nutrition. *Ztschr. f. Biol.*, 1870, *6*:305–401.

106. Walker, A. R. P., *et al.* Studies in human mineral metabolism. I. The effect of bread rich in phytate phosphorus on the metabolism of certain mineral salts with special reference to calcium. *Biochem. J.*, 1948, *42*:452–62.

107. Watt, B. K., *et al. Composition of foods: Raw, Processed, Prepared,* rev. ed. USDA Agri. Handbk No. 8, 1963.

108. Winitz, M., *et al.* Studies in metabolic nutrition employing chemically defined diets. I. Extended feeding of normal human adult males. *Am. J. Clin. Nutr.*, 1970, *23*:525–45.

109. Wotecki, C. E. Uses and limits to the use of RDA for diet planning and food selection. Speech delivered to the Food and Nutrition Board, National Research Council, Washington, DC, December 13, 1982.

110. Wretlind, A. Standards for nutritional adequacy of the diet: European and WHO/FAO viewpoints. *Am. J. Clin. Nutr.*, 1982, *36*:366–75.

24
CHAPTER

Optimal Dietary Recommendations: A Public-Health Responsibility

Degenerative diseases, such as diabetes, heart disease, hypertension, and breast and colon cancer, are still widely assumed by many to be a natural aspect of getting older as the body "degenerates." If this is true, we are confronted with explaining why these diseases are essentially limited to the most developed and, theoretically, the most scientifically advanced populations in the world. In my view, these conditions are not diseases, but symptoms of chronic metabolic injury resulting from the highly processed, artificial diet eaten in developed areas, principally from the excessive amounts of cholesterol and fat consumed.

A toxin is any substance that when taken in excess can cause death. Cyanide, present in lima beans, is rarely reported as the cause of adverse effects when consumed in this food. It can be assumed that the amount of cyanide in lima beans is far below the toxic level. In contrast to cyanide, iron is necessary to maintain life; but even so, excess iron intake can cause iron overload of the liver and result in death. In Africa, among the Bantu, the use of iron pots furnishes 3 to 5 times as much iron as the amount specified in the US Recommended Dietary Allowances (RDA) In these days of megavitamins, this may not seem much, but the excess reaches a toxic level creating iron overload of the liver in 75 percent of the males and 25 percent of the females, resulting in unnecessary deaths.

In the amounts in which they are consumed in Western countries, cholesterol and fat reach toxic levels. It is this toxicity that I hold responsible for the degenerative diseases —pathological processes resulting from aberrations in the intake and metabolic processing of lipid and cholesterol.

In 1955, when my cholesterol level hovered around 300 mg/dl, fueled by my daily ingestion of 700 mg of cholesterol, physicians assured me that it was in the high normal range, that my diet was excellent, and that stress and heredity were my principal heart-disease risk factors. Nevertheless, I soon developed coronary insufficiency so advanced that I was advised to completely limit all exercise. In retrospect, this circumstance may have been fortunate, saving me from a possible infarct resulting from the vigorous tennis matches in which I engaged at the time.

For 20 years prior, I had been closely following the epidemiology of cardiovascular and other degenerative diseases in the medical literature, though I had not been applying this information to my own lifestyle. I had concluded that atherosclerosis is essentially nonexistent in populations with adult cholesterol levels below 150 mg/dl. A feature common to all these populations seemed to be a cholesterol intake of less than 100 mg a day.

During the late 1940s and early 1950s, Keys reported the findings of more than 25 investigations; without exception, he found heart disease to be rare in these low-cholesterol-consuming populations.[11] Of particular interest were Keys's analyses of populations—especially the Japanese—who lost their immunity to heart disease when they migrated to areas in which cholesterol and fat intake were higher, and adopted the new diet.

The Japanese are heavy smokers, yet this well-established heart-disease risk factor seems to be of significantly less importance in the presence of a low-cholesterol and low-fat diet. Although they are number one among the developed nations in salt intake, hypertension, and strokes, the Japanese incidence of heart disease is the lowest among the developed nations. A 10-percent-fat diet keeps the average cholesterol level of this population at 150 mg/dl.

In the United States, where the mean population cholesterol level exceeds 200 mg/dl, both smoking and hypertension substantially contribute to the development of heart disease. Perhaps the low Japanese cholesterol levels are protective against the development of atherosclerosis in spite of these risk factors.

Among the populations that seem immune to heart disease is one close to our southern borders. Fifty thousand Tarahumara Indians, living in the isolation of the Sierra Madre Occidental mountains in northern Mexico, are part of a natural dietary experiment that has been going on for the past 2000 years. Their athletic stamina, as indicated by the ability to run up to 200 miles, has attracted the attention of a number of scientists. One of them, William E. Connor, has conducted a number of investigations of their diet and general health. He found no evidence of deaths from cardiovascular disease and concluded that their diet is typical of other populations among which heart disease is virtually nonexistent. Of their total caloric intake, fat makes up 10 percent (P/S = 2.0); protein, 13 percent; and carbohydrates, 75–80 percent. The diet provides 15–20 g/day of crude fiber, only 75 mg/day of cholesterol, and meets all nutritional requirements. Adult cholesterol levels among the Tarahumaras range from 100 to 140 mg/dl.[5,6]

In 1955, when I decided to change my high-cholesterol, high-fat dietary lifestyle, I adopted a diet nutritionally identical to the Tarahumara and other similar diets, though I endeavored to prepare the food in a manner pleasing to my Western-trained tastes. This is the same diet I have been recommending for 25 years, although for those with cholesterol levels of 250 mg/dl or greater, I found it was more effective to limit cholesterol intake to 15 mg a day, until serum levels dropped below 140 mg/dl.

In less than 3 years on this type of diet, my cholesterol level dropped to 100 mg/dl, and it has remained in that range for 25 years. In the last 6 years, my dietary recommendations have been incorporated into the nutritional service at the Longevity Centers, and cholesterol levels there, on an average, drop 27 percent in 3–4 weeks.

Serum cholesterol levels of people who come to the Longevity Centers—mostly white Americans—drop quickly on a diet nutritionally similar to the Tarahumara diet; conversely, when Tarahumara are given American intakes of cholesterol, serum cholesterol rapidly rises toward American levels.[12] The response seems universal.

Framingham data early indicated that "normal" cholesterol levels in the United States were normal only for a country where heart disease is rampant. Even the early Cleveland Clinic angiographic data[14] destroyed the "normal" cholesterol-level concept. Among 723 men 17 to 39 years old, significant (>50%) coronary lesions were found to be directly related to cholesterol level even within the "acceptable" limits of serum cholesterol (Table 1).

TABLE 1
SIGNIFICANT CORONARY LESIONS ASSOCIATED WITH
SERUM CHOLESTEROL LEVELS[14]

Serum cholesterol (mg/dl)	Significant lesions (> 50%) Percentage of total cases
<200	20
201–225	38
226–250	48
251–275	60
276–300	77

This growing mass of epidemiological evidence—all pointing in the same direction—was further illuminated by the findings of Brown and Goldstein, who were able to show the mechanisms involved in setting the safe limits of circulating serum cholesterol. To quote Michael Brown: "Why, therefore, is western man oversaturating his receptors and depositing LDL cholesterol in his arteries?" To lower plasma levels of LDL (to ideal levels) requires a diet of less than 100 mg of cholesterol daily and thus excludes all meat products and eggs, "a diet which I would never eat, which allows almost nothing except nuts and berries."[4] I phoned Dr. Brown and said, "I have bad news for you: nuts are not on my diet—too high in fat. All that's left is berries." It did not take long to explain that the marvelous recipes adapted from American and foreign cuisines would give him a wide-ranging fare free of the risks of high cholesterol and high fat intake. The question that arises is *Why is there such reluctance to change the atherogenic diet?*

Henry Blackburn wrote a splendid article,[3] "The Public Health View of Diet and Mass Hyperlipidemia," whose thesis can be summarized in three sentences: "Atherosclerotic CHD is a public health phenomenon of affluent cultures. Population comparisons suggest that mass hyperlipidemia is a prime requisite for mass atherosclerosis. On the basis of available evidence, the habitual diet of a culture is, in turn, the chief factor leading to hyperlipidemia." Blackburn divides the world into four categories according to cholesterol levels, as shown in Table 2.

TABLE 2

RELATIONSHIP OF MEAN POPULATION CHOLESTEROL LEVEL
AND INCIDENCE OF ATHEROSCLEROSIS [3]

Mean population cholesterol level (mg/dl)	Incidence of atherosclerosis
120	Rare
160	Minimal
190	Reduced
220–280	Epidemic

He selects a mean population cholesterol level of 160 mg/dl as the best compromise (minimal CHD, and good palatability), and states: "Population total cholesterol averages above 200 mg/dl are found incompatible with optimal cardiovascular health for populations." Other expert groups have concurred with this general position. The American Health Foundation Conference on "Health Effects of Blood Lipids: Optimal Distributions for Populations" made an optimal recommendation of 160 mg/dl.[16]

But what Blackburn recommends to the U.S. public with its average serum cholesterol of 220 mg/dl is the American Heart Association (AHA) diet: 30 percent fat and 300 mg cholesterol—because, he points out, large-scale studies have shown it is able to produce cholesterol drops of 6–7 percent. A quick calculation indicates that a 7-percent drop from 220 mg/dl still leaves those hapless individuals with excessively high levels of 205 mg/dl, which Blackburn himself stated is incompatible with optimal cardiovascular health. To achieve the ideal, a mean population cholesterol level of 160 mg/dl, requires a drop of 27 percent. On my recommended diet, this 27-percent cholesterol reduction occurs in a month.[8]

The hopelessness of the position of those who cannot see beyond the AHA diet is apparent also in a statement made by AHA spokesman Scott Grundy that the AHA diet could only reduce the mean cholesterol level of U.S. men to 200 mg/dl. He goes on to say: "Yet despite such a change, half the male population would have cholesterol concentrations over 200 mg/dl. Many workers believe that levels over 200 mg/dl are still too high for adequate prevention of atherosclerotic disease. Thus, it is doubtful that atherosclerotic disease in our society can be obliterated by diet control alone, and additional measures will have to be taken to rid the American population of this disease. The methods are currently not available and will have to be developed through new research."[9]

The conclusion that diet alone cannot reduce the mean serum cholesterol level below 200 mg/dl is true with the AHA diet, of course. But Grundy asserts that this 30-percent-fat, 300-mg-cholesterol diet is the most effective diet for lowering cholesterol level—which is not true. Since the AHA diet does not work, he blames this on "genetics" and says new methods not currently available will have to be developed through new research.

While health professionals knowledgeable about the dietary basis of CHD are unable to face up to the magnitude of the dietary changes that must be made to achieve adequate lowering of serum cholesterol, they are willing to use hypocholesteremic drugs that have been discredited because of the possible excess cancer risk they introduce; to subject hyperlipidemic patients to an ileal bypass that will reduce cholesterol level little more effectively than a diet with less than 10 percent fat and 100 mg of cholesterol; and to continue to make dietary recommendations of 300 mg cholesterol and 30 percent fat when during 20 years of trials this diet has failed to reduce cholesterol levels adequately.

Worse yet, it should be noted that these dietary recommendations when first made to the nation in 1961 had not been adequately tested. Pearce and Dayton, who directed the 8-year Wadsworth Veterans Administration AHA diet trial with 846 men, commented, "It is important to remember that no population under study has been consuming a diet high in polyunsaturated fats over long periods of time."[15] After the Wadsworth study, Dayton said not only that he would not recommend a high-polyunsaturated (PUFA) diet to most of his patients, but that a diet of 10 percent fat would be his choice. In the official report, the investigator wrote: "The diet tested in this program was selected for purely pragmatic reasons: we did not believe we could mount and sustain a trial of any other type of lipid-lowering diet in this institution. Epidemiological studies favor the conclusion that a low-fat diet is perhaps the promising path to longevity."[7]

Though high-PUFA diets fail to reduce the risk of heart disease, they may *enhance* the risk of cancer. The 1982 National Academy of Sciences report *Diet, Nutrition, and Cancer* concluded that a relationship between fat and cancer was most persuasive.[13] T. C. Campbell, one of the authors of the report, stated that if a diet is high in PUFA, total fat should be less than 20 percent of total calories because of the possible increased cancer risk. So convinced is Campbell of the danger of excess fat that he stated: "The relationship between diet and cancer, in my opinion, is now more persuasively established than the one between diet and heart disease."

What, then, was the recommendation that flowed from this observation? Campbell continued: "We decided to come up with a reasonable, practical number, something the whole population might work toward. So we recommended a reduction in fat intake from a current 40% of total calories to 30%, although I would suggest getting it down to about 20%. In China, where I was in June, it's only 9%. So you can go down to 20% and not experience problems."

But the public recommendation is 30 percent! Cancer and

heart-disease researchers are alike in their tendency to treat the public as though they were incapable of accepting an optimal dietary recommendation.

My experience with 10,000 people who have been through my centers and millions who have read or heard about my diet belies this underestimation of a large part of the public. Why shouldn't everyone who wishes to follow an optimal diet be informed of the facts and be encouraged to make the necessary lifestyle changes?

When people achieve rapid health improvement, as very many do on an optimal diet, they become motivated to continue permanently so as to maximize health gains and avoid regressing. My diet, combined with exercise, has been effective not only with patients with cardiovascular symptoms but with non–insulin-dependent diabetics, 75 percent of whom are off insulin in 4 weeks, including some who had been taking it for 20 years.[2] In 4 weeks, 85 percent of hypertensives on drug therapy are off medication, with normal blood pressure, on this same diet/exercise regimen. In 3 weeks, cholesterol and triglycerides drop 25–30 percent on the regimen. Compliance, considering the difficulties in pursuing this kind of dietary lifestyle in a milieu in which not even health authorities encourage it, is surprisingly good; over a 5-year period, compliance varies between 50 and 75 percent.[1]

If health-care authorities recommended that cholesterol intake not exceed 100 mg/day and fat intake not exceed 10 percent of total calories, the benefits experienced by those who follow my program could be experienced by millions more. The benefits would extend not only to sick people; healthy, active people would also gain. Many world-class athletes are on my diet and are experiencing thrilling new, higher levels of performance. In the October 9, 1982, Triathlon in Hawaii, 5 of these athletes will have been identified as being on the Pritikin diet.* It is encouraging from a public-health viewpoint that all these athletes adopted the new

---

* Of a field of 850 athletes, those on the Pritikin diet came in first, second, and fourth, setting a new course record of 9 hours 8 minutes. The first-place winner has been on the diet for 4 years. The third-place winner, who was not identified as being on the Pritikin

dietary lifestyle from reading my books or by word of mouth. I became aware of them only when I was contacted by one of their group. The event is grueling, consisting of a 2½-mile open ocean swim, a 112-mile bicycle race, and a 26-mile marathon run, all in continuous sequence.

The experts, already in agreement on the biochemical goals, are now beginning to agree on the guidelines: cholesterol intake needs to be under 100 mg/day and fat intake not over 10 percent. Leading investigators—Seymour Dayton in CHD, T. C. Campbell in cancer, and J. W. Anderson in diabetes—are all looking respectfully at a 10-percent-fat diet, or are already using it.

New health recommendations from authoritative sources are also moving slowly in the direction of advocating optimal fat and cholesterol intakes. These are encouraging trends; but there are still many problems to be overcome in terms of facilitating widespread enactment of these dietary goals. Only by replacing "compromise" by "ideal" can we ever hope to achieve the optimal diet for maximum quality and duration of life.

REFERENCES

1. Barnard, R. J., Guzy, P. M., Rosenberg, J. M., and O'Brien, L. T. Effects of an intensive exercise and nutrition program on patients with coronary artery disease: 5-year follow-up (Abstract). *Med. Sci. Sports Exercise*, 1982, *14*:179.

2. Barnard, R. J., Lattimore, L., Holly, R. G., Cherny, S., and Pritikin, N. Response of non–insulin-dependent diabetic patients to an intensive program of diet and exercise. *Diabetes Cure*, 1972, *5*:370–74.

3. Blackburn, H. The public health view of diet and mass hyperlipidemia. *Cardiovasc. Rev. Rep.*, Aug. 1980, 433–42; Sept. 1980, 361–69.

4. Carpenter, M. "Healthy" receptors can't handle even "normal" lipid. *Med. Tribune*, 1980, *21*:3, 19.

diet, is a younger brother of the athlete placing second. Since the contest started 4 years ago, only 4 athletes other than the Pritikin winners have completed the race in under 10 hours.

5. Cerqueira, M. T., Fry, M. M., and Connor, W. E. The food and nutrient intakes of the Tarahumara Indians of Mexico. *Amer. J. Clin. Nutr.*, 1979, *32*:905–15.

6. Connor, W. E., Cerqueira, M. T., Connor, R. W., Wallace, R. B., *et al.* The plasma lipids, lipo-proteins, and diet of the Tarahumara Indians of Mexico. *Amer. J. Clin. Nutr.*, 1978, *31*:1131–42.

7. Dayton, S., Pearce, M. L., Hashimoto, S., Dixon, W. J., and Tomiyusau, U. A controlled clinical trial of a diet high in unsaturated fat in preventing complications of atherosclerosis. *Circulation*, 1969, *40*: Suppl. 2, 1–63.

8. Diehl, H., and Mannerberg, D. Hypertension, hyperlipidaemia, angina, and coronary heart disease. In *Western Diseases: Their Emergence and Prevention*, Trowell, H. D., and Burkitt, D. P. eds. Cambridge: Harvard Univ. Press, 1981, p. 400.

9. Grundy, S. M. Saturated fats and coronary heart disease. In *Nutrition and the Killer Diseases*, Winick, M., ed. New York: Wiley, 1981, p. 76.

10. In the war against cancer the latest weapons are fruits and vegetables. *People*, July 12, 1982, 65–68.

11. Keys, A., Kimura, N., Kusukawa, A., Bronte-Stewart, B., *et al.* Lessons from serum cholesterol studies in Japan, Hawaii, and Los Angeles. *Ann. Int. Med.*, 1958, *48*:83–94.

12. McMurry, M. P., Connor, W. E., and Cerqueira, M. T. Dietary cholesterol and the plasma lipids and lipoproteins in the Tarahumara Indians: A people habituated to a low cholesterol diet after weaning. *Amer. J. Clin. Nutr.*, 1982, *35*:741–44.

13. National Research Council, Committee on Diet, Nutrition and Cancer. *Diet, Nutrition, and Cancer*. Washington, DC: National Acad. Sci. 1982, pp. 5–20, 5–21.

14. Page, I. H., Berrettoni, J. N., Butkas, A., and Sones, F. M. Prediction of coronary heart disease based on clinical suspicion, age, total cholesterol and triglyceride. *Circulation*, 1970, *62*:625–45

15. Pearce, M. L., and Dayton, S. Incidence of cancer in men on a diet high in polyunsaturated fat. *Lancet*, *I*:464–67.

16. Wissler, R. W., Armstrong, M., Bilheimer, D., *et al.* Conference on the health effects of blood lipids: Optimal distributions for populations. *Prev. Med.*, 1979, *8*:715–32.

25
CHAPTER

Runners' Deaths
By
Miles H. Robinson, M.D.

It is widely believed that running protects against heart attacks, and this belief has motivated many people to join the ranks of joggers. One of the most prominent advocates of this theory is T. J. Bassler,[1] a pathologist and long-distance runner, who 10 years ago asserted that "no active marathoner has ever died of myocardial infarction."* In 1978, he was reported advising that running would protect against a heart attack for 5 years in those who could run a sub-4-hour marathon and refrained from smoking.[2] As recently as 1982, Bassler was quoted as saying that if deposits were previously present in the arteries, running a total of 16,000 kilometers will remove the plaques and restore a free flow of blood in the arteries.[3] Furthermore, he reputedly declared that "when the level of vigorous exercise is raised high

---

* The word "infarct" is from the Latin, meaning to stuff into. The heart tissue, damaged by an inadequate supply of blood from clogged arteries, appears stuffed with dead and dying cellular material.

enough, the protection from coronary† heart disease appears to be absolute."' A great many joggers and other athletes have depended on this highly optimistic philosophy.

However, in 1980, Bassler acknowledged in a scientific journal that "No serious researcher should ever say that marathon running provides complete immunity from coronary-heart disease." He stated that the "Bassler hypothesis" was only that "the marathoner's life-style will protect against the aging process. Your ability to cover 42 km on foot is the best index of your life-style. No death in a marathon runner should be overlooked. Meticulous autopsies, such as those reported by Noakes *et al.*, provide the only way to evaluate this hypothesis."⁴

Thus, there seems to be a marked discrepancy between what Bassler says for popular consumption and what he admits in scientific publications. As a runner himself, he naturally has a great emotional temptation to believe that running *per se*, which has many physical and psychological benefits, can also prevent the insidious clogging of arteries. This damage has been overwhelmingly demonstrated, in animal experiments and by epidemiological studies of human populations, to be closely associated with the very high intake of fat and cholesterol in the modern Western diet.

Dr. J. B. Handler and colleagues⁵ at the Naval Regional Medical Center in San Diego strongly disagree with assertions that running protects against heart attacks:

> Unfortunately, statements regarding the protective value of running have been made in the medical literature and have been widely circulated among runners. These assertions are not only inaccurate but potentially dangerous. They foster the tempting illusion of invincibility in the runner, encourage denial of premonitory symptoms, and replace a measure of common sense with self-delusion. The misinformed runner may forgo the warm-up period, skirt medical check-ups, or attempt to "run through" angina pectoris.

---

† "Corona" is the Greek word for crown. The network of main arteries that nourish the heart muscle lies like a crown on the outside surface of the heart.

Handler cited a case of a 48-year-old marathon runner who had been active in competitive athletics since childhood, and for 8 years had been averaging 50–60 miles per week. He had successfully completed 7 marathons, as well as other shorter and longer competitions, and usually finished in the top 10 percent of his age group. His total blood cholesterol was 185 mg %, of which the level of HDL (high-density lipoproteins) was 51 mg % (mean for his age: 45 mg %), and there was no family history of heart trouble. He had smoked 7–10 cigarettes a day prior to, but not since, taking up the running program. He had never had any heart symptoms; but after 8 years of running he developed chest pain on exertion. A treadmill test showed characteristic signs of loss of blood flow to the heart muscle, and an X-ray of the coronary arteries (angiogram) revealed a 99-percent blockage of a major branch of these arteries.

Leaving aside previous reports of coronary disease in runners who were not well conditioned, or in whom risk factors were operative, Handler considers this case unequivocal evidence that a long-distance marathon runner's lifestyle (nothing was said about nutrition) is not necessarily protective against the progression of coronary heart disease.

There have been numerous poignant letters in the lay press of fatal heart attacks while jogging. Jim Shettler, 42, a runner for 25 years and winner of the National AAU Masters 25-kilometer run, died while on a short run, the day after running 23 hilly miles.[6] Jim Dooley, 37, the city official who oversaw the expansion of Anaheim Stadium for the Los Angeles Rams, died while jogging near his home.[7] Robert Clarke, 49, a physiologist, died when he stopped to rest before continuing up a hill on his regular 3–4-mile daily run.[8] Colonel Giles Hall, 50, USAF Director of Health Professions Recruiting for the Air Force in Randolph, Texas, a daily jogger for 20 years, died while jogging.[9]

Dr. Robert Summers, longtime administrator of the Miami Heart Institute, dropped dead while jogging.[10] Dr. Edward Lauth, 46, a proponent of a jogging program that he had helped a local heart association to institute, died while jogging around Miami Beach's La Gorce Country Club.[10] Dr. David Doroff, 49, a clinical psychologist active throughout his life, joined the jogging boom in 1978, completed an

18-mile training run for the New York City Marathon, scored negative on an exercise test administered by his cardiologist, and dropped dead of a heart attack in his office. Autopsy revealed two of the coronary arteries 90 percent occluded, and the third 60 percent blocked.[1]

One of the most prominent marathoners was Congressman Goodloe Byron, who died suddenly while on a 15-mile training run in 1978. According to his wife, he knew his heart was impaired, but believed in Bassler's theory, and "saw running as his way to stay alive."[12]

Vuori *et al.*[13,14] examined the circumstances surrounding 2606 sudden deaths, and found that 73 percent of them had been caused by acute or chronic coronary-artery disease. At least one-third were associated with physical or psychological stress. Sudden deaths in connection with sporting activities or regular daily routine were rare, but there was a considerable risk of sudden death associated with strenuous physical exercise in subjects with manifest or *latent* cardiac disease, especially if there had been no gradual increase in exercise and training.

Pain in the front or back of the chest that develops during running is a serious sign which should be investigated. Noakes and Opie,[15,16] from the Ischemic Heart Disease Laboratories of the University of Cape Town and Groote Schuur Hospital in South Africa, describe the case of a 35-year-old runner with these symptoms who died suddenly 2 hours after a short period of surfing during which he felt breathless. He had had a 3-week period of exertional chest pain with ST-depression on a treadmill test. Opie also described 2 other men who dropped dead, one a 19-year-old who died during a marathon. The other died suddenly after a 6–8-mile run, having previously undertaken several 20-mile runs. At autopsy, both of these had coronary obstruction, markedly so in the second case.

Opie's review of 21 sudden deaths in athletes[17] found that 18 had died of heart attacks either during or after sport, and that there was firm or strongly suggestive evidence of coronary heart disease in 16 and suggestive clinical evidence in 2. As a group, these subjects tended to be smokers; to have a family history of early heart attacks; and to have had antecedent symptoms of chest pain or pressure, fatigue, or blackout. Psychological factors were thought to be important in 8, since hormones of the adrenaline family may precipitate myocardial ischemia and arrythmias. From his careful review of the literature (35 references), Opie concluded that the benefits of exercise have to be balanced against a small risk of sudden death, a risk that is very serious if there is chest pain, pressure, or undue tiredness before, during, or after sport.

Regarding the effect of acute emotional disturbances, P. Reich and his colleagues[18] at Harvard studied 117 patients of whom 62 had survived cardiac arrest and 55 had suffered symptomatic ventricular tachycardia. Twenty-five of these patients were experiencing acute emotional disturbances during the 24 hours preceding their attack.

L. E. Lamb,[8] formerly professor of medicine at Baylor and Chief of Clinical Sciences at the USAF School of Aerospace Medicine, emphasized that most American men over 40 years of age have a *silent* disease of coronary-artery obstruction which may not prevent marathon running or even show up in electrocardiograph-treadmill testing.

Then one day a little fatty-cholesterol deposit bursts like a pimple or tears and a clot may form in the artery. After that occurs if you exercise, then you may indeed work your heart muscle beyond its blood supply and a fatal heart attack may occur. . . . Most of the young US army men who died while exercising had clots in a coronary artery that had been there for a day or longer before the exercise even occurred. . . . As many as one-third of all heart attacks are silent.

Lamb pointed out that exercise may not cause a heart attack, and exercise may not prevent a heart attack. He firmly believed that "safe exercise" would help to prevent heart disease, but that unwise use of exercise could be dangerous, and that the way to improve the safety of exercise is to relieve or reverse the disease in the coronary arteries. He cited the work of Wissler on monkeys, Brant and colleagues on humans, and 3 decades of worldwide epidemiological studies, all of which suggest that "major diet changes can result in reversal of coronary artery disease."

Lamb recommended that until the blood cholesterol and

blood pressure in a middle-aged man have remained at optimal low levels for 3 months, together with a ban on smoking, the only unsupervised exercise that should be permitted is walking and light calisthenics, and this should *never* be done at a pace so fast that it prevents carrying on a conversation at the same time.

Waller and Roberts,[19] at the National Heart, Lung and Blood Institute, studied clinical and autopsy data on 5 white male runners aged 40 to 53 years, 2 of whom had been marathon runners. None had clinical evidence of cardiac disease before becoming a habitual runner, and all of them died while running. At autopsy, all had severe (greater than 75 percent) atherosclerotic luminal narrowing of their major coronary arteries. Of the 5, at least 4 had had hypercholesterolemia, which was greater than 300 mg % in 3 of the men; 240 mg % in one; and no figure available for the 5th man. These high blood cholesterols indicate the high-fat, high-cholesterol diet of these men.

Two subjects had had hypertension, one had had angina pectoris, and none had clinical evidence of an acute myocardial infarct. Only 1 had had symptoms, which consisted of episodes of pain beneath the sternum with radiation to the left arm after he had run about 13 km. This pain would disappear after about 100 ft of walking, and he could then run another 19–26 km without further pain. He was the only one with a positive stress test, consisting of ST-depression without pain. He had had no angina when he started running at age 39, but it had appeared 8 years later, 2 years before his death.

Four of the 5 runners had healed (clinically silent) myocardial infarcts. The authors concluded that "coronary heart disease appears to be the major killer of conditioned runners aged 40 years and over who die while running."

G. Sheehan,[20] medical editor of *Runner's World* magazine, recently stated that men who have taken up running to prevent a heart attack may find it to have been a waste of time. He referred to a 5-year study in the press, done at Methodist Hospital in Houston, which reports that a large proportion of men aged 40 to 60 who were long-distance runners developed evidence of coronary heart disease. The authors of this study, T. L. DeBauche *et al.*,[21] found that of

41 men who had been marathon runners for at least 2 years, 5 had positive stress tests at the beginning of the investigation; 13 developed positive tests by the end of 3 years; and 18 had positive tests at the conclusion of the study. None of the men had chest pains or other heart-related symptoms, and all were able to maintain the same level of fitness throughout the 5 years. Sheehan concluded that running may not prevent heart disease, but (rather optimistically) that heart disease does not prevent running, either.

W. Kannel,[22] director of the NIH Framingham study, believes that "the key to the prevention of sudden deaths remains the reduction of risk of coronary attacks," especially since 60 percent of these deaths occur in persons who have manifested no prior indications of coronary disease known to either the patients' families or their physicians.

Cantwell and Fletcher[23] report on 2 patients who suffered severe cardiac complications while jogging in organized exercise programs. An acute myocardial infarct developed in one, while the other had a cardiac arrest.

What are the statistical risks of a heart attack for joggers as compared with nonjoggers? P. D. Thompson et al.[24] studied 12 men who died during jogging in the state of Rhode Island from 1975 to 1980. In 11 of these the cause of death was coronary heart disease (CHD), while 1 died of an acute gastrointestinal hemorrhage. The prevalence of jogging among men aged 30 through 64 in Rhode Island was determined by a random-digit telephone survey. The incidence of death during jogging was 1 death per year for every 7620 joggers, or approximately 1 death per 396,000 man-hours of jogging. It is of great importance that this rate is 7 times the estimated death rate from CHD during more sedentary activities in Rhode Island. The authors suggest that exercise contributes to sudden death in *susceptible* persons, but that the risk is small and does not justify routine exercise testing of healthy subjects before exercise training.

What makes a heart susceptible to a heart attack? Now we are getting down to the nitty-gritty. Except for Lamb's reference to animal, clinical, and worldwide epidemiological work suggesting that major dietary changes can reverse coronary disease, none of the foregoing reports, whether made by medical professionals or by laymen, have shown any real interest in what the runners were accustomed to eat before they died.

Yet there is ample scientific evidence that except for a few persons who have an unusual hereditary ability to manage excess fat and cholesterol, the hearts of most Americans are much more susceptible to heart attacks than they need be, simply because evolution did not design the arteries of the heart or of any other human organ to cope with the modern Western diet.

It is, therefore, unreasonable to promote running as a major protection against heart attacks while ignoring the basic protection of a low-fat, low-cholesterol diet, which is the most important factor in the preservation of arterial health. In the light of what we know today, the familiar saying that "we are as young as our arteries" is more meaningful than ever before.

REFERENCES

1. Bassler, T. J., *Lancet,* 1972, *2*:711.
2. Restak, R. M., *New York Post* (magazine section), October 29, 1978, pp. 13, 17.
3. Sumner, J., *The Age,* Sydney, Australia, October 16, 1982.
4. Bassler, T. J., *N. Eng. J. Med.* 1980, *302*:57–58.
5. Handler, J. B., *et al., JAMA,* 1982, *248*:717–19.
6. Henderson, J., *Runner's World,* September 1976.
7. Dodson, M., *Los Angeles Times,* June 12, 1981.
8. Lamb, L. E., *The Health Letter,* 1979, *13*:1–4.
9. *Aviation, Space, and Environmental Medicine,* June 1979, p. 656.
10. Sackler, A. M., *Medical Tribune,* October 18, 1978, p. 18.
11. Bloom, M., *Medical World News,* November 27, 1978, pp. 66–76.
12. *The Jogger,* 1978, *X*:1, 5.
13. Vuori, I., *et al., Cardiology,* 1978, *63*:287–304.
14. Danilevicius, Z., *JAMA,* 1978, *240*:1754–55.
15. Noakes, T. D., and Opie, L. H., *Medical World News,* June 27, 1977, p. 53.
16. Opie, L. H., *N. Eng. J. Med.,* October 30, 1975, *293*:941–42.
17. Opie, L. H., *Lancet,* 1975, *1*:263–66.

18. Reich, P., *et al.*, *JAMA*, 1981, *246*:233–35.

19. Waller, B. F., and Roberts, W. C., *Am. J. Cardiol.*, 1980, *45*:423.

20. Sheehan, G., *Runner's World*, 1982.

21. DeBauche, T. L., *et al.*, in press.

22. Check, W. A., *JAMA*, 1981, *246*:581–89.

23. Cantwell, J. D., and Fletcher, G. F., *JAMA*, 1969, *210*:130-31.

24. Thompson, P. D., *et al.*, *JAMA*, 1982, *247*:2535–38.

    Pritikin Programs
    Santa Barbara, CA 93108

Special Services
Available
for the Reader

The lay reader may request information on:
- Nutrition and diets for all ages and activities.
- Availability of Pritikin foods in your area.
- In-residence 13-day and 26-day medically supervised east and west coast centers. These programs are ideal for people on medication or with a weight problem. You learn a new way of life and feel the benefits while you are there. The majority of those on medication no longer require their drugs in 2 to 4 weeks during their stay. Five-year follow-up studies indicate that very few return to their medications.

(Please send self-addressed stamped envelope.)

Physicians and other health professionals may request:
- Scientific evidence of the effect of the Pritikin diet on various diseases.
- Reprints of any of our published studies.
- Copies of unpublished studies.
- Printed diet guides for your patients.

THE PRITIKIN PROMISE

You may also request having your name added to our mailing list for new information. Write:

Pritikin Programs
P. O. Box 5335
Santa Barbara, CA 93108

Acknowledgments

This book reflects the devotion of many cherished staff members and would not have been possible without their valued contributions. Nan Bronfen, Director of Nutrition Research for the Pritikin Research Foundation, and Nell Taylor, my secretary since the inception of my work as director of the Longevity Centers, helped immeasurably in the writing, research, editing, and collating of the manuscript. Important technical suggestions and assistance were provided by Miles H. Robinson, M.D., author and researcher, who also contributed the chapter titled "Runners' Deaths." Ilene Pritikin, my wife and close associate in my nutritional work, was responsible for the menu and recipe sections and the material on preparing the diet. My thanks to her co-workers: Esther Taylor, who worked closely with Ilene in testing and developing the recipes and who created many of them; and Janet Trent, who contributed to writing the recipes and helped organize the recipe work.

We are indebted also to the Pritikin cooks all over the country, professional and amateur, who shared their treasured recipes with us. While it is not practical to mention them all, I am especially grateful to: Dr. and Mrs. John A. McDougall of Kailua, Hawaii, who teach patients to cook for good health, and contributed some of their fine recipes; the late Rose Stebbins, who conducted a class on Pritikin cooking at the College of the Redwoods in Eureka, California, and generously shared her own and her students' best recipes; Ruth M. Barnard, of the Vita-Mix Corporation, who was so helpful; and Robin Rifkin, home economist and Pritikin cooking teacher. Harold Kridler, Heidi Minnick, and Susan Huntington also lent valuable assistance in the recipe work. I owe special thanks to my editor, Frederic W. Hills, whose splendid cooperation and suggestions were invaluable.

Illustrations for the food and exercise sections were done by Robin Harris Brisker. Scientific drawings were done by Nell Taylor.

General Index

adipose tissue, 57
  linoleic acid in, 66
  see also fats
Adsuar, Gloria G., 25–26
aerobic exercise, 142–43
afternoon fatigue, 120
Agricultural Revolution (1800s), 437
Agriculture, U.S. Dept. of, 14, 31, 440
Air Force, U.S., 63
airplanes, meals on, 168–71
alcohol, 127
  consumed after athletic activity, 62–63
  as diuretic, 63
alcoholism, 19
Aldomet, 107
"Always Say Diet" (Clapp), 67
American Diabetes Association, 14
American Health Foundation Conference, 482
American Heart Association (AHA), 37, 67, 114, 451, 482–83
American Meat Institute, 469
American Medical Joggers Association (AMJA), 62
amino acids, 28, 455–60
ammonia, 55
Anderson, James W., 441, 486
angiography, 113
animals, speed vs. endurance of, 56
apneic events, 63
apple juice, 182, 218
apples, 180
Armstrong, Duane, 101
arrowroot, 180
arthritis, 36
Ashe, Arthur, 4
asparagus, 206, 224, 225
atherosclerosis, coronary, *see* heart disease
athletic people, 53–61
  alcoholic beverages and, 62–63
  average percentage of body fat in, 66
  carbohydrate requirements of, 54–55, 57–59
  coronary atherosclerosis-related deaths in, 63–65, 92–102, 488–95

  dehydration and, 55
  fat requirements of, 56–57, 64–67
  fluid replacement for, 60–61
  increased endurance of, 56
  injuries of, 63
  mineral requirements of, 60–61
  protein requirements of, 53–56
  testimonials from, 68–77, 83–90
  vitamin requirements of, 59–60
  world-class, 78–91

baby lima beans, 222
backpacking, 175
Baker, Irwin, 48–50, 97
banana sandwiches, 169
Bantu tribe, 478–79
barley, 221
Barrows, C. H., 463
Bassler, Tom, 62–66, 93, 96, 488–89
beans, 205
  cooking practices for, 221–22, 224
  flatulence and, 165–66
  recommended intake of, 193
  seasonings for, 225
bean sprouts, 224
Beck, Claude, 99
Becker, John, 22
Beddor family, 76–77
beer, consumed after athletic activity, 62–63
beets, 207, 224, 225
Bergersen, F. J., 462
Berman, Irwin, 26
berries, whole (grains), 221
beta-endorphins, 11
Biener, Minnia, 42–44
biliary obstruction, 448
Blackburn, Henry, 482–83
black-eyed peas, 222
blender, electric, 177
blood:
  agglutination of, 115
  components of, 8, 9–10
  oxygen supply in, 7–8
blood pressure, high, *see* hypertension
blood sugar levels, 9–10
  emotional health and, 11

501

Index

protein (*cont.*)
  function of, 28
  "incomplete," 455
  lifespan and, 12–14
  in mother's vs. cow's milk, 35
  nitrogen balance and, 455–59, 467
  overconsumption of, 28–29, 454–70
  for pregnant women, 161, 461–62
  RDA of, 29, 464
  requirements of, 454–70
protein-efficiency ratio (PER), 455–56
protein powder, 34
prothrombin, 448
psychotherapy, exercise vs. drugs in, 12
"Public Health View of Diet and Mass Hyperlipidemia, The" (Blackburn), 482–83
pulse rate:
  in exercise program, 144
  test for, 116
push-ups, 149

racehorses, 56
racquetball, 143
rats, amino acid studies on, 455–56
RDA (recommended dietary allowance), 439, 478
  of protein, 29, 464
  of vitamin A, 444
  of vitamin C, 30, 32
  of vitamin E, 447
"rebound scurvy," 31
Recommended Dietary Allowance, 467
red bush tea, 213
Reddy, V., 455
red-vented bulbul bird, 30
Reich, P., 492
restaurants:
  in foreign countries, 169–74
  maintaining diet in, 108–09, 166–68
Richards, Arne, 64
Richardson, D. P., 459–60
Richardson, Hilda, 73–74
rickets, 446
Roastaroma, 213
Roberts, W. C., 93, 493
Robinson, Miles H., 488–95
Rogers, Bill, 81
romaine lettuce, 183–84, 206, 224
Rose, W. C., 456–57
Rosenberg, H. R., 456
Rosenthal, Monroe, 87–88
Rumania, protein RDA in, 454
Royce, Stephen, Jr., 101
Runner's World, 81, 493

running:
  alcoholism and, 19
  coronary atherosclerosis-related deaths in, 63–64, 92–102, 488–95
  incentive for, 22
  see also athletic people
rye, whole, 221

safflower oil, 67
salad dressings, 180
  dairy-free, 186
Salazar, Alberto, 81
salt, *see* sodium
sandwiches, suggestions for, 208–10
sapsago cheese, 179, 187
Scheff, John, 87
scoliosis, 74
Scott, Dave, 79–80
scurvy, 31, 32
sea salt, 181
selenium, 33, 36
Sheehan, George, 97, 493
Shettler, Jim, 95–96, 98, 100, 490
shoes, for exercise, 145
Shorter, Frank, 81
sleep, 12
smoking, 127–28, 129
snacks, 210–12
  for children, 159
sodium:
  in commercial products, 181–82
  dietary reduction of, 218
  in sweat, 60–61
soil depletion, 36
sour cream, mock, 187
soy sauce, 181
Spanish, ordering food in, 169
spices:
  fresh vs. stale, 183
  for seasoning vegetables, 225
  shopping list for, 189–90
spinach, 37, 206, 224, 225
split peas, 222
sprue, 448
squash, 206, 207, 224, 225
Stanford University, 31
starches, obesity and, 37
starvation, protein used in, 28
steatorrhea, 448
Stephenson, Dennis, 93–94
Stevens, Charles, 70
Stevens, Jack, 83–85
Stevens, Maisie, 83, 85
stock, cooking, 186, 218
sugar, 182
  brown vs. white, 36
  emotional health and, 11
  energy from, 37

508

Index

Index

Recipe Index

Index

Index

Index